20 | 20

Thinking

A Lynn Sonberg Book

AVERY

A MEMBER OF

PENGUIN PUTNAM INC.

NEW YORK

20|20

Thinking

1,000 POWERFUL STRATEGIES TO SHARPEN YOUR MIND,
BRIGHTEN YOUR MOOD, AND BOOST YOUR MEMORY

Maggie Greenwood-Robinson, Ph.D.

Foreword by Hunter Yost, M.D.

Every effort has been made to ensure that the information contained in this book is complete and accurate. However, neither the publisher nor the author is engaged in rendering professional advice or services to the individual reader. The ideas, procedures, and suggestions contained in this book are not intended as a substitute for consulting with your physician. All matters regarding health require medical supervision. Neither the author nor the publisher shall be liable or responsible for any loss, injury, or damage allegedly arising from any information or suggestion in this book. The opinions expressed in this book represent the personal views of the author and not of the publisher.

The recipes contained in this book are to be followed exactly as written. Neither the publisher nor the author is responsible for your specific health or allergy needs that may require medical supervision or for any adverse reactions to the recipes contained in this book.

While the author has made every effort to provide accurate telephone numbers and Internet addresses at the time of publication, neither the publisher nor the author assumes any responsibility for errors or for changes that occur after publication.

Most Avery books are available at special quantity discounts for bulk purchase for sales promotions, premiums, fund-raising, and educational needs. Special books or book excerpts also can be created to fit specific needs. For details, write Putnam Special Markets, 375 Hudson Street, New York, NY 10014.

AVERY

a member of
Penguin Putnam Inc.
375 Hudson Street
New York, NY 10014
www.penguinputnam.com

Figure I, "The Human Brain," on page 3 © 2003 Lippincott Williams & Wilkins. All rights reserved.

Library of Congress Cataloging-in-Publication Data

Greenwood-Robinson, Maggie.
20/20 thinking : 1,000 powerful strategies to sharpen your mind, brighten your mood,
and boost your memory / Maggie Greenwood-Robinson ; foreword by Hunter Yost.
p.   cm.
"A Lynn Sonberg book."
Includes bibliographical references (p.417) and index.
ISBN 1-58333-153-0
1. Thought and thinking.   2. Emotions.   3. Emotions and cognition.
4. Memory.   5. Mnemonics.   I. Title
BF441.G745   2003   2002026249
158.1—dc21

Printed in the United States of America
1   3   5   7   9   10   8   6   4   2

Book design by Meighan Cavanaugh

To my husband, Jeff, the greatest love of my life

Acknowledgments

Special thanks to the following people for their work and contributions to this book: my agent Madeleine Morel, 2M Communications, Ltd.; Lynn Sonberg of Lynn Sonberg Books; the staff at Prentice Hall and Avery; and my husband, Jeff, for love and patience during the research and writing of this book.

Contents

Part Three

Part Four

Part Five

Part Six

SMART CHOICES AND BEST SOURCES *371*

Foreword

by Hunter Yost, M.D.

20/20 Thinking is a book that enlightens, empowers, and informs. In clear and straightforward language, it provides practical and scientifically documented tools to help you deal with everyday issues of memory and mood, as well as more serious conditions of depression, anxiety, dementia, and drug abuse.

Traditionally, the language of medicine and psychiatry is filled with such words as "deficit," "negativity," "mood disorders," "attention deficit disorder," and "personality disorders"—terminology implying that something is wrong. Rarely do you find in conventional medical literature language that speaks to the resiliency, competency, or potential for rejuvenation that lies within all of us. *20/20 Thinking* is hopeful and upbeat, humanizing our mental and emotional processes and encouraging us to feel comfortable on our own journeys toward self-improvement. This book takes a refreshing non-pathological view on improving mental functioning naturally—through nutrients, humor, prayer, creative play, meditative activities, music, and positive social interactions.

You can read this book for information on a specific area of interest or use it to improve your overall lifestyle in terms of healthy brain practices. In fact, you can use it to help you take control of all aspects of your mental life in a multitude of ways never before collected and published in one book. The discussion of nutritional influences on mental functioning is especially important, providing information and hope for people who may be unaware of medically proven alternatives to prescription drugs.

20/20 Thinking fits nicely with current "out of the box thinking" appearing in scientific research about how the brain works. This research says that our brain functions may not be confined inside the bony structure called our skull. For example, you'll see how a neurotransmitter (brain chemical) made by the endocrine system and released by the nervous system has receptor, or entry, sites on white blood cells. And you'll learn how hormones originating in the liver and released by the endocrine system have receptors on the immune and nervous systems. In other words, you'll discover that there are no clear-cut divisions among our nervous, immune, and hormonal systems. They are seamlessly interwoven in a weblike complex that determines who we are and how we think and create.

20/20 Thinking can also help you and your doctor get to the bottom of what might be troubling you or making you ill. This goes along with a guiding principle in Chinese medicine known as "roots versus branches," meaning the doctor should look for root causes for an illness that manifests itself as diverse symptoms, or branches of a tree. These branches may appear unrelated and may be treated symptomatically by the unsophisticated practitioner without ever getting to the root cause.

A prime example of a root cause of illness is homocysteine, an amino acid produced in our bodies from dietary sources of another amino acid, methionine. Elevations of blood homocysteine are associated with depression, dementia, heart disease, and some cancers. This substance is directly toxic to the nervous system, it damages blood vessels, and it can alter genetic expression. Homocysteine elevation is often caused by insufficient folic acid, B_{12}, and B_6 in the diet or a genetic variation present in a third of the population that prevents the conversion of dietary folic acid to its active form in the body.

Although your doctor can order a test that measures your homocysteine level, there is no drug treatment for elevated homocysteine. The only treatment is to supplement your diet with increased amounts of folic acid, B_{12}, and B_6—a treatment substantiated by hundreds of medical journal articles over the past decade. This "root cause" demonstrates how lifestyle, diet, and genetics converge to affect our mental functioning and our overall health.

In this Internet era of virtually unlimited access to information, the informed public is often ahead of the medical profession about how to prevent health problems and enhance well-being. Resistance to change is often slow in medicine even when the scientific documentation is present. Some medical researchers estimate that it can take as long as fifteen years for new information to be incorporated into the daily practice of the average doctor. *20/20 Thinking* is for people who don't want to wait that long! Prescription drugs are appropriate for some people, *but* there is so much more to consider.

Perhaps this book can help open new dialogues between patients and their physicians. In fact, *20/20 Thinking* should be read not only by the general public but also by all health professionals, including psychiatrists, neurologists, primary care physicians, nurses, psychologists, and social workers. It is their job, after all, to help patients improve the quality of their lives, and this book is aimed at doing exactly that for anyone who wants to function at his or her best mentally and emotionally.

Dr. Yost is in private practice in Tucson, Arizona, specializing in functional and nutritional medicine. He is board certified in psychiatry and neurology. Prior to 1996, he was a practicing psychiatrist.

20|20

Thinking

Introduction:

You're the Boss of Your Brain

Atop the spinal cord, not unlike a flower upon its stem, sits the most complex and amazing object on Earth: the human brain. This moist, pinkish-gray organ has been dubbed the human control center because it regulates all that we do: thought, reason, intuition, emotion, sight, hearing, touch, movement, speech, memory, creativity—everything, in fact, that makes us human.

In all its complexity, the brain and the nervous system it supports are quite vulnerable. Obstructions to the brain's blood supply can cause strokes. Degeneration of brain cells leads to illnesses such as Alzheimer's disease and Parkinson's disease. Problems in mental and emotional processing, governed largely by brain chemicals, can interfere with productive living.

You might wonder then: With all the things that can go wrong, why is it that some people stay so mentally sharp and healthy long into their golden years? Is it luck or is it genes?

Neither, entirely. Many decades of research into the brain have revealed that *you are very much in control of your mind, mood, and memory—and in the preservation of your mental faculties for as long as you live.* In fact, you might be thrilled to know that the older brain is actually better developed and sharper at emotional tasks. That's certainly something to look forward to!

The secrets to lifelong mental fitness involve some relatively simple changes in lifestyle and psychological outlook, most of which are covered in this book. Even if you applied only a handful of the suggestions presented here, you'd be well on your way to a sound mind and body in your seventies, eighties, and beyond—and are more likely to lead a long, happy, and satisfied life as a result.

To appreciate the wondrous workings of the brain and how you can keep them intact, it first helps to understand its intricacies, namely its major structures and how they function in mind, mood, and memory. That said, we'll get started on a short anatomy lesson but one that will help you understand the key brain terms used throughout this book.

Your Amazing Brain and How It Works

Structurally, the brain is composed of many anatomically distinct regions. (See Figure 1 on page 3.) Although each region has a different function, several usually work together to contribute to any particular task. And if one area of the brain becomes damaged, another can take over for it. This amazing adaptability of the brain is technically known as "neuronal plasticity."

A rather dramatic example of this can be found in patients who undergo an operation called a radical hemispherectomy, in which one entire side of the brain is removed in order to cure a brain-damaging type of seizure. In patients who have this operation, the intact side takes over completely for the missing side.

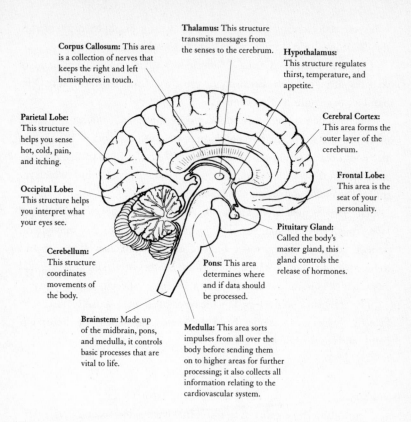

Thalamus: This structure transmits messages from the senses to the cerebrum.

Corpus Callosum: This area is a collection of nerves that keeps the right and left hemispheres in touch.

Hypothalamus: This structure regulates thirst, temperature, and appetite.

Parietal Lobe: This structure helps you sense hot, cold, pain, and itching.

Cerebral Cortex: This area forms the outer layer of the cerebrum.

Frontal Lobe: This area is the seat of your personality.

Occipital Lobe: This structure helps you interpret what your eyes see.

Cerebellum: This structure coordinates movements of the body.

Pituitary Gland: Called the body's master gland, this gland controls the release of hormones.

Pons: This area determines where and if data should be processed.

Brainstem: Made up of the midbrain, pons, and medulla, it controls basic processes that are vital to life.

Medulla: This area sorts impulses from all over the body before sending them on to higher areas for further processing; it also collects all information relating to the cardiovascular system.

FIGURE 1. THE HUMAN BRAIN.

THE CEREBRUM

There are three main regions of the brain. The largest is the cerebrum, where thinking and complex tasks such as speaking, reading, and conscious movement are controlled. The cerebrum is divided into two mirror-image hemispheres, left and right. Oddly, the left hemisphere is linked to the right side of your body; the right hemisphere, to your left side. The left hemisphere controls speech and language and deals with logic. It also helps you do things in a particular sequence, such as tying your shoes or backing your car out of the driveway. The right side deals with emotion, intuition, creativity, visual skills, and spatial abilities. If you were redecorating a room in your house, for example, you'd picture the decor in your head with your right hemisphere.

One hemisphere is usually dominant, so if you're right-handed, chances are your left hemisphere governs. Likewise, if you're left-handed, your right half is dominant.

The two hemispheres are connected by the *corpus callosum*, a bundle of nerves that keeps the two halves in touch with each other. Without it, you could read and understand the word "horse" (using your left hemisphere), but you would not be able to see a horse in your mind (which requires the use of your right hemisphere).

The two hemispheres are subdivided into four lobes each: *frontal lobes*, involved in reason, emotion, judgment, and voluntary movement; *parietal lobes*, which register feelings of hot and cold, as well as pain and itching; *occipital lobes*, which contain the centers of vision; and *temporal lobes*, which contain centers of hearing, listening, speech, and memory.

The cerebrum is enveloped by the *cerebral cortex*, a wrinkly outer surface that picks up messages from the senses and sends out the brain's commands to the body.

THE BRAINSTEM

Connecting the cerebrum to the spinal cord is the second major part of the brain, the brainstem. It controls basic bodily functions such as breathing and heart rate. At the center of the brainstem lies a conglomeration of nerve cells called the *reticular formation*, where the brain's most important decisions are made. Here, the millions of messages arriving at the brain are decoded in order of importance.

A structure called the *pons* connects the cerebellum (see Figure 1 on page 3) with the cerebrum and joins the hemispheres of the cerebellum. Its job is to monitor the data sent to your brain and to determine where, or if, this data should be processed.

Have you ever entered an area where a stench or strong smell was so overpowering that you couldn't stand it? Then, after being there just a few minutes, you no longer noticed the stench? It hasn't gone away, but the pons has stopped relaying bad-smell messages.

THE CEREBELLUM

Just behind the top of the brainstem is the third major region of the brain: an apricot-sized structure called the cerebellum, dubbed the "little brain." If you go for a stroll in the park, climb the stairs, or stand in line to buy concert tickets, your cerebellum is controlling your balance, coordination, and movement. The cerebellum also has a left and right half.

THE LIMBIC SYSTEM

Within the cerebrum, cerebellum, and brainstem are many other special regions of the brain. One of these is the limbic system, where most of your emotional processing takes place. For example, the limbic system activates the blush on your face when you're embarrassed, tears when you're sad, and the jumpy feeling you get when scared. The limbic system consists of five major structures in the brain: the thalamus, hypothalamus, hippocampus, basal ganglia, and amygdala.

The Thalamus

The thalamus is a two-lobed structure located deep within the brain at the base of the cerebrum. It acts as a "sorter" for messages going to the cerebrum. The thalamus can tell you, for example, that something cold is touching your body, but only the cerebrum can decide which part of the body and what kind of object is touching it. In addition to temperature and touch, the thalamus interprets pain and pressure and is also involved in memory.

The Hypothalamus

Just below the thalamus is the hypothalamus, a small area located in the middle of the brain. The hypothalamus is the body's control center for regulating thirst, appetite, and body temperature. It also controls the functioning of the pituitary gland, the so-called "master gland" of the body because it governs the thyroid gland and other glands of the body through the secretion of chemicals called hormones. The hypothalamus also functions in rage, aggression, pain, and pleasure.

The Hippocampus

Deep within the brain is a horseshoe-shaped structure called the hippocampus. Its job is to help you learn and remember. More specifically, the hippocampus takes sensory information from the thalamus and emotions from the hypothalamus to create short-term memory.

The Basal Ganglia

The basal ganglia are clusters of neurons found at the base of the cerebrum. Primarily, they help control well-learned activities such as walking.

The basal ganglia is one of the brain structures connected with the frontal lobe through the *substantia nigra*, a black moustache-shaped area named after the Latin phrase for "black mass." It appears black because its cells contain the pigment melanin, the end product of a brain chemical called dopamine after it has gone through a number of chemical reactions. Cells in the substantia nigra produce dopamine.

The Amygdala

One of the basal ganglia is a group of cells about the size of a chickpea called the amygdala. The term, derived from the Latin word for "almond," describes the organ's shape. As with most structures in the brain, there are two amygdalae: one in the left side of your brain and one in the right.

The amygdala is involved in mood and emotions, particularly the acquisition and expression of fear and anxiety. It also helps you vividly recall emotionally charged events from your past.

More specifically, the amygdala is like an alarm center in your brain. It takes input from your senses and orchestrates your reaction to it. Suppose you're walking down a dark alley and see a man coming toward you, wielding a knife. Your heart starts beating rapidly, your facial expression contorts into a look of panic, and you scram.

Each response—the rapid heartbeat, the facial expression, the flight—was activated by the amygdala the instant it received visual cues signaling danger. Put another way, the amygdala interprets the significance of a threatening situation, then organizes your emotional and bodily response to that threat. It communicates with other regions of the brain, particularly those that control breathing, heart rate, the release of hormones, and other responses.

THE NERVOUS SYSTEM

Your brain is connected to the rest of your body by the nervous system, which sends, receives, and processes nerve impulses throughout your body. Nerve impulses tell your muscles and organs what to do and how to react to the environment. There are three interconnected parts of the nervous system:

- The *central nervous system* (CNS) consists of the brain and spinal cord, which carries messages between your brain and the rest of your body. Overall, the CNS dispatches nerve impulses and analyzes information from your sense organs (ears, eyes, and so forth).
- The *peripheral nervous system* (PNS) is composed of nerves that spread out from the spinal cord like branches on a tree to every part of the body. The job of the PNS is to carry nerve impulses from the CNS to your muscles and glands.

  Of the forty-three main nerves of the PNS, thirty-one are spinal nerves. The rest are cranial nerves located in your neck. Cranial nerves do not pass through the spinal cord but go directly to your brain and include nerves that connect to your eyes, ears, nose, and tongue.
- The *autonomic nervous system* (ANS) controls breathing, heartbeat, digestion, blood pressure, and other bodily functions that go on or work automatically. The ANS is divided into two different parts: the *sympathetic* and the *parasympathetic* nervous systems.

  Consisting of nerves that branch off from your brain and the base of your spine, the parasympathetic system is controlled by the brainstem. This system sends signals to tell your body to slow down and work at a normal pace.

The sympathetic system consists of nerves that shoot off from the spinal cord between your neck and the small of your back. Under orders from the hypothalamus, it accelerates the body and its functions when your body needs to be active or is under stress. By producing opposite effects, the two systems keep the body in a balanced state.

THE CELLS OF THE NERVOUS SYSTEM

Every part of the nervous system (including the brain) is made up of nerve cells, technically known as *neurons*, as well as *glial cells*, which are supporting cells. Most of the cells in your body have a short life span and constantly are being replaced with new ones. Neurons, on the other hand, are long-lived.

A neuron is a starlike structure carrying signals that allow you to move, hear, see, taste, smell, remember, and think. Structurally, it has a nucleus in the middle and a long tail called an *axon* that stretches out from the cell body. Branching out from the cell body are tentaclelike structures called *dendrites*, after the Greek word for "tree."

Both axons and dendrites help transmit nerve signals through the neurons. Dendrites are receiving stations for incoming nerve signals. These nerve signals rush along the axon. At the far tip of the axon, the nerve ending, the axon has other dendrites that relay the message on to the dendrites of other neurons.

With use, neurons coat their axons with a white, fatlike covering called *myelin*. As more neurons are activated—say, through learning—more myelin is put down over the axon as a cover. And the more myelin covering an axon, the faster the transmission of messages. Multiple sclerosis is a disease related to the destruction of the myelin covering, or myelin sheath, of axons.

Neurons transmit messages both electrically and chemically. Within the neuron, messages are relayed through the movement of an electrical charge referred to as an impulse.

Communication between neurons also occurs chemically, at the *synapse*, a tiny gap that forms a connection between neurons. The transmitting neuron releases a messenger chemical called a *neurotransmitter* across the synapse. The neurotransmitter links up with compatible "receptors," tiny sites in the dendrites of the receiving neuron. This process works much like a key in a lock. The locks are the receptor sites; the key is the neurotransmitter. Like a lock, the receptor accepts only one kind of neurotransmitter. When the neurotransmitter fits, it is allowed entry into the neuron. This changes the chemistry of the receiving neuron's membrane, setting off electrical charges that relay the message along the length of the neuron.

Synapses do not pass on every nerve signal. If they did, you'd be bombarded by signals. At some synapses, the receiving neuron relays the signal—a process called "excitation"—and at others, they block the signal—a process called "inhibition."

Because neurons are the largest cells in the body, they rely on supporting cells, the glial cells, for their survival. The term "glial" comes from the Greek word meaning "glue." This name reflects one of their chief functions: to hold the moist mass of the brain together.

Yet glial cells do much more. Some glial cells supply neurons with food and energy. Others remove waste material of dead cells within the brain following damage and protect neurons against toxins. Still others encase nerve fibers to provide electrical insulation. A newly discovered function of glial cells is to give neurons the go-ahead to start constructing new synapses. Not only that, glial cells help neurons maintain the synapses they've built.

Glial cells outnumber neurons ten to one—and for good reason. A neuron that loses contact with its supporting glial cells will lose its synapse and die.

6 CRITICAL BRAIN CHEMICALS AND WHY THEY'RE IMPORTANT

Governing your mind, mood, and memory is a regular ebb and flow of brain chemicals known as neurotransmitters. Released by the neuron that is transmitting the signal, they carry messages from one neuron to the next by spewing out from the tail end of one neuron to another across the synapse.

The billions of cells in your brain use roughly 100 neurotransmitters. Of these, six are the most important.

ACETYLCHOLINE

Manufactured from a B vitamin called choline, this neurotransmitter is involved mostly in learning and memory. It has been under intense investigation in Alzheimer's disease. In this disease, there is a loss of acetylcholine from the synapses. One of the ways physicians have tried to combat this disease is by prescribing drugs that block an enzyme called acetylcholinesterase that breaks down acetylcholine.

DOPAMINE

Found in every nook and cranny in the brain, dopamine's chief function in the body is to initiate normal muscle movement. Yet this is not all it does. Dopamine triggers the euphoria and infatuation associated with the first blush of romantic love. It also influences attention and the ability to concentrate. Essentially, dopamine is a pleasure-producing neurotransmitter; at high levels in the brain, it makes you feel good. Imbalances in dopamine levels lead to Parkinson's disease, schizophrenia, mood disorders, and other brain disorders.

EPINEPHRINE

Better known as adrenaline, epinephrine is derived from the amino acid tyrosine. In response to stress, epinephrine increases heart rate, raises blood pressure, and increases levels of blood sugar (glucose)—all reactions that prepare your body for "fight or flight." Another of epinephrine's jobs is to increase fatty acids in the bloodstream so that your body can use them for fuel.

GABA

Technically known as gamma-aminobutyric acid, GABA is the brain's natural tranquilizer. Made from the amino acid glutamine, GABA is an "inhibitory" neurotransmitter. It prevents anxiety messages from being transmitted from neuron to neuron. When the brain doesn't produce enough GABA, depression, anxiety, and panic attacks can set in.

NOREPINEPHRINE

As one of the brain's "alert" neurotransmitters, norepinephrine prepares you for action in threatening situations. It also helps regulate blood pressure and maintain your ability to concentrate.

Norepinephrine is made from the amino acids phenylalanine and tyrosine in the body. Overproduction of this neurotransmitter can lead to irritability, anxiety, and insomnia.

SEROTONIN

Known as the "happiness neurotransmitter," serotonin is associated with tranquility, calm, and emotional well-being. Serotonin is produced in the body from the amino acid tryptophan found in protein foods. At night, the pineal gland in the brain converts serotonin to the sleep hormone melatonin.

Low levels of serotonin may increase the risk for depression or suicide. Brains of women produce two-thirds as much serotonin as those of men. This may explain why women are more prone to depression than men are.

39 FASCINATING FACTS ABOUT YOUR BRAIN

1. The human brain weighs approximately 3 pounds.
2. Nearly 85 percent of your brain's weight is water.
3. The human brain is about the size of a grapefruit.

4. The size of the brain is not related to intelligence.

5. Almost all neurons are generated during prenatal life. While growing in the womb, a human baby can develop more than 100,000 neurons in just one minute.

6. The nervous system appears about eighteen days after conception.

7. After birth, a baby's brain begins a growth spurt, which continues to around the age of ten.

8. At age five, a child's brain is already nine-tenths of its adult weight.

9. The human nervous system has 100 billion neurons—roughly the amount of stars in the Milky Way galaxy.

10. These 100 billion neurons are surrounded by about 10 trillion synapses.

11. Between the ages of twenty and seventy-five, it is estimated that an average of 50,000 neurons atrophy, or die, each day.

12. This loss of neurons does not correspond with a loss of function; the brain compensates by forming new branches (dendrites) and new synapses.

13. By the age of seventy-five, the weight of your brain will be reduced by one-tenth and the flow of blood through your brain reduced by nearly one-fifth.

14. Nerve cells, which include those in the brain, are the largest cells in your body. Some are so long that they stretch from your toes to your brain.

15. Axons (the "tail" of nerve cells) range in length from 0.04 inches to 1 yard.

16. There are more than 100 different neurotransmitters (brain chemicals) in your body.

17. Human brains have gotten bigger. Your brain weighs about 8 ounces more than your great grandmother's brain.

18. Spread out, your cerebral cortex (the outer layer of the cerebrum) would cover your office desk.

19. Your brain uses up about 20 to 30 percent of the calories you eat every day.

20. Your brain uses nearly a quarter of your body's oxygen every day.

21. Every minute, about 1 quart of blood flows through your brain.

22. The central nervous system, which includes your brain and spinal cord, transmits messages to more than 600 different muscles.

23. Even while you're asleep, 50 million nerve messages are being sent back and forth between your brain and various parts of your body, every second.

24. Nearly 100 million pieces of data race up your spinal cord every minute.

25. Brain messages can travel at speeds up to 360 mph.

26. After sending a signal, a nerve cell is ready to send another in less than 0.001 second.

27. Your brain retrieves most of its information from visual sources.

28. Brain cells receive thousands of incoming signals every second.

29. The human brain is more complicated that any computer on Earth. In fact, the most sophisticated computer is only as smart as a rat's brain.

30. The color of the brain is pinkish-gray.

31. The brain has the consistency of soft margarine.

32. If you were able to take a whiff of your brain, it would smell like blue cheese.

33. The brain grows by making new connections between brain cells. Axons grow new branches, and new synapses are formed. As the number of connections increases, your brain becomes more adept at complex thinking.

34. The processing speed of your brain declines by about 1 percent a year from age twenty-five on.

35. The brain does not feel pain because there are no sensors for pain within the brain. How, then, do you explain a headache? Headaches occur when blood vessels in the brain, not the brain itself, become swollen, inflamed, or abnormally constricted.

36. Information stays in your short-term memory no longer than just a few minutes.

37. Your short-term memory can store no more than nine pieces of information at one time.

38. By the time you're eight years old, your long-term memory has stored more information than a million encyclopedias.

39. Information can stay in long-term memory for weeks, months, years, or for the rest of your life.

Part One

THE FOUNDATIONS OF

GREAT MENTAL FITNESS

Imagine your life if you could:

- Build your brainpower into a tower of strength so formidable that you're never at a loss for creative and productive thoughts.
- Put an end to blue moods, once and for all, and feel upbeat practically all of the time.
- Expand your powers of recall so that you never fear losing your memory again.
- Unleash an explosion of mental energy so powerful that you experience the joy of life you were meant to have.

Impossible? Not at all. And you're about to find out why. In the part that follows, you'll learn why delicious foods, natural supplements, and simple physical and mental exercises hold the most powerful secrets to unbelievable mental fitness.

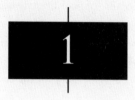

How to Boost Your Brainpower

You're about to discover the universe of brain health that awaits you in some of the most obvious places, like the supermarket, health-food store, gym—even your own bedroom!

You'll be introduced to some remarkable foods that lead to laser-sharp thinking; brain-boosting natural supplements; simple exercises that keep you mentally energized; and sleep secrets that will revitalize your mind.

There's just one catch: The key is to take this information to heart—do it, live it—if you want to experience its incredible rejuvenating power on your brain.

15 Lifestyle Secrets

Your mind does not have to turn to mush, your moods need not swing, and your memory does not have to fade. In other words, you're not destined for mental deterioration just because you're getting older. Senility is not synonymous with aging. In most people, mental faculties begin a downhill slide because of poor lifestyle habits. As discouraging as this may sound on the surface, it reveals some powerfully positive news: You can boost your brainpower and fend off mental decline well into your golden years by living a healthier life. Here are 15 best bets for protecting your mind, mood, and memory for the rest of your life.

EAT SMART

A healthful diet, devoid of highly processed foods, supplies your brain with the nutrients and energy it needs for optimal functioning and psychological health. A brain-restorative diet is one that includes at least three servings of fruits and five servings of vegetables daily, several servings of whole grains, moderate amounts of lean proteins (fish, poultry, lean red meat, and dairy products), and some fat.

Also, forgo the usual three square meals a day and eat more frequently—four or five smaller meals a day. Smaller meals are easier to digest and keep your brain and body constantly energized and nourished. By contrast, large meals sap your physical and mental energy by diverting nutrient and oxygen-carrying blood to your digestive tract rather than to your brain.

REDUCE DIETARY FATS

Even though they're all the rage now, high-fat diets may impair brain function over time. That's the finding of a recent animal study, in which researchers discovered that high-fat diets slowed the animals' ability to learn new tasks and damaged their memories. How? According to researchers, high-fat diets may starve the brain of its major energy supply—glucose, which is abundant in carbohydrates but not in fats. Fat-laden diets may also make brain cells less responsive to insulin, a hormone that helps usher glucose into cells for nourishment and energy.

Here are some pointers for slashing the fat in your diet:

- Make sure dietary fat does not exceed 30 percent of your daily calories. To translate this recommendation into meaningful terms, a 2,000-calorie diet should contain about 65 grams of fat a day.
- Read food labels for the fat content per serving. The grams of fat are listed under Nutrition Facts on any food package that provides a nutrition label.
- Choose lean cuts of good- or choice-grade meat and eat portions that are no larger than the palm of your hand. Lean cuts include round, sirloin, and flank. Chicken, turkey, and fish are always leaner meat choices. Among these leaner proteins, fish is a superior choice and deserves its reputation as brain food. It contains healthy fats that protect brain cells and preserve memory.
- Get rid of the fat you can see. When preparing and eating meats, make sure to trim all visible fat and skin, and use cooking racks to bake, broil, grill, steam, or microwave to avoid melting the fat back into the meat.
- Be wary of cold cuts. When eating lunch meats, select low-fat or fat-free chicken or turkey breast rather than high-fat bologna or salami.
- Go skim. Choose low-fat or skimmed products rather than whole milk and include them two to three times each day.
- Hold the butter. Opt for reduced-fat margarines and spreads rather than regular butter or margarine.

DRINK UP

Water may very well be the ultimate "neuronutrient" when it comes to the health of your brain. We need water to think, learn, stay alert, and feel good mentally. In fact, drinking enough water each day is one of the easiest, smartest moves you can make for preserving the health of your brain.

For one thing, water peps up your mental performance. Ever wonder why you feel mentally sluggish during the day? It could be that you're dehydrated, which technically means you're running low on water. In a study of subjects' abilities to perform mental exercises after experimentally induced dehydration, a fluid loss of only 2 percent of body weight caused a whopping 20-percent reduction in arithmetic skills, short-term memory, and the ability to visually track an object. Also, severe dehydration results in mental confusion and disorientation.

For another, water is an unsung hero when it comes to mental well-being. That's because water hikes up serotonin—the brain chemical involved in regulating mood, anxiety, stress, depression, pain, and memory. Some cutting-edge research with lab rats suggests that dehydration reduces levels of this feel-good chemical in the brain. By contrast, when animals were given sufficient water, serotonin levels rose. The lesson here: Water may turn out to be one of our best all-natural uppers yet!

To maintain peak mental capacity, drink eight to ten glasses of pure water every day. This will prevent dehydration.

Sodas don't count, either. Consider this: More than 70 percent of an 8-ounce glass of water is absorbed by the stomach, and only 6 percent of the same amount of soda is absorbed. Plus, diet soft drinks contain artificial sweeteners and other chemicals. How these additives affect the brain is unclear. For these reasons, water is the preferred choice for the fluid your brain needs.

If it's tough to swill plain water, you might opt for some of the new "smart waters." These are herb-fortified waters, containing such popular brain-enhancing herbs as ginkgo biloba, Siberian ginseng, or St. John's wort. Generally, herbal waters have a hint of flavor but without sugar, calories, or carbonation.

CONTROL ALCOHOL INTAKE

Alcohol is a drug that can cause memory loss when abused. In fact, chronic alcoholism can cause a type of amnesia in which the brain is unable to form new memories.

Moderate drinking (one to two drinks a day), however, has been shown to improve memory, problem solving, and reasoning ability, according to a study at Indiana University that tracked 4,000 male twins for twenty years.

Even so, moderate drinking carries risk, says the National Institute

on Alcohol Abuse and Alcoholism. These risks include stroke, motor ve-
hicle crashes, cancer, and birth defects.

LIMIT OR AVOID OTHER
BRAIN-DRAINING DRUGS

These include antihistamines, blood-pressure medications, and some
antidepressants—all of which tend to cloud thinking and impair memory. Look into gentler alternatives, such as herbs and other dietary supplements, before resorting to prescription drugs. Do so with the okay of
your physician or psychiatrist.

Another word of warning: Don't mess with the popular club drug
Ecstasy, or *MDMA* (3, 4-methylenedioxy-methamphetamine). Studies
show the drug impairs memory and damages brain mechanisms responsible for sleep, mood, and learning. These impairments can linger for
more than two years after you stop taking the drug. Even one-time use
can produce brain changes. Scientists are looking into whether the effects
of taking Ecstasy are permanent.

STAY PHYSICALLY ACTIVE TO
KEEP YOUR BRAIN ACTIVE

Exercise encourages blood flow to all parts of the body, including
your brain. A steady supply of fresh oxygenated blood to your brain will
keep you more alert and sharpen your thinking. Some proof: A study
conducted at Scripps College in California revealed that regular exercisers think better, remember better, and have quicker reaction times than
people who don't exercise. Thus, a simple routine of brisk walking can
improve your concentration, thinking speed, organizational skills, and
ability to answer complex questions.

PLANT A GARDEN

Down through the ages, gardening has long been considered not only a
hobby but a healing therapy as well. Ancient Egyptian physicians had their

mentally disturbed patients take long strolls in a garden. In the Middle Ages, monks cultivated gardens to soothe illnesses among their brethren.

In essence, gardening is a mind-body activity that can actually alter the course of physical and mental illness—a beneficial effect that has been verified by scientific studies. Research shows that frequent contact with nature, including gardens, accelerates recovery from surgery, reduces dependence on painkillers, reduces depression and hostility, and fights stress.

Because it is an activity that requires focus, gardening takes your mind off your cares and thus promotes greater emotional well-being. Not only that, working in the garden qualifies as exercise, which stimulates your body and brain.

USE IT OR LOSE IT

Your brain cells communicate with one another through fiberlike branches called dendrites. When brain cells are stimulated, dendrites grow and more synapses are created, increasing the number of connections between cells. This improves your memory, attention span, and ability to learn.

One of the best ways to build new connections is to use your brain. Some suggestions: Learn a language, solve crossword puzzles, do a jigsaw puzzle, memorize poetry, learn a musical instrument, or become a tutor.

Numerous studies show that people who regularly challenge their bodies and brains are less likely to lose cognitive function later in life—and may even reduce their chances of getting Alzheimer's disease.

GET EDUCATED

Some research, though not all, has found that having an intellectually challenging occupation or more education helps you stay mentally sharp as you get older. Case in point: A large-scale study of 1,200 people in their seventies revealed that their level of education predicted their cognitive function better than any other factor that was analyzed. In other words, the more educated members of the group were mentally sharper than their less educated counterparts.

The complexity of your grammatical usage also indicates how well your mind and memory are functioning, according to University of Kentucky investigators. They analyzed the early autobiographies of a group of nuns and, to their amazement, discovered that elderly nuns who showed symptoms of Alzheimer's disease had expressed themselves with simple sentences when they were younger. Through further research, the investigators found that by reading the nuns' autobiographies and analyzing sentence structure, they could predict—with up to 90-percent accuracy—which nuns would show signs of Alzheimer's disease sixty years later. The study does not explain why this is so, only that exercising your brain capacity appears to afford protection against this disease.

VARY YOUR INTERESTS

Scientists who study the brain and cognition have discovered that people with a variety of interests are more likely to preserve their cognitive skills. In practical terms, this means that you should pursue a variety of hobbies or try something you ordinarily wouldn't do. If you're a computer programmer, for example, you might take up painting, while an artist might take an accounting course.

TUNE IN TO CLASSICAL MUSIC

Listening to complex musical arrangements, such as those composed by Mozart or other classical composers, stimulates circuits in your brain that may improve your thinking and mental performance.

STAY CONNECTED

Piles of research reveal that people who have a network of friends and loved ones are less likely to get depressed or lonely—two conditions known to zap mental performance. If you're a loner, look for ways to get involved. Volunteer, join a house of worship, or become a member of an organization in which you're interested.

SLEEP WELL

Bad sleep damages memory and learning ability, and scientists believe that memory loss attributed to old age may be related to poor sleep. In addition to standard good-sleep advice such as maintaining a regular sleep schedule, it's important to keep your room well ventilated, eliminate or reduce sleep-robbing substances such as caffeine and alcohol, sleep on a mattress that is supportive and comfortable, exercise regularly, and eat a nutritious diet.

MARRY SMART

Being married to a smart spouse helps prevent mental decline. That's the finding of research demonstrating that people who marry smart are more likely to retain their intellectual abilities as they age.

SMARTEN UP, LIGHTEN UP WITH THE COMPANY YOU KEEP

Having positive thinkers as friends improves your outlook on life, according to psychology experts. Similarly, hanging out with smart people improves your intelligence. That's because we tend to become like the people with whom we spend the most time.

Further, socializing with midlife peers who are going back to college, learning to play musical instruments, or training for triathlons helps us believe that we too can succeed at new endeavors. Psychologists call this attitude "self-efficacy," which means a strong belief in ourselves and in our capability to accomplish our hearts' desires. With high self-efficacy, we have the power to adopt lifestyle habits that will improve the health of our brains and bodies. So seek out high-efficacy friends, and their can-do attitude will rub off on you!

6 NUTRIENTS TO EAT EVERY WEEK

More than any organ in your body, your brain relies on a minute-to-minute supply of nutrients for healthy functioning. And those nutrients have a critical influence on how your brain performs its chores, from thinking to remembering to processing the innumerable pieces of information coming in from the external environment. The right foods can have an enormous impact on your mental capabilities, alertness, problem-solving ability, memory, mood, reaction time, and more. Here's a look at six "smart" nutrients you need every week.

CARBOHYDRATES

From the oatmeal you eat for breakfast to the baked potato you eat for dinner, carbohydrates are the most important nutrient fuel for your body, and your brain thrives on them. During digestion, carbohydrates are broken down into glucose, also known as blood sugar. Glucose circulates in your blood to the brain and nervous system where it provides energy. It also aids in the synthesis of neurotransmitters such as serotonin, norepinedrine, and acetylcholine. If your brain cells are deprived of glucose, your mental power will suffer. Because your brain controls your muscles, you might even feel weak and shaky.

Studies have found that the higher the concentration of glucose in your blood, the better your memory and concentration. And when you're learning a new task, your brain begins to rapidly use up glucose. Scientists believe that glucose may activate the release of acetylcholine during learning to produce improved memory retention. Further, because glucose is needed to synthesize serotonin, eating carbohydrate foods is mentally soothing.

To feel your best mentally and physically, it's preferable to select natural, unrefined carbohydrates such as whole grains, fruits, and vegetables. Refined carbohydrates such as rolls, cakes, and cookies are laden with too much sugar. Sugar is rapidly released into your system, driving your blood sugar up too high and giving you a quick "rush" followed by a fast "crash" as blood sugar plummets. Low blood sugar has a depressant effect on the body and makes you feel blue.

ANTIOXIDANTS

Your brain consumes more oxygen than any other organ in your body. Thus, it is highly vulnerable to oxidation, a tissue-damaging process that occurs when oxygen reacts with fat. The byproducts of this reaction are devilish molecules called free radicals that attack bodily tissues, particularly cell membranes, and lead to disease.

Fortunately, though, oxidation and the free radicals it produces can be neutralized by antioxidants, which are available from food and supplements and are found naturally in the body. The chief vitamin antioxidants are vitamin C, vitamin E, and beta-carotene; the chief mineral antioxidants are selenium, copper, zinc, and manganese.

The best way to increase your supply of antioxidants is to eat plenty of fruits and vegetables every day—at least five servings of vegetables and three servings of fruits daily. Include a variety of green, orange, yellow, and purple fruits and vegetables in your diet. Although you should eat nuts, seeds, and oils sparingly, have some of them every day to ensure an optimum intake of vitamin E. Here are the twenty-one top antioxidant foods:

1. Beets
2. Concord grape juice
3. Grapes (red)
4. Berries (all types)
5. Red peppers
6. Spinach
7. Prunes
8. Citrus fruits
9. Sweet potatoes
10. Carrots
11. Winter squash
12. Tomatoes
13. Onions

14. Broccoli
15. Asparagus
16. Cabbage
17. Brussel sprouts
18. Beans (all types)
19. Watermelon
20. Wheat germ
21. Nuts

TABLE 1.1
Supplementing with Antioxidants

For nutritional insurance, it's wise to supplement your diet with a one-a-day type multivitamin–mineral antioxidant formula. In addition, you may wish to take other antioxidants to help maintain brain health. Supplementation suggestions are listed below. For more information on brain-protective supplements, see the section titled "Smart Supplements" later in this chapter.

ANTIOXIDANT	BRAIN-PROTECTIVE ACTIONS	DOSAGE
Vitamin C	Protects neurons against free-radical damage; helps manufacture norepinedrine, an important neurotransmitter; improves memory performance.	250 milligrams daily
Vitamin E	Protects neurons against free-radical damage; guards against degenerative brain diseases.	400 IU daily
Alpha-Lipoic Acid	Works in partnership with other antioxidants to terminate free radicals; protects neurons against damage.	20 to 50 milligrams daily

OMEGA-3 FATS

No doubt, you have heard the term "omega fats" used to describe different types of essential fats—fats you must obtain from food because your body can't make them on its own. "Omega" refers to the chemical structure of the fat and is simply a way of classifying essential fatty acids.

Found mostly in fish, shellfish, and plants, omega fats have become best known for their good deeds in cardiovascular health, where they have been found to lower blood pressure, reduce cholesterol, thwart dangerous blood clotting, and protect against irregular heartbeat.

However, they are vital for optimum brain health. Mounds of scientific evidence reveal that omega-3 fats combat depression, improve intellectual performance (particularly in children), rebuild the fatty membranes of brain cells, and protect against stroke.

Omega-3 fats come in three varieties: alpha-linolenic acid (ALA), eicosapentaenoic acid (EPA), and docosahexaenoic acid (DHA). Alpha-linolenic acid is found mostly in plant foods such as flax, soybeans, and vegetables. From these foods, it is converted to EPA and DHA in your body. EPA and DHA are also found in fish, where they are "preformed." This simply means that they don't require conversion from alpha-linolenic acid and thus are better utilized by the body. You can thus obtain EPA and DHA directly from fish and shellfish.

To obtain ample omega-3 fats, the current recommendation is to eat two to three fish meals a week. Just a 4-ounce portion of salmon twice a week, for example, serves up about 5 grams of omega-3 fatty acids, the amount recommended by most health-care practitioners.

Not all fish supply the same amount of omega-3 fats, however. It's best to choose fattier fish such as salmon, tuna, mackerel, or sardines most of the time, since they contain the most omega-3 fats. If you're not a fish-eater, eat 1 tablespoon of flaxseed oil each day instead. Flaxseed is the richest plant source of alpha-linolenic acid. Or supplement with DHA. For more information on supplemental DHA, see "3 Healthy Fats That Power Your Brain" on page 33.

FOLIC ACID

This nutrient is one of three B-complex vitamins that reduce a brain- and heart-damaging protein called "homocysteine" in your body. Others are vitamin B_6 and vitamin B_{12}. Homocysteine is technically an amino acid, high blood levels of which can damage the inner walls of your arteries, causing them to narrow and thicken. Scientists suspect that high homocysteine levels trigger 10 to 15 percent of all heart attacks.

But what hurts your heart may also hurt your brain. High homocysteine levels have been linked to:

- *Stroke.* Homocysteine gums up carotid arteries, the blood vessels on either side of your neck that carry oxygen to your brain—a finding confirmed by researchers in the well-known Framingham Heart Study. The oxygen, nutrient, and blood supply to brain cells can thus get choked off if there are high homocysteine levels in your body, leading to a brain-damaging stroke.
- *Alzheimer's disease.* Investigators have learned that people with Alzheimer's disease have higher homocysteine levels than those without the disease. This suggests a link between Alzheimer's disease and homocysteine.
- *Mental and mood disorders.* Folic acid also helps maintain normal levels of serotonin, the brain's "happiness" neurotransmitter. Deficiencies can lead to depression, dementia, and schizophrenia. In a study of depressed patients on lithium (an antidepressant), supplementation with folic acid for one year dramatically relieved depression.

The best sources of folic acid are dark-green, leafy vegetables. Whenever possible, these should be eaten fresh and raw because storage and cooking destroy as much as 80 percent of the vitamin. Lima beans, cauliflower, liver, meats, eggs, and nuts also supply folic acid.

THIAMINE (VITAMIN B₁)

Among its other functions, thiamine helps manufacture acetylcholine, one of the brain's major chemical messengers. A scarcity of this nutrient impedes your brain's ability to use glucose, sapping the energy required to perform mental activities. A deficiency also overexcites brain cells, and they keep firing until the frazzled cells die off. Thus, a nutritional shortage of thiamine is likely to impair your mental performance.

Yet many people are deficient in this vitamin. Eating foods low in thiamine, cutting calories to lose weight, overcooking foods, and abusing alcohol are just a few of the practices that cause deficiencies or destroy thiamine in the body. Alcohol, in particular, depletes bodily stores of thiamine. Alcoholics are known to have problems with short-term memory.

The best food sources of thiamine are legumes and whole grains.

VITAMIN D

The brain seems to have a special need for vitamin D, a nutrient that is vital for a healthy nervous system but is one that many Americans, particularly those over age fifty, don't get enough of. That's alarming, since memory loss and Alzheimer's disease can occur with a vitamin-D deficiency.

The link between this nutrient and Alzheimer's disease has been discovered in a number of scientific investigations. In a review of Alzheimer's patient records, University of Kentucky Medical Center researchers found that those with low blood levels of calcium and phosphorus—which can be caused by a shortage of vitamin D—suffered from early onset Alzheimer's disease. (Vitamin D helps maintain a normal ratio of calcium and phosphorus in the blood and helps transport calcium in and out of bones.) In a study of aging rats, the same research team observed that those supplemented with vitamin D had more nerve cells in the hippocampus area of their brains. The hippocampus is the seat of memory and the portion of the brain damaged by Alzheimer's disease. These and other studies have led researchers to believe that vitamin D protects brain cells and maintains brain health.

Most of your vitamin D requirements can be met by exposure to sunlight and by eating such foods as vitamin D–enriched dairy products.

2 Proteins That Improve Your Thinking

For needle-sharp thinking throughout the day, boost your diet with protein, a nutrient essential to physical and mental performance. Protein helps the brain synthesize neurotransmitters; builds and repairs tissue; keeps your immune system functioning up to par; helps carry nutrients throughout the body; has a hand in forming hormones; and is involved in important enzyme reactions such as digestion.

As a general rule, Americans overindulge in protein, so it's best to make the healthiest choices. These include lean beef, poultry, fish, eggs, dairy products, and legumes such as soybeans, kidney beans, and pinto beans, to name just a few.

All proteins are valuable to your brain, but there are two in particular with special qualities for preserving your thinking cap.

EGGS

Eggs are not nasty nutritional villains as they've often been cast. Eggs, in fact, are one of the best nutritional sources of choline, an essential nutrient used to manufacture the neurotransmitter acetylcholine needed for normal brain function. An ample supply of choline in your diet helps prevent cloudy thinking.

In addition, choline is vital for the normal development of memory. In animal experiments, rat pups fed choline in the womb or during the second week of life show lifelong memory enhancement. Because of these findings, researchers feel that adequate choline intake during human pregnancy is monumentally important, too.

Eggs are such an excellent dietary source of choline that you'll want to consider eating three or four a week as part of an all-around brain-healthy diet. But don't go overboard by eating more than that allotment. Eggs are loaded with cholesterol, which in high bodily levels has been implicated in heart disease and Alzheimer's disease.

YOGURT

The next time you're hankering for an afternoon snack, reach for some yogurt. In a study conducted at Tufts University, college-aged men were able to solve more arithmetic problems in significantly less time after snacking on yogurt than after consuming a diet soft drink.

Yogurt is a great snack because it is high in both protein and energy-producing carbohydrates, a combination that provides an even release of energy for mental and physical vigor. In addition, yogurt is packed with vitamin D and the B-complex vitamins, all brain-friendly nutrients. What's more, it contains the live active yogurt culture *acidophilus* and other friendly bacteria that help digest food and have protective effects against many diseases.

The Mental Merit of Mixed Meals

For mental balance and energy, it's always a good idea to eat mixed meals—that is, a combination of protein and carbohydrates. This helps deliver steady amounts of tryptophan, an amino acid, to the brain. Found mostly in animal proteins, tryptophan is a precursor to the neurotransmitter serotonin.

The amount of tryptophan that reaches the brain depends not on the amount of protein you consume but on the total amount of protein *and* carbohydrates you eat. Here's the reason: Protein foods contain amino acids other than tryptophan and in larger amounts. To reach the brain, these amino acids must cross the "blood-brain barrier," a protective network of tightly knit cells lining the blood vessels of the brain. These cells are trusty, vigilant receptionists who screen substances for entry into the brain and bar the door to unwelcome toxins. Those substances that do get in are ferried across the blood-brain barrier by special carrier molecules. Like a passenger vying for a seat on a crowded bus, tryptophan has to compete with five larger amino acids for a ride over. Consequently, not much tryptophan enters the brain, so very little serotonin is synthesized in response to a high-protein meal.

However, if carbohydrate foods are eaten with protein foods, the carbohydrates help deliver more tryptophan to the brain. Carbohydrate triggers the release of the hormone insulin, which drives amino acids right into brain cells. Thus, eating high-carbohydrate meals—*not* high-protein meals—ships tryptophan into the brain where it can be ultimately converted into serotonin. Mixed meals thus provide just the right balance of nutrients to support healthy brain function.

3 HEALTHY FATS THAT POWER YOUR BRAIN

Although it is the most demonized of all nutrients, you need some fat in your diet to survive. In fact, there are a slew of "good" fats with astonishing powers to outwit disease and keep your brain healthy for a lifetime.

DHA

To protect your brain cells, boost your smarts, and ease your mind, serve up foods rich in an omega-3 fatty acid called docosahexaenoic acid, or DHA, for short. DHA is plentiful in fish but is also found in flaxseed, red meat, and eggs. It is also the most abundant omega-3 fatty acid in breast milk.

Considered a building block of the brain, DHA is required for normal brain development as well as for mental well-being and visual functioning. DHA is also a constituent of cell membranes. One of its primary jobs is to protect the fluidity of brain cell membranes to ensure the normal transmission of nerve signals.

DHA has numerous brain-boosting benefits. For example, low levels of DHA are linked to depression. Researchers reported in the *American Journal of Clinical Nutrition* noted that the documented increase in depression in North America in the last century parallels the dwindling consumption of DHA over the same time period.

Some researchers speculate that DHA, because of its importance in human brain tissue, may help prevent degenerative brain diseases such as dementia, memory loss, and Alzheimer's disease. In fact, a study conducted at Tufts University discovered that a low level of DHA is a significant risk factor for these brain diseases. DHA may also bring about memory improvement, according to animal studies.

Children who were breast-fed as infants generally have higher intelligence and greater academic achievement than infants who were formula-fed, according to studies spanning more than twenty years. The common denominator is believed to be the DHA found in breast milk. Formula is generally low in DHA.

Another potential use of DHA lies in treating schizophrenia, a destructive distortion of thinking in which a person's interpretation of reality is severely abnormal. Substantial evidence shows that chemical abnormalities in the brain cause schizophrenia. A growing number of researchers are convinced that one of these abnormalities may be caused by low levels of DHA in brain cells and in red blood cells.

You can increase your supply of DHA by eating more fish (the current recommendation is two to three fish meals a week), incorporating 1 tablespoon a day of flaxseed oil into your diet or by taking DHA supplements. (High-DHA fish are listed in Table 1.2.)

The recommended dosage of DHA supplements is 100 milligrams a day for healthy adults who obtain some DHA from fish and other sources. If you eat little or no fish, 200 milligrams a day is recommended.

MONOUNSATURATED FATS

Protect the blood vessels in your brain by including monounsaturated fats (found primarily in olive oil, canola oil, and nuts) in your diet. The Framingham Heart Study, a long-term study monitoring the health status of men and women from Framingham, Massachusetts, found that men whose diets contained higher levels of monounsaturated fats had the lowest risk of stroke. Saturated fat (found in meats and dairy products) was also discovered to be protective. But polyunsaturated fat (found mostly in vegetable oils) had no effect.

TABLE 1.2
Omega-3–Rich Fish

Seafood is the richest source of omega-3 fatty acids in our food supply. The following types of fish are the highest in omega-3 fatty acids.

Sardines, in sardine oil	3.3 g	Striped bass	.8 g
Atlantic mackerel	2.5 g	Florida pompano	.6 g
Atlantic salmon	1.8 g	Pacific halibut	.4 g
Atlantic herring	1.7 g	Catfish	.3 g
Pacific herring	1.7 g	Cod	.3 g
Bluefin tuna	1.6 g	Flounder	.2 g
Lake trout	1.6 g	Haddock	.2 g
Anchovy	1.4 g	Red snapper	.2 g
Atlantic bluefish	1.2 g	Swordfish	.2 g
Pink salmon	1 g		

Adapted from: Nettle, J. A. 1991. Omega-3 fatty acids: Comparison of plant and seafood sources. *Journal of the American Dietetic Association* 91:331–337; Connor, W. E. et al. 1993. N-3 fatty acids from fish. *Annals of the New York Academy of Sciences* 14:16–34.

To increase the monounsaturated fats in your diet, try snacking on a few olives or nuts during the week, cook with olive oil or canola oil, and prepare salad dressings with olive oil.

LECITHIN

Let lecithin boost your mental vigor. Lecithin is a phospholipid—a fat that contains a molecule of phosphorus. This chemical structure makes the phospholipids soluble in water so that they can travel in and out of the lipid-rich membranes of cells. Manufactured in the liver, lecithin is found in nervous tissue, primarily the myelin sheath (the protective covering for the nerves); in egg yolks, soybeans, and corn; and as an essential constituent of animal and vegetable cells. It helps process cholesterol in the body. As a supplement, lecithin comes in capsules, granules, and liquid form.

A small, unpublished study hints that taking 2 tablespoons of lecithin daily may help prevent memory lapses. In this study, 117 healthy adults were tested on their ability to remember names and find misplaced items. Those supplementing with lecithin had the biggest memory gains.

In another study, mice fed a lecithin-rich diet had much better memory retention than did mice on regular diets. The lecithin-supplemented mice took much longer returning to cages where they had received a mild electric shock, indicating that they had remembered their bad experience. In addition, their brain cells, when examined under a microscope, showed fewer signs of aging.

Investigators believe that lecithin may aid memory by supplying the brain with choline, an essential nutrient that helps produce acetylcholine, the memory neurotransmitter. Lecithin is the richest source of choline.

Here's another plus for lecithin: Normally, as your brain ages, its cell membranes stiffen and lose their ability to take in and release neurotransmitters and send messages. This leads to memory loss and mental confusion. A lecithin-rich diet, however, appears to prevent hardening of cell membranes, according to various studies involving lecithin.

Something else also happens. Aging brain cells lose "dendritic spines," chemical receptor areas that play an important role in transmitting messages. With fewer dendritic spines, messages get distorted and lost. Animal experiments, however, show that aging lecithin-fed mice have as many dendritic spines as younger mice.

To tap into the memory-boosting benefit of lecithin, sprinkle 1 to 2 tablespoons of lecithin granules on cereal, salads, or yogurt. One tablespoon supplies 250 milligrams of choline. The recommended daily intake of choline is 425 milligrams for women and 550 milligrams for men. See Table 1.3 on page 37 for information on supplementing your diet with fats.

TABLE 1.3 Supplementing with Fats		
To increase your intake of brain-protective fats, consider taking the following supplements.		
SUPPLEMENTAL FAT	BRAIN-PROTECTIVE ACTIONS	DOSAGE
DHA	Protects neurons; prevents depression; guards against degenerative brain diseases; improves memory; promotes intelligence.	100 milligrams daily if you eat fish; 200 milligrams daily if you eat no fish
Flaxseed Oil	Is a good source of brain-protective DHA.	1 tablespoon daily
Lecithin	Improves memory; guards against brain aging; supplies the brain with choline.	1 to 2 tablespoons of lecithin granules daily

2 SURPRISE FLUIDS FOR PEAK MENTAL FITNESS

You may think of your brain as a blob of gray matter, but, in reality, it is a moist mass composed of 75-percent fluid. Some of this fluid envelops the brain and protects it from harm by acting as a shock absorber. Because there is such a large turnover of bodily fluids every day, fluid must be replenished constantly to keep your brain and other organs in peak working order. The best way to do this is to drink plenty of fluids every day—but not just any fluids. What follows is a look at the two fluids—besides water—you absolutely need for peak brain fitness.

CAMELLIA SINESIS:
YOUR BRAIN'S CUP OF TEA

Green tea comes from the leaves and leaf buds of *Camellia sinesis*, an evergreen tree from Asia. Sipping a cup or two of green tea daily may save your brain cells from free-radical attacks. Free radicals are cellular aggressors that cripple cells, ultimately causing degenerative diseases such as Alzheimer's disease and accelerating the aging process.

Here's the deal: Several important animal studies conducted within the last six years have discovered that beneficial chemicals called "catechins" in green tea mount a formidable defense against free-radical injury to brain cells. Overwhelmingly, this research indicates that catechins may prevent the destruction of brain cell membranes, snuff out free radicals in the brain, and generally protect against brain-cell damage. What this means is that catechins may be able to keep the health of your brain well up to par. Incidentally, green tea is richer in catechins than black tea.

You can reap the benefits of green tea in the conventional way—with a serving of brewed or iced tea—or by popping a pill of green tea extract. One cup of green tea contains roughly 100 milligrams of catechins. Depending on the supplement, a single pill may contain as many health-building chemicals as four cups of brewed green tea. If you choose to supplement, follow the manufacturer's recommendations for dosage.

Green tea also contains some caffeine. That's a nice bonus since caffeine boosts mental alertness and stimulates creativity. Caffeine, however, aggravates certain health problems, including ulcers, high blood pressure, and insomnia. But unless you're sensitive to caffeine or have trouble sleeping, green tea or extracts containing it are very safe and quite valuable to your body and brain.

Research shows that catechins have other benefits. They may protect against certain cancers, enhance cardiovascular health, and boost fat burning.

JUICE UP YOUR BRAIN FITNESS

A glassful of juice a day may protect against one of the scariest consequences of aging—stroke. A stroke is a disturbance to the brain's blood supply, caused by a blood clot or by bleeding into the brain. Stroke is the third leading cause of death and the number-one cause of disability among adults. Fortunately, though, 80 percent of all strokes are preventable, and drinking certain types of juices appears to be key.

Citrus Juice

In a groundbreaking study of 110,000 men and women, researchers at Harvard discovered that drinking a glass of orange or grapefruit juice every day reduced the risk of a blood-clot stroke by 25 percent. That's a powerful payoff.

So strong is the evidence for juice's antistroke benefit that the U.S. Food and Drug Administration (FDA) has ruled that Tropicana Products, makers of orange juice and other food products, can now claim that its orange juice helps reduce the risk of stroke and high blood pressure. That's because orange juice is high in potassium, an artery-protective nutrient. What's more, orange juice and other citrus juices pack a wallop with vitamin C and folic acid—two good-for-your-brain nutrients.

Another advantage: Juices are an excellent source of brain-nourishing fluids. Orange juice, for example, is nearly 90-percent water.

Purple Grape Juice

According to a study conducted at Tufts University, swigging a cup or two of purple grape juice daily for a week to ten days reduces a process known as "platelet aggregation." This is the tendency of platelets— oval disks in the blood—to stick together and potentially form abnormal clots that can contribute to stroke and heart attack. The research found that purple grape juice reduced stickiness by an amazing 77 percent—an inhibitory effect that was even stronger than aspirin, a known clot buster.

FRESHLY SQUEEZED OR COMMERCIAL?

Clearly, for easy-to-get protection against stroke, drink juice as a regular part of your diet. The question is: Which is better for you—freshly squeezed juice or its store-bought counterpart?

Freshly squeezed juice is often touted as a better source of nutrients than commercial juices—and it usually is, but only if you drink it immediately after squeezing. Nutrients are quickly lost from fresh juice if it is allowed to loll around in the refrigerator for too long.

Commercially prepared juices that are frozen and refrigerated properly are only slightly lower in nutrients than fresh juice. So you're not really missing out if you opt for convenience and drink commercial juices.

A Recipe to Quench the Brain

There are a number of nutrients that research shows can protect brain cells, energize thinking, and enhance memory. These include green tea catechins and vitamin C for cell protection; glucose (sugar), the chief brain fuel; ginkgo biloba, a proven "smart nutrient"; and water, which boosts mental performance. These nutrients are ingredients in the following recipe.

The Brain Quencher

10 green tea bags
10 cups boiling water
1 small can frozen lemonade concentrate (6 fluid ounces)
2 cups orange juice
2 teaspoons vitamin C powder
8 drops liquid ginkgo biloba extract

In a large pitcher, poor boiling water over the tea bags. Let the tea steep. When the liquid has cooled completely, remove tea bags. Add the remaining four ingredients and mix well. For extra sweetness, simply add some sugar. Serve over ice. Makes 8 to 10 servings. Store in the refrigerator for up to one week.

4 Eating Plans to Sharpen Your Thinking

Wouldn't you love an elixir that bolsters your brainpower, manages your mood, sharpens your concentration, and boosts your memory?

You've got it—food. That's right. Food is one of the most powerful prescriptions you have for maximizing your brainpower. By simply eating the right foods, you can control your mind, mood, and memory. The four sample menus featured here show you how.

Each sample menu includes breakfast—a meal you must never miss. When you get up in the morning, you've been on a fast for about eight to twelve hours. During sleep, the amount of energy-giving glucose in your blood drops, so you need to restore it by eating breakfast. The best breakfast for boosting brainpower includes a combination of carbohydrate, protein, and some fat. Because protein and fat are digested more slowly, they help your blood glucose stay elevated longer.

Compared to those who skip the morning meal, people who eat breakfast:

- can do more work.
- maintain their mental efficiency throughout late morning.
- demonstrate faster reaction time.
- have sharper memories.
- think better.
- have a more positive mood.
- feel more calm.

Those are the conclusions of mounds of research, including a famous collection of studies known as the Iowa Breakfast Studies conducted in the early 1950s.

With each of these menus, be sure to drink eight to ten glasses of water a day.

THE BRAINPOWER DIET

On a day when you're on the go—writing a report in the morning, meeting with a client at lunch, and giving a presentation at 2 P.M.—you need to fuel yourself for the long haul. That requires the right food to provide all-day stamina, fight mental slumps, process information, and still be energized for after-work activities such as working out and enjoying your family.

A great brain-boosting diet incorporates multiple meals throughout the day to keep your energy levels high, along with slow-digested food combinations to sustain mental pep and prevent low blood sugar. A typical day's menu looks like the following.

BREAKFAST
1 cup orange juice
2 eggs, scrambled
1 bran muffin
1 cup skim milk
1 cup coffee

MID-MORNING SNACK
3 tablespoons almonds
3 tablespoons raisins

LUNCH
3 to 5 ounces tuna
Large bed green leafy lettuce
Sliced tomato
2 tablespoons reduced-fat Italian dressing
1 banana or other piece of fruit
1 cup coffee

MID-AFTERNOON SNACK
1 high-protein nutrition bar

DINNER

4- to 5-ounces grilled steak

½ cup cooked carrots

1 cup cooked cabbage

1 medium baked potato with 2 tablespoons low-fat sour cream

1 cup fruit-flavored yogurt

The Nutrient Strategy of the Brainpower Diet

- The bran muffin, tuna, milk, almonds, raisins, and cabbage are all high in various B vitamins, known to enhance mental energy. The orange juice and green leafy salad are both loaded with folic acid, a B vitamin important for mental well-being.
- The eggs are rich in choline, required to help synthesize the neurotransmitter acetylcholine, which is involved in memory retention.
- This menu is naturally high in protein, found in eggs, skim milk, tuna, yogurt, the nutrition bar, and steak. Protein foods contain an amino acid called tyrosine, which promotes clear thinking.
- The milk, yogurt, tuna, steak, and green leafy vegetables are chock-full of iron, which helps your brain obtain the oxygen it needs for peak functioning. Iron is also deposited in a part of your brain that stimulates and maintains alertness. The orange juice contains vitamin C, which increases your body's absorption of iron. Thus, ample dietary iron is required to help you stay mentally focused.
- The lunch in this menu is purposely designed to be low in carbohydrate and high in protein—a combination that helps you keep your mental edge throughout the rest of the day.
- The coffee at breakfast and lunch contains caffeine, which helps counter mental fatigue and stimulates creative thinking.
- The fruits and vegetables in this menu are rich in antioxidants, which protect your brain cells from free-radical destruction. These foods are also loaded with potassium, a mineral that helps prevent mental fatigue.

- This menu is also relatively low in fat to help prevent cognitive decline.
- The higher amount of carbohydrate at dinner (the potato and fruit-flavored yogurt) provides glucose, used by the brain to produce serotonin. Adequate levels of serotonin help you sleep better and get the rest you need for the next day of vigorous mental demands.

THE GOOD-MOOD DIET

Perhaps you've got the doldrums and need a lift. Some experts believe you can eat to defeat a bad mood, as long as you select the right foods—those that have a positive effect on brain chemistry. Here's a sample menu that will help banish the blues.

BREAKFAST
1 bagel
½ cup cooked oatmeal, sprinkled with 1 tablespoon flaxseed
   and 1 tablespoon sunflower seeds
½ cup skim milk
½ grapefruit

MID-MORNING SNACK
1 cup fruit-flavored yogurt

LUNCH
Seafood pasta: 1¼ cups pasta topped with ¼ cup seafood
   and ¾ cup marinara sauce
1 small spinach salad with 1 tablespoon ranch dressing

MID-AFTERNOON SNACK
1 granola bar
1 banana

DINNER

4 to 5 ounces grilled salmon

½ cup brown rice with ½ cup red beans

½ avocado with 1 tablespoon Italian dressing

BEDTIME SNACK

½ cup frozen yogurt or sherbet

1 cup chamomile tea

The Nutrient Strategy of the Good-Mood Diet

- The breakfast featured here is high in carbohydrate, which increases bodily levels of serotonin, the neurotransmitter responsible for elevating your mood.
- The flaxseed, salmon, and seafood pasta all contain mood-stabilizing omega-3 fatty acids, which play a role in mental well-being by raising levels of serotonin in the brain.
- The pasta suggested for lunch approximates five times as much carbohydrate as protein—a proportion that has been found in research to prevent serotonin levels from dipping too low.
- The tomato-based marinara sauce is rich in selenium, a mineral needed in the diet to prevent depression. Other depression-defeating nutrients include vitamin C, in the grapefruit; folic acid, in the spinach and avocado; vitamin B_{12}, in the fish and dairy products; niacin, in the vegetables and dairy products; and calcium and vitamin D, also in the dairy products. Brown rice is high in thiamine, a B vitamin that helps reduce mood-sapping fatigue.
- The protein-rich foods in this menu—fish, dairy products, sunflower seeds, brown rice, and red beans—supply various types of good-mood amino acids. The fish, beans, sunflower seeds, and oats (in the oatmeal and granola bar), for example, are high in tryptophan, a building block of serotonin. These same foods are also rich in tyrosine and phenylalanine, two amino acids that keep bad moods at bay.

- The frozen yogurt or sherbet in the bedtime snack is high in glucose, which has a near-immediate effect on the production of serotonin, a mood-lifting neurotransmitter. Chamomile tea contains sedative compounds that induce sleep and relaxation.

THE ATTENTION-SURPLUS DIET

You may be up against a deadline, scheduled to take an afternoon test, or driving long hours to your destination. In such situations, you need laser-sharp focus and quick response time. So the next time you must stay mentally alert, try this menu.

BREAKFAST
Western omelet (2 eggs, 1 ounce cheese, 1 tablespoon each chopped green
    pepper, onion, and tomato)
1 slice whole-wheat bread with 1 pat butter or margarine
1 cup Concord grape juice
1 cup coffee

MID-MORNING SNACK
8 ounces glucose-electrolyte sports drink
1 medium apple

LUNCH
4 ounces grilled chicken salad (2 to 3 cups mixed salad vegetables,
    including 1 tomato, cut into wedges)
2 tablespoons reduced-fat French dressing
1 cup coffee

MID-AFTERNOON SNACK
1 medium pear
2 tablespoons almonds

Dinner

4 to 5 ounces grilled shrimp
½ to 1 cup cooked mixed vegetables
1 medium sweet potato
1 cup skim milk

The Nutrient Strategy of the Attention-Surplus Diet

- The apple, pear, almonds, and tomatoes are loaded with boron. Research indicates that people given additional boron score higher on tests that measure attention and memory.
- Sipping a glucose-electrolyte sports drink is a good idea when you need to pay attention to a task or event at hand. Research shows that rising levels of glucose are associated with faster information processing and better recall. Another good source of glucose is the whole-wheat toast.
- The lunch in this menu is low in carbohydrates. Here's the reason: Too many carbs at lunch impairs attention span and reaction time. To increase alertness, stick to high-protein lunches.
- In addition, keep your lunch on the moderate-to-light size. Large meals have been found in studies to promote momentary lapses of attention. What's more, fat at lunch should be minimal since high-fat lunches produce slower reaction times.
- Have coffee with lunch if you want to abolish post-lunch mental slumps. Coffee is a source of caffeine, which boosts alertness.
- The large salad at lunch contains potassium. If you don't get enough of this mineral in your diet, you may have trouble concentrating.
- The grape juice, sweet potato, and other vegetables are chock-full of brain-protecting antioxidants. Concord grape juice, in particular, is one of the most antioxidant-rich foods you can have.
- Overall, this menu is high in protein. Protein-rich foods supply tyrosine, which has been linked in studies to increased alertness. The shrimp supplies iron and selenium, two minerals that boost concentration and enhance brain health.

THE MEMORY-BOOSTING DIET

Feeling like the absent-minded professor lately? Fortunately, you can bring back a faltering memory by boosting your diet with memory-boosting foods. A typical menu to un-muddle your mind looks like this.

BREAKFAST
½ cup cream of wheat, sprinkled with 2 tablespoons wheat bran
    and 1 tablespoon lecithin granules
2 eggs, any style
½ cup blueberries
1 cup green tea, iced or hot

MID-MORNING SNACK
8 ounces tomato juice blended with 1 tablespoon brewer's yeast
3 tablespoons almonds or walnuts

LUNCH
Tuna salad on a bed of green leafy lettuce
1 banana
1 cup green tea, iced or hot

MID-AFTERNOON SNACK
2 rice cakes or whole-wheat crackers
2 ounces sliced turkey with hot mustard
1 cup skim milk

DINNER
12 baked oysters
½ cup brown rice
1 cup cauliflower
8 ounces fruit-flavored yogurt

The Nutrient Strategy of the Memory-Boosting Diet

- Eggs, dairy products, and lecithin are excellent sources of choline for producing acetylcholine, the memory neurotransmitter.
- Blueberries have been identified in recent animal studies as a fruit that enhances short-term memory. The fruit is well endowed with antioxidants and phytochemicals (plant chemicals) that protect the brain against degeneration. Tomato juice and green leafy vegetables also contain important antioxidants. (For more information on blueberries, see the following section.)
- Folic acid is present in brewer's yeast and green leafy lettuce. Among its many other duties in brain health, folic acid helps prevent dementia.
- Brewer's yeast and brown rice are top sources of thiamine (vitamin B_1), which is required for the synthesis of acetylcholine and is involved in improving learning capacity.
- Tuna, turkey, whole wheat, eggs, brewer's yeast, bananas, and cauliflower all contain vitamin B_6, which helps boost long-term memory.
- Tuna is high in docosahexaenoic acid, or DHA, a key memory-enhancing fat.
- Oysters, tuna, and wheat bran are loaded with zinc, a mineral that plays a vital role in memory formation and retention.
- The fish, poultry, and brewer's yeast in this menu provide the B vitamin niacin, which dilates blood vessels so that more blood, oxygen, and nutrients can reach and nourish your brain.
- Nuts such as almonds and walnuts are good sources of vitamin E, which appears to protect against degenerative brain diseases such as Alzheimer's disease.
- Drinking green tea is recommended for memory preservation. It protects against cognitive decline in the elderly by reducing bodily levels of homocysteine and cholesterol. Both substances are associated with elevated amounts of beta amyloid peptides, proteins that form plaques in the brain and lead to Alzheimer's disease.

A Berry for the Brain: The Amazing Fruit That Fortifies Your Mind

Want to rejuvenate your brainpower? Eat blueberries as a regular part of your diet.

Blueberries may squelch the loss of short-term memory that occurs with age, says a Tufts University study conducted with rats. Much like people, rats become more forgetful as they get older, unable to find their way through mazes they once knew how to navigate. But when fed extracts of blueberries for two months, they actually improved their ability to navigate through mazes! Not only that, the rats' balance, coordination, and running speed improved. In similar tests, strawberries also worked, but not as well.

Scientists speculate that antioxidants in blueberries reduce inflammation, a process that may harm brain tissue as we get older. Blueberries are among the richest fruit sources of antioxidants.

The take-home message here is look for ways to fill your diet with more blueberries. Here are some ideas:

- Eat ½ cup of fresh blueberries most days of the week. Serve them over cereal or in yogurt.
- Bake them into muffins, pies, or cobblers.
- Use them in green salads, tossed with vinaigrette dressing.
- Mix them with other fruits for a tasty fruit salad.
- Blend them into smoothies and frosties. (See "Brain-Boosting Blueberry Frosty" below.)

BRAIN-BOOSTING BLUEBERRY FROSTY

1 8-ounce container non-fat, non-sugar vanilla yogurt
⅓ cup skim milk (liquid, not powder)
½ cup frozen blueberries

Place all ingredients in a blender and puree until smooth. Pour mixture into a tall glass and eat with a spoon. Makes 1 serving.

IRON AND BORON:
BRIGHTEST MINERAL SUPERSTARS

Revving up and restoring your mental powers may be as easy as getting enough of two important minerals: iron and boron. Deficiencies of either can affect brain function.

IRON

Iron is an essential mineral for the healthy upkeep of your central nervous system. Unfortunately, iron deficiency is the most prevalent nutritional disorder in the world, one that has serious repercussions for brain health.

Over the past few decades, a catalog of studies conducted with children and adults indicates that iron deficiency:

- interferes with the brain's normal production of dopamine, a neurotransmitter involved in normal muscle movement and in the production of pleasure.
- harms motor activity, which involves normal muscle movement and coordination.
- impairs cognition (learning and memory).
- reduces attention span.

Therefore, it's important to make sure you get ample iron, particularly from your diet. Here are some suggestions for ways to fortify your diet:

- *Try to keep or add some meat to your diet.* With the exception of some fortified foods, liver is the richest source of iron. But if you can't stomach the taste of liver, beef is your next best bet. Eating a 3- to 4-ounce portion of lean beef two to three times a week gives your iron levels a real boost. Chicken and turkey contain appreciable amounts, too.
- *Eat iron-fortified, ready-to-eat cereals.* This is particularly important if you're a vegetarian.
- *Eat fruits and vegetables that are high in iron.* Green leafy vegetables like kale and collards and dried fruits like raisins and apricots are all good plant sources of iron.
- *Enhance your body's absorption of iron.* You can do this by combining high iron-containing foods with a rich source of vitamin C, which helps the body better absorb iron. For instance, drink some orange juice with your iron-fortified cereal with raisins for breakfast. Or sprinkle some lemon juice on kale or collards.
- *Take an iron supplement.* Pregnant women, marathon runners, and people with digestive diseases or other conditions that cause blood loss or poor mineral absorption are candidates for iron deficiency. Only a doctor can diagnose iron deficiency, so be sure to obtain the advice of your physician prior to supplementing. Self-medicating with large doses of iron is risky.

The daily reference intake (DRI) for iron is 18 milligrams for women and 8 milligrams for men. The amount of iron found in various food sources appears in Table 1.4.

TABLE 1.4
Dietary Iron

Best Food Sources	Iron Content per Serving
Fortified cereals (1 cup)	7 to 24 milligrams, depending on brand
Liver (4 ounces)	7 milligrams
Oysters (6)	6 milligrams
Lean beef (4 ounces)	4 milligrams
Raisins (1 cup)	3 milligrams
Collard greens (1 cup)	2 milligrams
Dark-meat chicken (4 ounces)	2 milligrams
Dark-meat turkey (4 ounces)	2.6 milligrams
Dried apricots (10)	1.65 milligrams
White-meat chicken (4 ounces)	1.5 milligrams
White-meat turkey (4 ounces)	1.5 milligrams
Kale (1 cup)	1.2 milligrams

Adapted from: Sizer, F., and E. Whitney. *Nutrition Concepts and Controversies*, 7th ed. (Belmont, California: West/Wadsworth, 1997).

BORON

As for boron, how alert you are may depend on how much of this mineral you consume. In one study, the more boron in the diets of the subjects, the better they performed on attention and memory tests. Specifically, the better performers were eating 3.2 milligrams a day; they performed 10-percent higher on tests when compared with a low-boron group.

Boron is found in prunes, apples, peaches, avocados, and nuts, as well as celery, carrots, and other vegetables. Although no DRI has been set for boron, leading mineral experts suggest that 1 milligram a day is a reasonable amount to consume. If you eat lots of fruits, vegetables, and nuts throughout the week, you'd already be consuming two to six times that amount of boron.

The amount of boron found in various food sources appears in Table 1.5.

TABLE 1.5	
Dietary Boron	
BEST FOOD SOURCES	**BORON CONTENT PER SERVING**
Prunes (½ cup)	21 milligrams
Peanuts (½ cup)	18 milligrams
Almonds (½ cup)	14 milligrams
Avocado (1)	11 milligrams
Red grapes (½ cup)	4.6 milligrams
Plum (1)	4.2 milligrams
Apple (1)	2.7 milligrams
Broccoli (½ cup)	2.5 milligrams
Celery (½ cup)	2.19 milligrams
Carrots (½ cup)	2 milligrams

Adapted from: Naghil, M. R. et al. 1996. The boron content of selected foods and the estimation of its daily intake among free-living subjects. *Journal of the American College of Nutrition* 15:614–619.

7 BRAIN-PROTECTIVE PHYTOCHEMICALS

In the past decade, scientists have discovered a cornucopia of new substances in food that have some amazing disease-fighting properties. They're called phytochemicals, which means "plant chemicals."

Unlike vitamins and minerals, phytochemicals don't have any nutritive value, but they do seem to protect against cancer, heart disease, and other illnesses. You can get all the disease-fighting power of phytochemicals by simply eating a variety of fruits, vegetables, and grains—and lots of them—every day.

Here's a brief rundown of seven important brain-enhancing phytochemicals and what they do.

ALLYLIC SULFIDES
Found in garlic, onions, and leeks, these plant chemicals may play a role in protecting against the loss of brain function in aging and enhanc-

ing memory, according to a number of studies. The reason? Allylic sulfides are powerful antioxidants that protect cell membranes from intrusion by free radicals. Plus, they fortify the body's own internally produced team of antioxidants, particularly in the brain.

CAROTENOIDS

Carotenoids are components of fruits and vegetables that neutralize free radicals, thus protecting cell membranes and brain cells against damage. The main carotenoids are beta-carotene, alpha-carotene, cryptoxanthin, gamma-carotene, lutein, and lycopene.

CATECHINS

In research with aged rat brains, catechins, which are found mostly in green tea, demonstrated the ability to snuff out free radicals and protect brain tissue. Catechins, therefore, may be important neuroprotective nutrients, particularly as we age.

ELLAGIC ACID

Plentiful in red and white grapes, ellagic acid prevents toxic chemicals from damaging cells. In research with rats, it blocked the action of an enzyme responsible for the development of brain cancer.

FERULIC ACID

Extracted from rice bran oil and available as a nutritional supplement, ferulic acid has recently been found to suppress the toxic action of "beta amyloid peptides" in the brains of mice. These peptides are harmful proteins that promote free-radical damage and inflammation in the brain and thus are considered conspirators in the development of Alzheimer's disease. Ferulic acid, therefore, may be helpful in preventing Alzheimer's disease.

Ferulic acid has also been shown to help normalize cholesterol and triglyceride levels, thus improving blood circulation, and to treat menopause symptoms, including moodiness.

FLAVONOIDS

These phytonutrients are abundant in the flesh of citrus fruits and berries. As potent antioxidants, they protect cells, including brain cells, from degenerative changes and may play an important role in preventing—even reversing—the devastating effects of oxidation on brain function. To get more of the brain-protecting benefits of flavonoids, eat whole fruits instead of drinking juice.

PHYTOESTROGENS

Prevalent in soy foods, these plant chemicals, which include genistein and isoflavones, may guard against the degeneration of brain function that can occur in postmenopause. When a woman undergoes menopause, her natural levels of estrogen dip considerably—a decline believed to increase the risk of Alzheimer's disease and dementia, since estrogen protects brain function. Studies show that estrogen replacement therapy dramatically decreases the risk of mental decline. However, not all women are candidates for this therapy. Therefore, phytoestrogens may provide a safe, natural alternative to prescription estrogen and thus help prevent mental slumps.

4 Easy Workouts to Pump Up Mental Fitness

What's good for your body is good for your brain—and that includes regular exercise. Exercise boosts the flow of oxygenated blood to your brain. With more oxygen traveling to your brain, you think more clearly and creatively. In a study comparing regular exercisers to couch potatoes, the exercisers were more decisive and better able to size up a situation.

Also, exercise involving complicated motor skills such as aerobic dance

affects mental agility, possibly by increasing the amount of oxygen deliv-
ered to the brain and stimulating the brain to develop new connections.
Animal studies have found that skill-type exercise creates new brain
synapses, special connections that help the brain process more information.

Exercise trains the mind in other ways, too. The neural processes that
control movement are slowed by age as brain cells shrink and messenger
systems work less efficiently. One noticeable result is a reduction in reaction time—unless you exercise. Reaction time refers to how long it takes
to respond to an unexpected situation—for instance, slamming on the
brake pedal when a pedestrian walks in front of your car or bolting out
of bed if you hear an intruder.

Many people who exercise regularly are less likely to experience slow-
downs in reaction time and are better able to keep their mental skills
sharp. Researchers at the University of Utah compared the brain-wave
activity of two groups of older people: one very active; the other, seden-
tary. What they found was that the brain waves of the active group more
closely resembled those of younger people.

Exercise also enhances the synthesis of neurotransmitters, which are
required for the rapid transmission of messages throughout the body.
Significantly, diseases such as Parkinson's and Huntington's are caused
or accompanied by a short supply of neurotransmitters in specific areas
of the nervous system. Thus, exercise could have a protective or therapeutic effect on these conditions.

That said, what kind of exercise should you do to maximize brain fitness? Any exercise is good; however, different types of exercise have different effects on the brain. The key is to pick an exercise that matches
what you need to accomplish in a particular day. Here are four examples
of brain-boosting workouts.

PLAN 1: THE NERVE-CALMING WORKOUT

Suppose you're giving a big presentation today, or you're scheduled
for your annual performance review. Prior to the event, ease the jitters
with an intense bout of aerobic exercise—the kind that gets your heart
pumping (running, jogging, or stationary cycling).

The reason why aerobic exercise calms the nerves is that it releases certain chemicals produced by the brain. The most well known are endorphins, which are responsible for reducing pain and heightening feelings of pleasure. The result is a general sense of mental well-being. Whenever regular exercisers are asked about the psychological benefits of working out, most say that it makes them feel better, that they can handle stress better, or that they feel more energetic.

PLAN 2: THE CONFIDENCE-BUILDING WORKOUT

Maybe today's the day you've got to announce a layoff, pitch a product to a new client, or negotiate a contract. Whatever the challenge, you need sky-high confidence, and one way to get it is to play a competitive sport—a match of tennis or racquetball, a game of basketball, a little sparring with a punching bag, for example. Competitive exercise—particularly if you win—stimulates the body to churn our more testosterone, a hormone that heightens feelings of aggression and gives you that on-top-of-the world confidence.

PLAN 3: THE SLUMP-BUSTING WORKOUT

You know the feeling: It's 3 o'clock in the afternoon and you're ready for a nap, especially after the stressful day you've put in at work so far. To rejuvenate, do some exercises in your office or right at your desk. Some examples include stretches or push-ups, even a walk up and down the stairs in your office building.

Why are such exercises so important? They relieve you of stress, which can cloud your mind and impair your memory. What's more, they get blood pumping to your brain.

PLAN 4: THE MEMORY-BOOSTING WORKOUT

For enhancing memory as you age, nothing beats pumping iron, also known as weight training, strength training, or resistance training. This form of exercise involves weight-bearing activity in which your muscles are challenged to work harder each time they're exercised. Examples of strength training include lifting weights, working out on weight-training machines, and exercising with special rubber cords or bands.

In a study conducted at the University of Berne in Switzerland, forty-six men and women (average age seventy-three) were randomly assigned either to a strength-training group or to a control group. The strength trainers exercised just once a week, performing eight different exercises, for eight weeks. By the end of the experimental period, the strength trainers experienced a big increase in cognitive function and memory. The benefits were long lasting, too. One year later, the researchers found that memory performance among the strength trainers remained high.

All it takes to get started on a strength-training program is to join a gym and enlist the help of a qualified instructor to teach you the ropes. You can work out at home, too. Two to three workouts, thirty to forty-five minutes each, will boost your mind, memory, and muscle.

SMART SUPPLEMENTS: 10 MIRACLE PILLS AND POTIONS THAT IMPROVE MENTAL ACUITY

With smart supplements, you can set your wits to work wonders. The supplements discussed below are particularly helpful if you're having trouble concentrating, thinking up great ideas, learning new information, or performing mentally.

Some important guidelines: Many smart supplements can be used concurrently (acetyl-L-carnitine and vitamin E, for example), but be careful about taking a handful of different products at the same time. It's unclear how well some combinations work. They may enhance the effects of each other or they may not.

You're better off trying one supplement at a time. Give each supplement several weeks to take effect before deciding whether it's improving your mental functions. If you're getting good results but they suddenly stop, your brain may have built up a tolerance for that particular supplement. In that case, "cycle" it, that is, go on and off the supplement. Take it for a couple weeks at a time, discontinue it, and then resume supplementation.

ACETYL-L-CARNITINE

If you want to spark your creativity, give your brain a dose of acetyl-L-carnitine, a derivative of the amino acid–like nutrient carnitine. Carnitine and acetyl-L-carnitine are both available as nutritional supplements. However, carnitine does not easily reach the brain; acetyl-L-carnitine does.

Researchers say there is strong evidence that acetyl-L-carnitine prevents mind and memory decline. For example, acetyl-L-carnitine:

- promotes the activity of two neurotransmitters—acetylcholine and dopamine—in the brain for clearer thinking.
- improves communication between the left and right parts of the brain, thus promoting creativity and sharper intuition.
- improves reflex speed and accuracy, according to a study conducted with adults whose mental processing was observed while they played a computer game.

For brain protection, experts recommend a dose of up to 1,000 milligrams a day. The supplement produces virtually no negative side effects. However, dosages that exceed recommendations cause gastrointestinal discomfort. Also, people with kidney disease or other illnesses should not supplement unless they first confer with a physician.

ALPHA-GLYCERYLPHOSPHORYLCHOLINE (ALPHA-GPC)

In the neighborhood of smart supplements, the new kid on the block is alpha-GPC, an antiaging supplement that has value in treating a host of brain problems, from stroke to senility. Alpha-GPC is rich in choline, an essential nutrient required for optimal brain function; and glycerol and phosphate, two substances that work with choline to protect and maintain cell membranes. Quite a bit of research has accumulated on alpha-GPC's merits as a mental rejuvenator. These studies show that alpha-GPC:

- improves performance on psychometric tests, which measure intelligence, emotional reactions, and behavior—in both healthy adults and Alzheimer's patients.
- boosts memory and cognition.
- activates the release of GABA, a neurotransmitter that produces calmness, in animal brains. This hints that alpha-GPC may be of value in treating anxiety and seizure disorders.
- speeds cognitive recovery in stroke patients.

Experts recommend a dose of 400 milligrams, taken three times daily. Available in tablets, capsules, and powders, alpha-GPC has few serious side effects. In clinical trials, however, some patients have experienced heartburn, nausea, vomiting, insomnia, and headache. These can be minimized by reducing the dosage.

ASHWAGANDHA (INDIAN GINSENG)

Stressed-out executives, students, the elderly, and others are looking to this herb to clear the mind, calm the body, promote restful sleep, and rejuvenate all bodily systems. It is derived from the root of a tall branching shrub cultivated in India and North America.

Ashwagandha's curative powers have been touted for thousands of years in India, but only recently has the herb been clinically tested. As they've deconstructed the root, scientists have isolated compounds known to relax the central nervous system and fight stress. Ashwagandha also contains numerous amino acids that can fortify the brain, including glycine, valine, and tyrosine. In a study at the University of Leipzig in Germany, an extract of ashwagandha positively affected the metabolism of acetylcholine in rats, and this could explain its positive effects on cognition.

Ashwagandha is available in dried-root form, powders, capsules, tablets, or liquid extract. Follow the dosage recommended on the label. No serious side effects have been associated with this herb. However, in large amounts, ashwagandha can cause irritation to mucous membranes or to the gastrointestinal tract. Do not take ashwagandha in conjunction with sedatives because the herb can exaggerate the effects of these drugs.

BACOPA MONNIERA

Among "smart" herbs, bacopa monniera is the leader of the pack, renowned for its reputed ability to improve your intellect and make you smarter. Used for more than 5,000 years in India, bacopa comes from the root of the Brahmi plant. It is believed to work by fortifying the immune system against stress (a mental mangler), stimulating the production of serotonin in the brain, and regenerating dendrites in brain cells.

Hard evidence for bacopa's reputation as a smart supplement comes mostly from animal and clinical studies. In one study, rats that were fed an extract of bacopa showed significant learning and memory enhancement in navigating a maze compared with control rats that were given no bacopa and rats given only Valium. Research into bacopa is continuing.

About 70 milligrams of the extract (once in the morning and once in the evening) is considered a reasonable dose. If you're taking the powdered dry root, the recommended dose is ½ teaspoon in the morning and ½ teaspoon again in the evening. Doses that exceed these recommendations may be harmful since bacopa contains plant chemicals whose action resembles that of strychnine, a poison.

CHOLINE

Present in all living cells, choline is synthesized from two amino acids—methionine and serine—with help from vitamin B_{12} and folic acid. Choline is very important to brain chemistry. Choline converts to acetylcholine in the brain. Research into choline indicates that it can improve performance on memory and intelligence tests.

Although choline is abundant in various foods, it's a wise move to consider supplementation. Here's why: Choline is one of the few nutrients that can penetrate the blood-brain barrier, which protects the brain from toxins and other unwanted visitors. Channels to the brain, however, are like limited access highways where nutrients have to compete for entry like cars trying to get on a road. After you eat a meal (eggs, for example), the choline and amino acids in that meal compete with one another for access to the brain. When taken in supplement form, however, choline has no competition and enjoys a direct route to the brain.

Supplementally, choline is available in various forms: regular choline, phosphatidylcholine, and lecithin. For enhancing cognitive function, experts recommend a dosage of 1,500 milligrams daily. To strengthen its effect, try taking choline with water, apart from regular meals. Certain forms of choline—namely, choline bitartrate and choline chloride—can cause diarrhea or produce a fishy body odor.

GINKGO BILOBA

Ginkgo biloba, derived from the leaves of an ornamental tree, is the reigning superstar among brain-enhancing supplements. It is particularly effective for combating the loss of mental capacity due to advancing age.

As we get on in years, oxygen blood flow to our brains slacks off, primarily because arteries begin to thicken and narrow—a condition medically known as atherosclerosis. Ginkgo improves and normalizes blood circulation to the brain and other organs. It accomplishes this by thinning the blood, enhancing the health and tone of blood vessels, inhibiting abnormal clotting, and fighting fluid buildup. Ginkgo also stimulates areas of the brain responsible for memory. These actions have been extensively verified by numerous clinical trials.

Ginkgo also protects cells against oxidative damage that normally occurs as our bodies burn oxygen to live. If not held in check by antioxidants, oxidation can corrode cell membranes in much the same way that rust forms on metal. A product of oxidation is free radicals, nasty molecules that attack bodily tissues. As explained in an earlier section, degeneration of brain function is believed to be linked to oxidative damage in brain tissue.

Normally, ginkgo works its mental magic over the long term. But it can be fast acting in high doses. For instance, a study of healthy young women found that those who supplemented with 600 milligrams of ginkgo extract one hour prior to taking a memorization test scored significantly higher than subjects who took no ginkgo.

The standard dose is 120 to 240 milligrams in two to three separate doses daily. It takes about eight weeks to see an improvement. Do not supplement with ginkgo if you are taking blood thinners. (For more information on ginkgo, see "Ginkgo Biloba" under "Other Amazing Anti-Alzheimer's Herbs" on page 317 in Chapter 14.)

GINSENG

Used for thousands of years in the East as a tonic to strengthen and restore health, ginseng has more recently been touted as a brain-boosting herb. Its active constituents are compounds called ginsenosides, which stimulate the brain's neurotransmitter activity and help it synthesize protein to function optimally.

Ginseng comes from the root of a medicinal plant in the ginseng family (Araliaceae). There are various types of ginseng, including those in the *Panax* classification and a botanical cousin called Siberian ginseng (*Eleutherococcus senticosus*), or "eleuthero," for short. Eleuthero's active constituents are substances known as eleutherosides, which differ in chemical structure from ginsenosides but have similar brain-boosting powers.

Panax ginseng is the Asian variety, also known as true ginseng or Chinese or Korean ginseng. It grows in the mountainous forests of eastern Asia and is the most widely used form of the herb. There are red and white *Panax* ginsengs as well. All ginseng roots are white when raw and peeled, but certain processing methods turn ginseng red.

Various clinical trials substantiate ginseng's ability to boost brainpower. In one study, college students who supplemented with two capsules of *Panax* ginseng a day showed improved concentration and better test scores than those who did not take the herb. Ginseng also improved accuracy and response time among proofreaders and telegraph operators—professions in which accuracy is required.

Taking *Panax* ginseng with ginkgo enhances mental functioning. In a fourteen-week study of 256 healthy adults (ages forty to sixty-six), this combo improved subjects' scores on computerized recall, recognition, and spatial tests by more than 7 percent. No such improvements were seen in placebo-takers. The daily doses used in the study were 200 milligrams of ginseng and 120 milligrams of ginkgo.

Panax ginseng and eleuthero are approved medicines in Germany. In fact, the German Commission E—Germany's equivalent of our Food and Drug Administration (FDA)—states in its monographs that these ginsengs can be used "as a tonic for invigoration and fortification in times of fatigue and debility, for declining capacity for work and concentration, also during convalescence."

Ginseng is available as teas and as powders, capsules, extracts, tablets, teas, and ginseng-flavored soft drinks. For *Panax* ginseng, the German Commission E recommends 1 to 2 grams daily of the powdered herb or equivalent for up to three months; eleuthero, 2 to 3 grams of the powdered root. Extracts of ginseng are recommended in many different doses; read the supplement label for exact instructions.

Side effects of ginseng supplementation are rare, and the herb is considered safe. However, excessive doses and long-term use may cause high blood pressure, nervousness, insomnia, painful breasts, and vaginal bleeding. People with high blood pressure should avoid ginseng.

GOTU KOLA

A member of the parsley family, gotu kola is a common weed, usually found growing in drainage ditches in Asia and orchards in Hawaii. Also available as a supplement, it is reputed to be an aphrodisiac, a wound healer, and a brain builder. One study found that mentally challenged children's intelligence scores and behavior patterns were improved when given the herb.

Herbalists like gotu kola because it exerts a dual effect. On one hand, it stimulates the brain for mental alertness. But it also contains two sedative compounds. So, by taking gotu kola, you can relax but stay mentally sharp at the same time.

Gotu kola comes in extracts and whole-herb forms. Follow the dosage recommended on the label. This herb may cause a skin rash or headache. Lower your dosage if you experience side effects, or stop taking the herb altogether.

Gotu kola is often combined with ginkgo, ashwagandha, and ginseng in brain and memory tonics. These supplements are billed as natural ways to help increase mental acuity and concentration and to fight memory loss and dementia.

NICOTINAMIDE ADENINE DINUCLEOTIDE (NADH)

Found naturally in the muscle tissue of fish, poultry, and beef, NADH is a cofactor (activator) of niacin (vitamin B_3) and plays an essential role in the energy production of cells. In the brain, increased concentrations help improve the production of neurotransmitters.

According to research, NADH:

- improves mental function.
- increases alertness and concentration.
- enhances mood.

NADH generally comes in dosages of 2.5 milligrams and 5 milligrams. Start with the lower dosage to see how you respond, then increase to the 5-milligram dose, if needed. Best taken in the morning on an empty stomach, NADH apparently works rapidly. You may begin to feel more alert within a few hours.

VITAMIN E

Vitamin E is highly recommended as a must-have nutrient for boosting brainpower. That's because it is a powerful antioxidant that works in brain cell membranes (and other cell membranes) to guard them against free-radical damage. This may be the reason vitamin E has been shown in research to slow the progression of Alzheimer's disease and to enhance performance on memory tests.

Vitamin E occurs naturally in vegetable oils, whole-grain cereals, seeds, dried beans, and green leafy vegetables—yet the content is not high. Consequently, many researchers feel that vitamin E supplements are more effective than foods as a means of getting adequate vitamin E.

Supplementing with 400 international units (IU) of vitamin E daily is an excellent way to get the protective amount.

Train Your Brain and Sharpen Your Senses with These 16 Mental Exercises

If you neglect your brain—that is, don't use it—expect foggy thinking, poor memory, and sluggish reasoning to set in. By contrast, though, stimulating your brain activates neural pathways, expands capillaries, triggers lively neurotransmitter activity, and builds connections for supercharged mental power. The result of all this activity is a brain that stays sharp and refuses to age. What follows are some easy-to-perform mental exercises that will give your noggin a great workout.

READ SMART

Pick up and read a challenging or engrossing novel, such as something by Charles Dickens or another one of the classics. The greater the reading challenge, the better your brain is stimulated.

REMEMBER WHAT YOU READ

If you're like most people, you easily forget the book—its plot and characters—shortly after you finish it. For better retention (and memory practice), study the table of contents and try to memorize it. Write down the key characters in the book (practice recalling their names), plus the significant events associated with their lives. Note the relationships among characters. You might even try outlining—a proven study strategy used by students who want to remember lesson material because it helps compartmentalize and retain information.

Refer to your notes or outline, trying to remember the information as if you're studying for a test. Then practice retelling the story to a friend.

DO PUZZLES

Crossword puzzles, acrostics, cryptograms, word jumbles, jigsaw puzzles—these keep your brain stimulated and powered up. Research shows that word-type puzzles build verbal skills and jigsaw puzzles build spatial skills.

DANCE

Take up dancing—ballet, tango, tap, line dancing—any form of dance that involves complex coordinated movements. As you concentrate and think through the movement, your brain produces more dendrite connections, those bridges between brain cells that help keep your brain young and active. In addition, the physical exercise involved in dance boosts the blood and oxygen supply to your brain. Exercise also increases the supply of "neurotrophins," natural substances that stimulate the growth of brain cells.

BOOST YOUR VOCABULARY

Each week, pick a new word from the dictionary. Review its definition and memorize its spelling. Try to incorporate it into your language, in both writing and speaking.

PLAY WITH WORDS

Pick a word with six or more letters. Then try to create as many additional words from those letters as you can in a specified time period, such as one minute. Take the word "magazine," for example. From that word, you might create "maze," "again," "gaze," "gain," "main," "mane," "enigma," and so forth.

MEMORIZE

One of the easiest ways to vitalize your mind is to embark on a regular program of memorization. Each week, commit something to memory—a short poem, quote, Bible verse, or other memory builder. Tape the passage to your mirror so you'll see it when you're getting dressed, or post it by your computer at work—just so that it's in front of you most of the time. In subsequent weeks, while you're memorizing new material, practice recalling the earlier stuff you memorized. Memorization stimulates your neural circuits, boosts blood flow to your brain, and keeps neurotransmitters active.

PLAY BOARD GAMES

Some of the best brain-teasing games include Scrabble™ (Milton Bradley), as well as Scattergories™ and Taboo™ (both by Hasbro), or Trivial Pursuit™ (Parker Brothers). Another is Stratego™ (Milton Bradley); it helps you recall which of your opponent's pieces have moved and which have stayed put.

Chess and bridge improve your powers of concentration, perception, and reasoning. All of these games and others like them are excellent for keeping your brain alert and your memory sharp.

PRACTICE THE NAME GAME

Here's a great memory builder: Every so often, look at a list of ten nouns (have someone create it for you). Read over the list for one minute, then try to remember as many words as you can. (See your doctor if it's difficult to recall more than one to three words without trouble.)

A variation: Have someone pick ten objects and arrange them on a tabletop. Study them for thirty seconds. Cover the objects, then try to remember as many as you can. Repeat this exercise during the week, but with different objects. Make it your goal to remember all ten. Once you've accomplished that, begin practicing the exercise with more than ten objects.

STRENGTHEN YOUR POWERS OF OBSERVATION

One reason our minds and memories get dull is because we haven't paid enough attention in the first place, so things don't get embedded in our memory banks. To recharge your mental powers, try this exercise: Pick up a home and gardening magazine or a remodeling magazine. (This exercise can be performed with any favorite magazine.) Look closely at a photo of a room, paying attention to details. Then close the magazine and try to remember everything you can about the picture. What was the color scheme? What was the layout? What type of furniture was in the room? What were the accessories?

Write down what you recall and read it aloud (this helps reinforce memory). Look at the photo again, checking for details you overlooked. Keep doing this exercise until you remember every detail about the room. With practice, you'll become a whiz at remembering detail.

FOSTER YOUR FOCUS

All of us could do with a better attention span. Here's an exercise to improve your concentration. Sit quietly, close your eyes, and listen to your surroundings—the hum of your computer, birds chirping outside your window, cars whizzing by. Then pick the loudest or most prominent sound and concentrate on it, blocking out everything else for an entire minute. Then move on to a different sound. Practice this exercise several times a week, and your powers of concentration will strengthen immensely.

DO MATH IN YOUR HEAD OR ON PAPER

Occasionally, forgo your calculator. Overused, calculators can make us mentally sluggish. The next time you have to tally up a tip or add up some simple numbers, figure it in your head. If balancing your check-book, do it on paper, without the help of your calculator.

STRETCH YOUR BRAIN

When stimulated, your brain actually stretches in size, thanks to the for-mation of new connections between brain cells. Here's a brain-stretching tip from Brainergy, Inc., a consulting firm that conducts brain-enhancing seminars: Turn a page of text upside down and try reading for three min-utes. This exercise helps sharpen your thinking. (For information on Brain-ergy, Inc., access the company's Web site at www.brainergy.com, or call 1-800-782-2200.)

Another similar exercise is to recite the alphabet backward until it be-comes rote. Practice this several times a week.

GO BACK TO SCHOOL

Scientists have peered into the brains of people who decided to return to school for more education. What they found is rather intriguing: The brain cells in back-to-schoolers become stimulated and active—a phe-nomenon known to help protect your brain from damage as you age. And, as pointed out earlier, people with education are less likely to de-velop dementia later in life.

ENRICH YOUR ENVIRONMENT

Having an environment that forces you to use your brain keeps your thinking razor sharp. The opposite of this is boredom, which dulls your senses and brings on depression. To enrich your environment, attend lec-tures, visit exhibits, join new groups, see interesting movies, and meet new people.

The importance of being in an enriched environment was first dis-covered in studies of rats, which were placed in cages with companion rats, mazes, and lots of toys to play with. The scientists observed that the brains of the stimulated rats were thicker due to an increase in dendrites. The rats also became better learners.

DO THINGS DIFFERENTLY

Although your brain never stops learning, it's essentially a lazy organ that will revert to automatic pilot when asked to do something the same way, time after time. Change your routine activities to stimulate your brain to form new connections and exercise different types of memory.

Some suggestions: Brush your teeth with your left hand (if you're right-handed, or vice versa), use your computer mouse with the opposite hand, read a newspaper article you wouldn't normally opt to read, or take a new route to work. Even rearranging the furniture in a room will challenge your brain and make it more responsive.

IMPROVE YOUR PERFORMANCE WITH MENTAL REHEARSAL

Long before the actual race, sales meeting, recital, speech, procedure, or new job, play it over in your mind, rehearsing every second of the situation or encounter in minute detail. Make the image so vivid that you can see, hear, feel, and smell your surroundings. Then visualize yourself winning, succeeding, performing without errors, and coming out on top. Practice this long enough, and the same success can be yours in real life.

Studies conducted for more than sixty years point to the fact that mental rehearsal—the practice of successfully carrying out an action in our mind—can maximize our performance and potential in nearly every aspect of life.

Why such a powerful effect?

Scientists have learned that the brain—specifically, the subconscious mind—can't tell the difference between real and imagined events. Mentally previewing and rehearsing a movement activates the same areas of the brain that are activated when you physically perform that movement—with the exception of the motor cortex, which triggers the neural circuits for muscle movement. So, in a sense, your subconscious mind is tricked into thinking that the image is reality.

WHAT YOU GAIN

The specific benefits of mental rehearsal are numerous. For example, mental rehearsal:

- helps you learn new skills.
- improves those skills after the initial learning phase and physical training.
- familiarizes you with the activity that lies ahead. When you're actually ready to perform, your brain senses that you've already done it—successfully. Thus, you're mentally primed for success.
- banishes "can't-do" thoughts from your mind. Mental rehearsal replaces such thoughts with images of success that gear you up for optimal performance. Performance anxiety is reduced as a result.
- achieves a more flawless and accurate performance. Studies with musicians have found that combining mental practice with physical practice leads to a more error-free performance and also improves speed and memorization of musical pieces. An Australian study found that basketball players who mentally rehearsed their free-throw shots improved their accuracy by 23 percent over players who didn't.
- increases response time, particularly when split-second decisions must be made. This has been shown in training exercises in which police officers visualize how to respond to deadly force situations such as the apprehension of armed suspects. Visualization reduces the trainees' reaction times and can increase the officers' odds of survival.
- bolsters self-image. Perhaps you've experienced some personal setbacks or failures. Then try visualization, recommended by psychologists to help their patients rebuild a stronger sense of

self. Think back to prior successes or to times when your life was going well. Project yourself into that image and begin to see yourself behaving and acting that way now.

HOW TO MENTALLY REHEARSE

For mental rehearsal to be effective, you have to be a good imager. Here's how:

1. Sit in a relaxed position or lie down in a quiet place.
2. Close your eyes and take several deep breaths through your nose. Continue breathing in this manner until you begin to feel very calm. Your mind can focus better when you're in a relaxed state.
3. Imagine in your mind's eye the movement required to successfully perform the task or activity. In other words, think in pictures. See yourself sinking a putt, dunking a free throw, delivering a dynamic presentation, making a brilliant sales pitch to a new client, performing magnificently in a musical recital, conducting a flawless surgical procedure, boldly asking for a raise—whatever you're up against or want to accomplish well. Be as detailed as possible in your imaginings, visualizing your performance exactly as you would like it to be.
4. Bring as many other senses into the rehearsal as possible, such as the smell and feel of your surroundings. Hear the sounds of your environment, too, even your own voice.
5. Practice mental rehearsal regularly. Experts suggest that you begin with daily ten-minute sessions.
6. Develop a positive-image reservoir that you can retrieve and replay in your mind when needed for successful performances. It's like having your own video library stored in your brain, ready to replay when you need it.

5 WAYS TO MAKE SMARTER DECISIONS

Should you switch careers?... Take a new job?... Get married?... Get divorced?... Buy a house?... Move away?... Sink money into an investment?... Go to grad school?... Hire the person you just interviewed?

Decisions. Decisions. Decisions. We're faced with them every day. Sometimes we make seat-of-the-pants decisions without realizing the consequences. Or we do the opposite, never making a decision, letting opportunities slip from our grasp.

Decision-making skills become increasingly important as we age. Scientists at the University of Iowa College of Medicine discovered that older adults, though healthy, may exhibit faulty decision making due to age-related damage to a part of the brain called the ventromedial prefrontal cortex, or VPC, for short. The VPC is responsible for the interface of decision making and emotion (decision making depends very much on your emotions).

When the VPC is impaired, people generally have trouble making decisions regarding social relationships and finances—which is why many seniors are more likely than their younger counterparts to fall prey to telemarketing schemes and other financial scams. Damage to the VPC is believed to be caused by aging and, quite possibly, by high blood pressure medication prescribed for many older patients.

No matter what the current state of your decision-making habits, you can reprogram your mind to make better choices, most of the time, in every area of life—personal, professional, and financial. Here's how:

GO ON A FACT-FINDING MISSION

To make a smart decision, become an expert on the situation at hand. Suppose your broker calls with a hot tip on a stock. Before taking the bait, do some research yourself—about the company, its performance, its long-range forecast, and so forth. Use all available resources—the Internet, the library, your broker, or other related sources—to find the information you need. Ask lots of questions and do lots of homework. By conducting a thorough analysis of the situation, you'll be better equipped to make a smart decision.

THINK FOR YOURSELF

While it's helpful to listen to other points of view, it's often too easy to let other people talk you out of a decision you know in your gut may be right. Letting others do your thinking for you is a major reason many people waffle on making decisions. Thinking and deciding for yourself, on the other hand, is personally empowering. It teaches you to be responsible and helps you deal more effectively with both day-to-day and long-term challenges. Plus, when it's your decision, you're more likely to implement it.

EVALUATE THE SITUATION
ACCORDING TO YOUR GOALS

Whether personal or professional, goals set the direction for our lives. Ideally, the decisions we make are stepping stones toward those goals. When faced with a decision, ask yourself if the choice you're about to make will help you meet your goals or send you on a path away from those goals.

LIST THE PROS AND CONS OF
A COURSE OF ACTION

It's instructive to see the consequences of a choice written out in black and white. Let's say you're trying to decide whether to apply for a job or to graduate school. Simply list the advantages and disadvantages of each on a sheet of paper.

Next, try to imagine the consequences of each decision: "What would happen if . . . ?" Or "Is this the best and most beneficial course of action?" Again, "Which course of action helps me meet my goals?" It's also considered smart decision making to consider the negative consequences of a course of action.

In a similar vein, you can brainstorm various alternatives without throwing out any ideas, no matter how offbeat or ridiculous. Generating alternative solutions opens the door to possibilities you might not have otherwise considered. Next, simply narrow down your alternatives according to which are the most feasible for your situation.

Most decisions have no "right" or "wrong" attached to them. But sometimes moral and ethical issues are involved. In those cases, rather than try to analyze the situation, you should weigh your options according to your personal moral, ethical, or spiritual code.

SLEEP ON IT

Most decisions don't have to be made on the spur of the moment. Take some time before making a decision. Relaxing, sleeping on, or getting away from the decision helps you gain valuable perspective. This also allows your unconscious to do some decision making and problem solving for you. That $5,000 sofa you wanted to buy yesterday may not look so desirable three days from now.

LEARN WHILE YOU SLEEP

Say you've got a big test tomorrow or need to memorize your lines for a play. Whatever you do, don't burn the midnight oil, cramming the night away. Get some shut-eye instead. That's the conclusion of boundless evidence proving that sleep is essential to learning.

In a Harvard Medical School experiment, for example, people who crammed through the night exhibited little improvement in their performance. The experiment worked like this: Twenty-four volunteers were trained in new tasks. Half the group was kept awake until the second night of the study; the other half was allowed to sleep. All the participants slept on the second and third nights of the study. On the fourth day of the experiment, those who had slept the first night performed better on the tasks while those who lost sleep the first night showed no improvement.

Similarly, a Canadian study found that students who studied hard for

an exam, then slept, retained more information than those who had
stayed up studying all night.

INSIDE THE SLEEPING BRAIN

When you learn a new activity or stimulate your brain in some way,
brain cells (neurons) begin firing in a specific pattern. Later, during sleep,
your brain replays what happened during the day and crystallizes memories. It does this by repeating and reactivating the same patterns of neuron
firing that occurred as you acquired a new skill or absorbed new information during your waking hours. This effect has been observed in rats—
whose brains are structured like human brains—and in human subjects
through the use of an imaging technology called positron emission tomog-
raphy (PET). PET can take three-dimensional pictures of brain activity.

Researchers using PET at the Massachusetts Institute of Technology
observed that sleeping rats dreamed about the mazes that they had been
learning to navigate while awake. PET scans showed that neuronal firing patterns associated with running the maze reappeared during rapid
eye movement (REM) sleep, the stage of slumber in which dreams occur.

What happens in rats' brains also occurs in human brains, according
to a study conducted at the University of Liege in Belgium. Scientists
took PET images of brain activity in seven people who were learning a
computerized task. The subjects were taught to press buttons in response
to symbols appearing on the computer screen.

The scientists observed brain activity during REM sleep in participants who had learned the task and discovered that the same brain areas
were activated, suggesting a link between sleep and memory processing.
According to the scientists, these findings suggest that REM sleep helps
deposit new learning into permanent storage.

SLEEP DEPRIVATION AND LEARNING

Sleep scientists feel that disrupting REM sleep can have a destructive
effect on the learning of new skills or information, since this is the sleep
stage that seems to be most involved in consolidating learned experi-

ences. Deprived of REM sleep, you're likely to lose mental focus and alertness. One study found that interrupting REM sleep sixty times in one night blocked learning entirely. (During sleep, you undergo several periods of REM sleep, usually occurring about once every ninety minutes and totaling about one and a half hours. In REM sleep, your eyes dart around rapidly as you dream.)

Scientists have recently discovered that non-REM (or non-dreaming) sleep is also important for learning and memory. As each REM period ends, you move into non-REM sleep, which has its own distinct stages, from the general drowsiness you feel as you begin to fall asleep to a very deep non-REM sleep. Non-REM sleep stages alternate with periods of REM sleep.

In a study of kittens, researchers at the University of California at San Francisco found that non-REM sleep significantly enhances brain plasticity in the same way that mentally challenging activities do when we're awake.

In this particular study, kittens that slept for six hours after receiving an environmental challenge (their vision was blocked in one eye for several hours) had twice as many beneficial brain connections as animals that were kept awake. The scientists point out that non-REM sleep, following a learning experience, helps build new connections critical to learning and memory.

OTHER AMAZING BRAIN-BOOSTING BENEFITS OF SLEEP

Other studies on sleep and learning have found that:

- Sleep helps us solve specific problems.
- Sleep strengthens and improves memories.
- REM sleep is critical for recovering from mental stress.
- Naps can make you smarter and more productive, which is why some companies encourage employees to take power naps during the day.
- Large amounts of sleep during early development influence how well a baby's brain develops, especially in regard to learning and memory.

9 Ways to Get Mentally Stimulating Sleep

With this scientific evidence in mind, we should all try to get more sleep, particularly to bolster our learning, retention, and memory. Here are some tips to help ensure memory-building sleep, night after night.

1. Go to bed at a regular time and maintain a regular sleep schedule.
2. Before resorting to prescription sleeping pills, try some gentle, sleep-enhancing herbs prior to bedtime. These include chamomile, valerian, and kava in tea or capsule form. (Kava, in particular, has been found to enhance non-REM sleep.) Follow the manufacturer's recommendation for dosage, and don't take herbs for an extended period of time.
3. Establish calming pre-bedtime activities. Some ideas: Take a hot bath, sip a mug of chamomile tea, or read your favorite book or magazine. By contrast, do not watch violent TV dramas, horror shows, or news programs before retiring. These can and do produce nightmares.
4. Eat a nutritious diet. A poor diet can interfere with sleep by causing digestive problems that keep you awake at night. Populate your diet with lots of fresh fruits and vegetables, whole grains, lean proteins, and dairy foods. Consider supplementing your diet, too; B vitamins, for example, have been shown to help alleviate sleeplessness.
5. Exercise regularly but moderately. Physical activity helps you slumber. But don't exercise too late in the day or in the evening because exercise revs up the metabolism and builds up natural chemicals in the body that have a stimulating effect on your system.
6. Keep your room well ventilated.
7. Cut out sleep-robbing substances such as caffeine and alcohol. (Eliminate coffee and caffeine-containing foods after midday.)
8. If you must get up at night, don't turn on any lights. Exposure to light in the middle of the night can block your body's production of melatonin, a hormone that regulates your sleep/wake cycle. It could be harder for you to fall asleep again.
9. Create a neat, restful sleep environment in your bedroom.

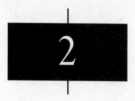

2

How to Manage Your Mood

A bad mood. Who needs it? Not you!

Without question, there's no bigger roadblock to peak brain fitness than a down-and-blue mood. But here's some uplifting news: You can banish the blues in some incredibly easy ways.

Did you know, for example, that there are blues-busting foods that are probably sitting in your pantry or refrigerator right now? Or that there are some herbs and other supplements that offer astonishing protection against bad moods? Did you also know that optimism—one of the unrecognized secrets behind brain fitness, happiness, and longevity—can be learned?

Here is your personal roadmap to the answers you're seeking—so that you can live life more fully, with an upbeat outlook and positive attitude toward the world around you.

STOCK YOUR PANTRY WITH
THESE 13 MOOD FOODS

You're feeling down in the dumps, but you don't know why. Instinctively, you reach for a piece of chocolate cake, polish it off, and wash it down with a glass of milk. Your mood lightens and you're back in good spirits.

Is food a "mood drug"?

Yes, to a certain extent. For more than forty years, scientists have known that food alters our brain chemistry in some rather astounding ways—it elevates mood, increases alertness, and improves our ability to think and remember. Basically, the protein and carbohydrate content of food affects the brain's synthesis of key chemicals in the brain, namely neurotransmitters, and these have a profound effect on mood and mental functioning. The neurotransmitters most affected by food intake are serotonin and dopamine. In addition, some foods contain feel-good chemicals of their own, which act like drugs to boost mood. Other foods are high in minerals that help the brain transmit its electrical impulses.

Remarkably, you can manipulate your brain chemistry to stay calm and upbeat simply by what you put on your plate, or you can indulge in foods that induce a natural high. Most of these foods are common, everyday staples. Here's a rundown.

BRAZIL NUTS

These tasty mega-nuts are packed with selenium, an antioxidant mineral with a windfall of health benefits, including the ability to boost mood. Grown in selenium-rich soil, a single nut supplies nearly twice the recommended daily amount of selenium—55 micrograms—so if you don't like popping pills, crunch down on a Brazil nut each day instead.

When researchers at the University of Wales gave fifty men and women a daily supplement of 100 micrograms of selenium (which equates to the amount in one Brazil nut), the subjects reported feeling more cheerful, with much-improved moods by the end of the five-week experiment. Those who were deficient in selenium at the beginning of the study experienced the most dramatic improvement in mood. Another study, conducted by the U.S. Department of Agriculture (USDA), found that men on a selenium-rich diet experienced significantly improved moods after just fifteen weeks.

Other selenium-packed foods include tuna, lean meat, organ meats, chicken, cottage cheese, fruit, and whole grains.

MILK

The calcium in milk and other dairy products is calming, particularly during episodes of premenstrual syndrome (PMS). That's the outcome of a study of thirty-three women conducted at Mount Sinai Medical Center in New York City, where researchers gave a daily 1,000-milligram calcium supplement to the subjects for three months. By the end of the study, 75 percent of the participants felt less irritable, nervous, or depressed and experienced fewer mood swings, compared with those taking a placebo.

It's relatively easy to get the same mood-lifting amount of calcium from food, as you can see from Table 2.1.

TABLE 2.1
A Day's Worth of Calcium

Food	Measure	Calcium Content per Serving
Orange juice, calcium fortified	1 cup	300 milligrams
Skim milk	1 cup	302 milligrams
Tofu	4 ounces	108 milligrams
Low-fat yogurt	8 ounces	415 milligrams
Turnip greens, cooked, chopped	1 cup	249 milligrams
	Total	1,374 milligrams

FISH

Fish is not only brain food; it's also mood food. Numerous studies show that consuming fish reduces the symptoms of depression.

By studying the differences between people who get depressed and those who don't—a type of research known as psychiatric epidemiology—scientists first discovered the fascinating link between omega-3 fats and mood. Epidemiological studies have found that countries with the highest rate of fish consumption have the lowest rates of depression. As a result, doctors and mental health experts are now suggesting that we eat more fish for protection against depression.

Exactly how omega-3 fats help alleviate mood disorders such as depression is a puzzle. But there are some clues. Some studies suggest that higher levels of essential fatty acids in plasma may lead to increased levels of neurotransmitters, particularly serotonin, and serotonin is the neurotransmitter most responsible for boosting mood.

TURKEY

Ever notice the calm you feel after gobbling down the gobbler at Thanksgiving dinner? Chalk it up to tyrosine, a key amino acid in turkey. Tyrosine is a precursor, or building block, to the neurotransmitters dopamine and norepinephrine, both involved in helping the body better cope with stress.

BEEF

Red meat is the best source of iron on the planet, and sufficient dietary iron is vital for preventing fatigue, the root cause of much moodiness, particularly in women. So to prevent fatigue-related blue moods, try to eat some lean red meat two or three times a week.

WHOLE-GRAIN BREAD

The attraction of whole-grain bread is its mixture of brain-pleasing nutrients, namely carbohydrates and amino acids, a combo that allows the most efficient delivery of tryptophan to the brain. Tryptophan is required for the synthesis of serotonin. A lack of tryptophan flowing into the brain can result in depression, increased sensitivity to pain, and wakefulness.

Whole-grain bread, a near-perfect blend of proteins and carbohydrates, practically ensures that your brain will get enough tryptophan to manufacture serotonin.

CHOCOLATE

You may not know that the Valentine's Day candy you eat every February is actually a conglomeration of natural chemicals that have a near-narcotic effect on your mood. One of these chemicals is theobromine, a stimulant similar to caffeine that can perk up your mental vigor. Another is phenylethylamine (PEA), a natural chemical that makes you feel lovey-dovey toward a person to whom you're attracted.

Chocolate also contains minute amounts of a substance called anandamide, which interacts with brain cells in much the same manner as tetrahydrocannabinol (THC), the narcotic in marijuana. But there's no way you can get high on chocolate unless you were to eat about 18 percent of your weight in chocolate in one sitting.

While you might not get a buzz from chocolate, you might feel more lovey-dovey. That's because chocolate also contains phenylalanine, an amino acid that produces feelings similar to those experienced during love and romance. Phenylalanine is found naturally in almonds, avocado, bananas, cheese, cottage cheese, nonfat dried milk, chocolate, pumpkin seeds, and sesame seeds.

It's no secret that chocolate candy also contains sugar, which produces a temporary energy boost. Chocolate also boosts brain levels of serotonin.

CINNAMON

It's everyone's favorite spice, and, remarkably, it can spice up your mood. Cinnamon prevents a condition called hypoglycemia, better known as low blood sugar. Hypoglycemia is a metabolic problem behind many a bad mood. When blood sugar plummets, so does mood. Cinnamon contains an active compound—methylhydroxy chalcone polymer (MHCP)—that helps improve the body's production of glucose.

So if you're plagued by low blood sugar blues, sprinkle a teaspoon of cinnamon on your cereal each morning to help you stay happy throughout the day.

SPINACH

Popeye the Sailor downed spinach for strength; now you can eat it for mental vigor. Spinach is loaded with the B vitamin folic acid, shown in research to be effective for easing depression. To get the mood-boosting benefits of folic acid, try to eat a cup of spinach or other green leafy vegetable several times a week.

HONEY

This syrupy sweetener is a treasure trove of natural tryptophan, the amino acid used by your brain to make serotonin, the happiness neurotransmitter. If you want to feel more relaxed after a stressful day or get a good night's sleep, spread a tablespoon of honey on a piece of bread or stir it into a cup of herbal tea.

BANANAS

If you're leading a hectic life with too much on your plate, there's one more thing to add to that plate: bananas. That's because bananas are well endowed with magnesium, a mineral depleted by stress. When you're chronically stressed out, your body starts churning out more stress hormones, high levels of which cause magnesium to be flushed from cells.

This can lead to all sorts of problems, including vulnerability to viruses and mood-sapping fatigue.

Research with chronic fatigue sufferers found that consuming a weekly gram of magnesium (the amount found in two bananas) resulted in increased energy. Other studies reveal that increasing magnesium intake alleviates anxiety and produces more restful sleep.

Other foods high in magnesium include nuts, beans, green leafy vegetables, and wheat germ.

ORANGES

To feel your absolute best, eat oranges and other citrus fruits on a regular basis. They are nature's best sources of vitamin C, a nutrient that increases levels of the neurotransmitter norepinephrine in your brain. Norepinephrine helps you stay alert, motivated, and thus less likely to experience the doldrums.

A short supply of vitamin C can make you feel irritable and blue, according to research. In a study of people with marginal deficiencies of vitamin C, researchers found that when subjects consumed amounts equivalent to the recommended intakes, they felt less cranky and depressed. Other research shows that vitamin C (400 milligrams daily) prevents fatigue. Scientists speculate that because vitamin C helps your body absorb iron, a lack of the vitamin can hinder iron absorption and thus lead to tiredness.

JALAPEÑOS

Want to feel happier pretty quickly? Serve up some hot salsa as a snack or hors d'oeuvres. Salsa and other hot foods are made with jalapeño peppers, which contain a natural ingredient called capsaicin. When your tongue burns after a dose of fire-alarm hot Mexican food, you have capsaicin to thank for the sensation. In response, your brain releases endorphins. These are responsible for reducing pain and heightening feelings of pleasure. The result is a general sense of mental well-being. The more hot peppers you eat, the greater the feel-good effect.

THE 6 HAPPY HORMONES:
PUT THEM TO WORK FOR YOU

When your mood has nose-dived and you feel like you've lost your joie de vivre, fluctuating hormones may be to blame. Hormones are chemical messengers produced by glands and sent out to various organs to stimulate the release of substances essential to the development and maintenance of life.

With age, levels of many hormones decline—a process that can start as early as age twenty-five—and this influences physical and mental health at each stage of life. An adverse consequence of declining and fluctuating hormones is a blue mood, that down-in-the-dumps feeling that seems to occur for no apparent reason. Fortunately, such mood disturbances can be treated. One way is by replenishing the body's supply of mood-modulating hormones (DHEA, estrogen, melatonin, pregnenolone, progesterone, and testosterone).

DEHYDROEPIANDROSTERONE (DHEA)

DHEA is a hormone naturally produced by the adrenal glands as well as by the central nervous system. In fact, it is the most abundant hormone in the bloodstream, concentrated mostly in brain tissues. Yet, the body's natural production of DHEA steadily declines after age thirty.

In the body, DHEA breaks down and is converted to both estrogen and testosterone. What its actual function is remains a mystery to scientists.

Supplemental DHEA appears to play a role in alleviating depression. In one study, men and women who took 50 milligrams of DHEA a day for six months experienced a dramatic improvement in their psychological well-being. In a similar study, 50-milligram doses taken for three months produced enhanced feelings of well-being, a better mood, a better ability to handle stress, and increased energy in men and women.

DHEA is readily available as a supplement, sold in pharmacies, grocery stores, health-food stores, and department stores. Some of these supplements come in the form of wild yam extracts that claim DHEA activity and potency but, in fact, have neither.

As for dosage, some experts believe that 5 to 15 milligrams for women and 10 to 30 milligrams for men are appropriate. If you're interested in supplementing with DHEA, consult your doctor first because the supplement may not be safe. The National Institute on Aging (NIA) has warned consumers that DHEA may produce such side effects as confusion, headaches, drowsiness, and liver damage, and may increase the risk of breast and prostate cancers. Additionally, the NIA feels that DHEA should be available by prescription only—a conviction shared by the FDA.

ESTROGEN

Estrogen is the collective name for a trio of female hormones: estradiol, secreted from the ovaries during your reproductive years; estriol, produced by the placenta during pregnancy; and estrone, secreted by the ovaries and adrenal glands and found in women after menopause. These naturally occurring estrogens are responsible for developing female sexual characteristics, regulating menstrual cycles, and maintaining normal cholesterol levels.

Fluctuating estrogen levels during the menstrual period, menopause, and postpartum period are responsible for the characteristic mood swings many women experience. Scientists suspect that these fluctuations directly influence levels of the happiness neurotransmitter serotonin. Under normal conditions, estrogen blocks enzymes that degrade serotonin, allowing more of the neurotransmitter to work in the brain and prevent depression. But during your period, after giving birth, or during menopause, estrogen levels fall and so do levels of serotonin. Thus, your brain chemistry is very sensitive to the ups and downs of estrogen.

If your mood swings are quite severe and other causes for your mood disorder have been ruled out, you may want to consider hormone replacement therapy (its mood-elevating benefits take about four to six weeks to kick in). The decision to do so, however, should not be made without serious deliberation. Worrisome side effects include vaginal bleeding, water retention, breast pain and tenderness, nausea, headaches, gallbladder disease, and mood disturbances. More serious risks include increased risk of uterine cancer (if estrogen is not combined with natural or synthetic progesterone), deep vein thrombosis, and breast cancer. Estrogen requires a prescription.

If estrogen replacement therapy is not an option, ask your doctor if a serotonin-boosting antidepressant such as fluoxetine (Prozac), paroxetine (Paxil), or sertraline (Zoloft) might be right for you. These drugs lengthen the amount of time that concentrations of serotonin stay active in the brain.

Natural alternatives to prescription serotonin boosters include 5-HTP and St. John's wort. Both have far fewer side effects than their prescription counterparts.

MELATONIN

Melatonin is a natural substance secreted by the pineal gland, located in the middle of the brain. Discovered in 1958, melatonin is available today as a supplement, produced synthetically or from animal sources. As many as 20 million consumers use melatonin, spending roughly $350 million on the supplement annually.

Melatonin's job is to set and regulate the internal clock that controls your body's sleep/wake cycle. It has been touted as a curative for sleep disorders, an antioxidant that protects cellular health, a youth restorer, and a mood booster.

Because people suffering from depression have trouble sleeping, melatonin has been shown to help improve the quality of sleep in these patients. Research with melatonin indicates that dosages of 1 to 3 milligrams taken one to two hours prior to bedtime are helpful in producing restful sleep. Melatonin has some untoward side effects, however, including aggravation of existing depression and next-day grogginess. Make sure you purchase melatonin made by a reputable manufacturer. Many brands contain impurities and tiny amounts of the actual hormone, according to researchers. Before supplementing, consult your doctor.

PREGNENOLONE

This hormone is a building block of numerous other hormones in the body, including DHEA, testosterone, and estrogen. There are high concentrations of pregnenolone in tissues of the nervous system. Scientists believe that it may improve mood, energy, and memory by enhancing the transmission of electrical messages in the brain and central nervous system.

Research shows that people with current depression or a history of the disease have lower-than-normal concentrations of the hormone in their cerebrospinal fluid. This suggests that increasing pregnenolone may help alleviate depression.

Supplemental pregnenolone is available without a prescription in tablets, capsules, liquid sublinguals, creams, and sprays. The dosage recommended by health-care practitioners is 5 to 10 milligrams daily. Check with your doctor prior to supplementing.

Pregnenolone should not be taken if you suffer from seizures because it antagonizes calming receptors in the brain. It may also cause changes in the menstrual cycle.

PROGESTERONE

Progesterone is a female hormone that helps regulate mood. It is responsible for breast development and for thickening and nourishing the womb lining in preparation for pregnancy. With menopause, progesterone production falls off by nearly 100 percent—one reason why mood swings are so prevalent during this stage of life.

To replace the progesterone that is lost, your doctor may prescribe a supplemental form of the hormone. Progesterone is given with estrogen if you have not had a hysterectomy. Estrogen taken alone greatly increases the risk of uterine cancer. Progesterone offsets that risk.

There are two forms of supplemental progesterone. One is the synthetic version, referred to as progestin, which is commonly found in birth-control pills and hormone replacement therapy. Examples of progestin products, along with their uses and side effects, are listed in Table 2.2.

TABLE 2.2

Progestins

BRAND NAME	TYPE OF PROGESTERONE	AVAILABLE DOSAGES	MAJOR USES	SIDE EFFECTS
Activella and Femhrt	Norethindrone acetate (combined with a form of estrogen)	1 mg (estrogen)/5 mcg (Norethindrone acetate)	Relieves symptoms of menopause; prevents osteoporosis in post-menopausal women.	Abdominal pain; breast tenderness and enlargement; depression; enlargement of uterine fibroids; headache
CombiPatch	Norethindrone acetate (combined with a form of estrogen)	Given through a slow-release patch applied to the skin	Relieves symptoms of menopause.	Abdominal pain, abnormal PAP smear, acne, back pain, breast pain, depression
Cycrin	Medroxyprogesterone acetate	10 mg 5 mg 2.5 mg	Treats hormonal imbalances; prevents abnormal growth of uterine lining in women taking estrogen.	Acne, life-threatening allergic response, blood clots, breast tenderness, depression, excessive hair growth
Depo-Provera	Medroxyprogesterone acetate	Given by injection	Balances out or reduces estrogen buildup that may promote tumor growth.	Acne, life-threatening allergic response, blood clots, breast tenderness, depression, excessive hair growth
Megace	Megestrol acetate	20 mg 40 mg	Treats severe, widespread endometrial cancer.	Nausea, vomiting, dizziness, headache, menstrual bleeding

Brand Name	Type of Progesterone	Available Dosages	Major Uses	Side Effects
Micronor	Norethindrone acetate	0.35 mg	Prevents pregnancy by changing the body's hormonal balance.	Weight gain, depression, fatigue, acne, hair loss
Ortho-Prefest	Norgestimate (combined with a form of estrogen)	1 mg (estrogen)/0.09 mg norgestimate	Relieves symptoms of menopause; prevents osteoporosis in post-menopausal women.	Headache, breast pain, abdominal pain
Provera	Medroxyprogesterone acetate	10 mg 5 mg 2.5 mg	Treats hormonal imbalances; prevents abnormal growth of uterine lining in women taking estrogen.	Acne, life-threatening allergic response, blood clots, breast tenderness, depression, excessive hair growth

The second form of supplemental progesterone is natural progesterone, a plant hormone derived from wild yams, soybeans, or peanut oil, that exactly duplicates the progesterone naturally produced in your body. Natural progesterone is generally used to treat symptoms of premenstrual syndrome (PMS) and to relieve irritability associated with menopause. It is a natural alternative to hormone replacement therapy but without the side effects associated with synthetic progesterones.

The best way to use natural progesterone is in a cream containing 400 to 500 milligrams of progesterone per ounce. The therapeutic dosage of progesterone cream is 20 milligrams a day.

Available without a prescription, the creams listed below are among the products that have been analyzed by Aeron LifeCycles and certified to contain more than 400 milligrams of natural progesterone per ounce.

- Angel Care
- Balance Cream
- DermaGest
- EssPro 7
- Femarone 17
- Fem-Gest
- Maxine's Feminique
- NatraGest
- Procreme
- Renascence Progesterone

An oral form of natural progesterone called Prometrium has recently become available by prescription. This type of progesterone comes in a "micronized" form, which means it is broken down into tiny particles to allow for a steady, even absorption of the medication.

In a British study, researchers found that oral micronized progesterone, taken for two months, significantly improved the mood of a group of premenstrual women, compared to a placebo. Like estrogen, supplemental progesterone is believed to preserve levels of the feel-good neurotransmitter serotonin. There are side effects to oral micronized progesterone, however. These include dizziness, abdominal cramping, headache, and breast pain.

Note: Avoid creams that say they contain diosgenin, a precursor to progesterone that is derived from wild yams. Your body cannot convert diosgenin into progesterone. Instead, look for products that say "progesterone USP" on the label or look for those that contain pharmaceutical-grade progesterone. Then you know you're getting the right stuff.

TESTOSTERONE

Secreted by the testes, testosterone is the hormone responsible for developing masculine characteristics. As with estrogen in women, testosterone levels in men taper off with age, although the drop isn't quite as abrupt as estrogen is in women. Testosterone supplementation for older men is being extensively researched as an antiaging treatment because it appears to build muscle and bone, reduce body fat, protect the heart, and boost sex drive.

Another potential plus for testosterone therapy: Preliminary research hints that it elevates mood. In ongoing studies with the hormone, men have reported a general improvement in their moods and mental well-being.

Interestingly, some mental health experts have suggested that a testosterone deficiency may be at the root of depression in some women—a theory put forth at the annual meeting of the American Psychiatric Association in 1998. (Women have about one-tenth the amount of testosterone as men.) With menopause, the natural production of testosterone declines by about half.

Testosterone deficiency in women shows up as decreased sensitivity in the nipples and clitoris, lowered sex drive, inability to reach orgasm, and a general feeling of being down in the dumps. If you have no history of depression and suddenly and without explanation, you get the blahs, you could be suffering from a short supply of testosterone. This can be properly diagnosed by your doctor. However, a deficiency may be difficult to treat, since there are few suitable medications on the market for women.

Although testosterone replacement therapy has the potential for reversing signs of aging and boosting mood, it is not without side effects. For men, these include low red blood cells counts; a shutdown in your body's own ability to produce testosterone (you become dependent on testosterone replacement therapy for the rest of your life); and accelerated growth of prostate cells.

For women, taking testosterone can result in the development of male secondary sex characteristics such as body hair and a low voice—side effects that are irreversible. One of the biggest dangers comes if testosterone is taken during the child-bearing years. Testosterone can masculinize a female fetus.

GET HEALTHY: BECOME AN OPTIMIST

Is your cup half full or half empty? Whether you're an optimist or a pessimist may have a profound effect on your health, well-being, and longevity.

That's the conclusion of a thirty-year study of patients at the Mayo Clinic in Rochester, Minnesota. While being treated for a variety of ailments, these patients were given a personality test, part of which measured optimism and pessimism.

After researchers followed up some thirty years later, they found that the glass-full optimists in the group had lived longer than expected based on their age and gender. The pessimists, on the other hand, had a shorter-than-expected survival rate—a 19-percent increase in the risk of death when compared to their expected life span. Researchers believe that an optimistic outlook strengthens the immune system and also motivates people to take better care of themselves.

This rather amazing study is just one piece of research in a growing body of evidence linking optimism with good health. Other research has found that:

- Pessimists have higher average daily blood pressures than optimists. (High blood pressure is a risk factor for heart disease and stroke.)
- Pessimists are more prone to increased anxiety and depression.
- Optimists report fewer health problems than pessimists. On average, pessimists come down with twice as many infectious diseases and make twice as many trips to the doctor's office as optimists do.
- Optimists recover more quickly after being sick or undergoing serious procedures such as coronary bypass surgery.
- Pregnant, optimistic women are less likely to suffer from postpartum depression.

• Optimists feel better about their own physical and emotional health—and take steps to protect it.

Clearly, if you have a positive outlook, you'll enjoy better health, greater happiness, and even a longer life. Becoming an optimist is certainly a goal worth striving for. But what if you're a perennial grouch? Is pessimism a trait you're born with, or can you change? Although some research says that pessimism is rooted partially in our genes, other studies have found that pessimism is a mental habit, one learned mostly from watching our parents deal with various situations. Say you have parents who are chronic naysayers. Chances are, you're also likely to view life negatively.

If pessimism is learned, then it can be unlearned. Put another way, optimism is a skill you can develop. Coined by the developer of positive psychology, Martin Seligman, Ph.D., learned optimism means learning to expect occasional difficulties, setbacks, and bad days but to not let them color your whole view of life or attitude toward yourself. Setbacks are not a result of some character flaw, but a temporary situation that will pass.

Here's how you can transform yourself from pessimist to optimist.

REWRITE YOUR INTERNAL SCRIPT

A lot of the stuff we tell ourselves about ourselves is a distortion of the truth, or not truthful at all. Challenge your negative thoughts by deciphering whether there's any truth in them. Suppose you've lost your job and say to yourself: "No company will ever hire me; I'll be unemployed the rest of my life." If you believe that, you may not even try to find a job.

Instead, challenge the truthfulness of your thinking by making logical statements: "I've had other jobs before, so I'll be hired again." Then take action to fix the situation. Optimists are action-oriented, solution-finding people.

CHANGE YOUR SELF-TALK

Your attitude can be easily polluted with negative words like "can't," "never," or "won't"; or put-downs, self-blaming, and other derogatory statements. The problem is that a steady stream of pollution can lead to self-doubt, anxiety, and, ultimately, depression. Positive thoughts are "can-do/will-do" inner conversations that build up rather than put down. The result can be a renewed, more upbeat attitude toward life.

One of the best ways to do this is to make a list of some of your typical negative messages or defeatist statements and replace those messages with flip-side positive messages. For example, replace a statement like "Bad things always happen to me" with "Good things always happen to me." Or replace "I made a big mistake" with "That was a valuable learning experience."

ANALYZE YOUR SETBACKS RATIONALLY

Everyone has setbacks—even optimists. A major difference between optimists and pessimists, however, is in how they respond to those setbacks.

A pessimist is convinced that setbacks result from permanent conditions ("I burned the cookies because I'm a terrible cook") and that good things come from temporary ones ("I got a raise because my boss was in a good mood today").

An optimist, on the other hand, knows that setbacks stem from temporary situations ("I burned the cookies because I wasn't paying attention") and that good things come from long-standing situations ("I got a raise because I'm good at my job").

Pessimists also tend to blame themselves, even if something wasn't their fault. A pessimist who got stood up by a date may blame herself, saying, "I'm not attractive enough. No wonder he didn't show up." By contrast, an optimist attributes the situation to poor manners on her date's part. She might respond by saying, "If that's an example of how he acts, I'm glad he didn't show up." An optimist feels powerful; a pessimist feels powerless.

Pessimists often spend too much time thinking about their setbacks or

about all the wrong things they did in the past. They tend to think of failure as a character flaw rather than as a faulty strategy or decision. If you
take this attitude toward failure, you'll have a hard time succeeding at anything.

Let's say you've tried to quit smoking on different occasions, but you
haven't yet quit. If you look at your unsuccessful attempts to quit as failures, then you're bound to repeat them. Further, you're likely to think of
yourself as a weak person. Even worse, you're likely to give up trying to
quit altogether.

Instead, congratulate yourself for all the times you've tried. Along the
way, you probably discovered many methods that really didn't work for
you. Thomas Edison was once asked about his many failures in his
search for a new storage battery—50,000 experiments before he achieved
results. "Results," replied the inventor. "Why I have gotten results. I
know 50,000 things that won't work."

So try thinking that those positive things you're doing now are all
steps on the path to becoming the person you were meant to be. Then believe you will succeed. That's the attitude of an optimist.

GET SOME PERSPECTIVE

Pessimists tend to catastrophize situations, turning the proverbial
molehill into a mountain. Or they worry about situations over which
they have no control. Both approaches to life are immobilizing and unhealthy. They make things worse than they really are.

The next time you find yourself mired in this type of thinking, ask
yourself: What is the worst thing that can happen? How likely is that to
occur? How much difference will this situation make in my life a year
from now? Am I even likely to remember it? This type of self-talk puts a
more positive spin on the situation.

FIND THE SILVER LINING

This involves a new way of looking at situations, an action psychologists call "reframing." Rather than feel discouraged by an unfortunate

turn of events, root out what you can learn from them and do better next time. Let's say you've been recently divorced. Maybe this is a good time to pursue activities you couldn't do while married, to find out what you want from a spouse, or to figure out what you'll do differently in future relationships. In other words, turn the bad into good.

Researchers at the University of California at Davis surveyed 2,000 people about bad experiences they had, including divorce, job loss, illness, death, and combat. Surprisingly, most respondents could point to the positives that emerged from their tragedies, from stronger relationships to renewed faith in God.

MOVE FROM DESTRUCTIVE TO CONSTRUCTIVE RELATIONSHIPS

Optimists tend to hang out with and attract other optimists. If you find yourself moving through a pattern of negative, abusive relationships, turn instead to people who will affirm and encourage you. If necessary, seek counseling to help you break free from your pattern of unhealthy relationships.

PRACTICE POSITIVITY

If you're not an optimist yet, start acting as if you were one. Respond to situations as an optimist would: Believe you'll succeed, see the silver lining in bad situations, change your self-talk, see the temporary results of setbacks, focus on your past successes, and so forth.

The "as if" principle works because it puts you in a new role. The more you act it out, the more comfortable you become in the role. Before long, you're not role-playing anymore.

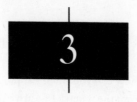

Positive Psychology to Improve
Your Frame of Mind

When Abraham Lincoln said, "Most people are about as happy as they make up their minds to be," he could have been talking about "positive psychology," a powerful new mental health therapy that is revolutionizing the way depression and other mental maladies are treated.

For decades, therapists tended to treat things that go wrong in people's minds, rather than things that go right. That approach began to change with the advent and acceptance of positive psychology, which focuses on people's happiness over their sadness and helps them move up the scale of happiness and contentment.

Bolstered by decades of research into what makes people happy, positive psychologists view happiness as a condition that must be actively pursued—an approach that would come as no surprise to Benjamin Franklin, one of the framers of the Constitution. After Franklin concluded a speech on the guarantees of the Constitution, a heckler shouted, "Aw, those words don't mean anything. Where's all the happiness you say it guarantees?" To which Franklin replied, "My friend, the

Constitution only guarantees the American people the right to pursue happiness; you have to catch it yourself."

7 Ways to Catch Happiness

With that in mind, how can you catch happiness? Here are seven recommendations taken from the tenets of positive psychology.

SHUN MATERIALISM

Much research into positive psychology has focused on the relationship between income and happiness. Among the findings: Yearning for material possessions harms the person doing the yearning, and people become obsessed (and unhappy) with what they don't own. The desire for material possessions also triggers spending, rather than saving, and overspending ultimately leads to anxiety and money worries.

For happiness and contentment, adopt a count-your-blessings approach to what you do own. Focus on how well your possessions meet your needs, not on how they compare to your neighbors' stuff.

PURSUE VOLUNTEERISM

Research shows that people who give to charity, contribute to their communities, and do volunteer work tend to be happier. In one landmark study of volunteerism, researchers found that those who helped regularly were less depressed and had a greater sense of calmness and well-being.

In fact, you can experience the same physiological changes when you help others as you do when you exercise. Heart rate and breathing decrease, and feel-good endorphins are released—all of which power up the immune system. This is the exact opposite of what happens when you're unhappy and stressed out.

BE GRATEFUL

Recent studies show that people with the attitude of gratitude—to others or to God—are happier. Further, they're in better health, more successful in their careers, and less depressed than the general population. To get in the gratitude mode, consider keeping a daily or weekly list of what you're grateful for.

FORGIVE OTHERS

People do things to us, and we to them. We may lie to, betray, or hurt others—and vice versa. These things are a sad, unfortunate fact of life. After being hurt, we can either carry the pain in our hearts or let it go. Holding the pain in, many experts theorize, leads to unhappiness and depression and inhibits the immune system, leaving you vulnerable to life-threatening illnesses such as heart disease and cancer. An unforgiving spirit can be physically and mentally destructive.

STOP VIEWING YOURSELF AS A VICTIM

Over the past few decades, society has seen a tendency among individuals and groups to describe themselves as victims—of poor parenting, oppression by a majority ethnic group, an uncaring government, and so forth. The problem with "victimology" is that it excuses away behavior and shifts blame for one's actions on someone or something else. Further, it engenders a sense of hopelessness, which makes people feel they've lost control over their lives, when in fact they have enormous personal freedom to guide their own destinies.

CULTIVATE POSITIVE EMOTIONS

This involves training yourself to identify the positives of a negative situation and the good that can come out of it. For example, let's say you've been diagnosed with a serious or chronic illness like diabetes. That will bring on a down spell pretty quickly. But then you see that the illness will force you to change your diet or your overall lifestyle in some way. That's one of the positives. Make decisions to see the positives when faced with a problem and experience fully the emotions they bring.

PURSUE HAPPINESS ACTIVITIES

Identify activities and pursuits that make you happy, then commit yourself to doing them. Perhaps you're in a dead-end job that seems to bring nothing but frustration or boredom. What would you really like to be doing? What were some of your dreams before your life got side-lined? The answers to such questions will force you to set concrete, achievable goals for yourself. Although your abstract and ultimate goal is to be more happy, happiness will be a byproduct of achieving a concrete goal like switching careers or immersing yourself in something you love.

HUMOR AND YOUR MENTAL HEALTH: 11 WAYS TO LAUGH AWAY YOUR PROBLEMS

Laughter has been called "the tranquilizer with no side effects." And for good reason. It stimulates the pituitary gland in your brain, which in turn triggers the release of tension-relieving endorphins, while reducing levels of stress hormones. Some of these endorphins stay in your system for up to twelve hours, producing an ongoing natural high.

When you laugh, you automatically draw in a deep breath. This expands your lungs and increases your blood and oxygen circulation, in much the same way as deep breathing or exercise does. The net effects are relaxation and a reduction of tension. (Anger and stress do the reverse.) In fact, laughter produces near-identical responses to those associated with progressive muscle relaxation, a widely used stress-relief technique.

And, with more oxygen reaching your brain, you're able to think more clearly. This is precisely why some corporate CEOs are bringing humor consultants into the workplace to increase creativity and productivity.

The Greeks may have been the first to use laughter as a cure for psychosomatic illness, a disease with bodily symptoms brought on by a mental or emotional disturbance. The earliest example of this comes from the annals of ancient history: Galen (A.D. 129–199), a Greek physician who practiced in Rome, was called in to treat the ill wife of a Roman aristocrat. She remained unresponsive to medical treatment until Galen whispered something funny in her ear that made her laugh. That laugh put her on the road to recovery and is the first recorded incidence of a psychiatric treatment used to heal an illness.

Laughter also serves a protective psychological function by distracting you from the negative side of a situation. Your mood is enhanced as a result. As the Roman philosopher Seneca put it, "It better benefits man to laugh at life than to lament over it."

For the same reason, humor can be useful in addiction therapy. "In the rehabilitation of persons recovering from substance addiction, humor can help them express negative emotions in a positive light, thus relieving feelings of despair and hopelessness," writes Brian Luke Seaward, Ph.D., in *Health Progress*. "Many addictions are related to low self-esteem. Although humor does not necessarily build self-esteem, the ability to laugh at oneself can be a crucial transition in the basic stages of recovery."

Laughter and humor promote other positive changes in the body. They stabilize blood pressure, massage inner organs, strengthen the immune system, and improve digestion. They may even help you live longer. For proof, look no further than some of our most famous—and long-lived—comedians: Bob Hope, Milton Berle, and George Burns.

So, how can you get in on the remarkable benefits that laughter and humor bring? Here are eleven suggestions.

BEGIN YOUR DAY WITH LAUGHTER

Abraham Lincoln always opened his cabinet meetings by saying something humorous, because he understood the stress-relieving power of laughter. One day, when he read aloud to his cabinet an anecdote he found funny, no one cracked a smile. Lincoln rebuked them: "Why don't you laugh? With the fearful strain that is upon me night and day, if I did not laugh I should die, and you need this medicine as much as I do."

READ OR WATCH FUNNY STUFF EVERY DAY

This includes reading the comics, renting a funny video, enjoying a comedy at the movie theater, or watching funny sitcoms. Other suggestions include:

- listening to a comedy routine on audiocassette on your way to work.
- attending a performance at a comedy club.
- reading funny cards at a stationery store.

POKE FUN AT YOURSELF WHEN
YOU DO SOMETHING SILLY

"People who see the humor in everyday occurrences are proven to feel less pain, feel healthier, and actually have more robust immune systems than others," says Athena du Pré, Ph.D., the author of *Humor and the Healing Arts* and a researcher who has studied the role of humor in health and healing for ten years.

KEEP A MENTAL CATALOG OF FUNNY EPISODES
THAT HAVE OCCURRED IN YOUR LIFE

"Like the time the rain came pouring into your tent while camping or the dog ate the Christmas ham," suggests du Pré. "Most funny things occur when things didn't go exactly as planned. Cherish these memories."

SHARE JOKES AND HUMOR WITH OTHERS

"You need not be hysterically funny," du Pré says. "Some people I meet say they don't use humor much because they aren't good at telling jokes. Relax. A smile or funny face is often enough to get people smiling."

SEEK OUT HUMOR THERAPY IF YOU MUST BE HOSPITALIZED

Many hospitals around the country, particularly those with oncology wards, have developed humor programs to help take patients' minds off their illnesses and ease depression. These programs include humorous books and videos, in-house humor cable channels, and other resources. Some hospitals even provide clowns to lift the spirits of hospitalized children.

USE HUMOR APPROPRIATELY IN HEAVY SITUATIONS

Humor will not make a severe problem go away, but it may put it in a better perspective. "In my hospice work, I have noticed that if there is laughter and humor at a funeral or wake, the bereavement period goes more easily," writes humor specialist Marion B. Dolan in *Caring Magazine*. "When survivors can share happy stories about the deceased, the grief is lessened and healing can begin."

ASSOCIATE WITH HAPPY PEOPLE

In your circle of acquaintances, identify those who make you laugh and spend more time with them.

KEEP A HUMOR NOTEBOOK

Whenever you come across a joke, saying, story, cartoon, or poem that tickles your funny bone, cut and paste it into a notebook. That way, you have access to funny stuff when you're alone and need a lift.

RENEW THE KID IN YOU

Preschoolers laugh about 450 times a day, while adults laugh only 15 times a day. As you go through life, try to see things through the eyes of a child and respond like a kid if you can.

FAKE IT

Even when you feign a chuckle or a giggle, your body reacts as if you expressed a sincere laugh because, either way, you still must take in a deep, relaxing, circulation-boosting breath.

DREAM UP A GOOD MOOD

Whenever you felt down in the dumps, your mother probably told you, "Things will look better in the morning." And she was right. A good night's sleep improves your mood.

Scientific verification of this comes from the Sleep Research Center at Rush-Presbyterian-St. Luke's Medical Center in Chicago, where researchers have studied dreams and mood. In one experiment, they divided a group of sixty mentally healthy volunteers into two groups: those having neutral feelings prior to bedtime and those feeling down in the dumps.

The researchers gave a mood test to both groups, monitored their sleep in the sleep lab, and administered a second mood test to the participants after they awoke in the morning. During the night, the researchers periodically awoke the volunteers to ask them about the contents of their dreams.

The down-in-the-dumps group felt much better in the morning; the neutral group had little change in their overall mood. These attitudes were reflected in the contents of the volunteers' dreams. Individuals whose mood improved overnight had negative dreams at the beginning of their slumber but fewer negative dreams as the night progressed. The contents of dreams did not change in people with neutral moods.

According to the researchers, these findings suggest that if you go to bed in a bad mood, your brain starts to actively process away the negativity; hence, the initial negative dreams followed by the more pleasant dreams—and ultimately working through the bad mood. In short, dreaming chases away the blues, overnight.

Doom Your Gloom: 5 Supplemental Amino Acids to Lift Your Spirits

Want to feel more upbeat, more of the time? Try supplemental amino acids. By definition, amino acids are linked-together pieces of protein that we get from food or that our bodies make on their own. They have far-reaching duties in the body—from building and repairing tissue to producing chemicals that make our brains function.

Amino acids are available in capsules, nutritional drinks, and sports nutrition bars. Isolated from animal protein, yeast protein, or vegetable protein, supplemental amino acids are used therapeutically to treat a host of physical and mental conditions. See Table 3.1 on page 113 for a quick look at these amino acids and read below for more information. See Table 3.2 on page 114 for information on two other, potentially promising amino acids.

GAMMA-AMINOBUTYRIC ACID (GABA)

GABA naturally tranquilizes the brain by preventing the transmission of anxiety messages from nerve cell to nerve cell. As a supplement available in capsules and tablets, GABA can be taken to simmer down anxiety much in the same way that prescription tranquilizers do.

The usual dosage is 200 milligrams taken four times a day. Too much GABA can increase anxiety, cause shortness of breath, and produce tingling or numbness in the extremities.

GLUTAMINE

Another brain fuel is glutamine, the most abundant amino acid in the body. In your brain, it is converted into glutamic acid, which is important for optimal brain health. Glutamine also elevates levels of GABA in the brain, which is vital for healthy brain function and mental activities.

This important amino acid also serves as a building block for proteins, nucleotides (structural units of RNA and DNA), and other amino acids, and is the favored fuel source for cells that make up your immune system.

Foods high in protein such as meat, fish, chicken, beans, and dairy products are also high in glutamine. Supplemental glutamine can be helpful in enhancing mental functioning, treating senility and schizophrenia, and fighting fatigue. The recommended dosage for glutamine varies, usually ranging from 500 milligrams to several grams daily. Both heat and acid destroy glutamine, so you should not take it with hot or acidic foods, such as vinegar.

Glutamine supplementation is well tolerated, with few side effects. People with liver or kidney disease or other preexisting medical conditions should not supplement with glutamine, however, because it can aggravate these conditions and interfere with their treatment.

PHENYLALANINE

A building block for brain neurotransmitters that elevate mood, this amino acid has sometimes been used to treat depression because it provides an amphetaminelike lift in mood. Because many people overeat when depressed, phenylalanine's antidepression properties are beneficial for maintaining a positive frame of mind while dieting. The amino acid is also believed to favorably affect memory and alertness.

Natural sources of phenylalanine include almonds, avocado, bananas, cheese, cottage cheese, nonfat dried milk, chocolate, pumpkin seeds, and sesame seeds.

Supplementally, phenylalanine comes in three forms, designated as L-phenylalanine, which is present in protein foods; its chemical mirror image D-phenylalanine, which is not normally found in food; and DL-phenylalanine, a combination of the two. L-phenylalanine is the most common form and is used as a building block for various proteins in the body. It can also be converted to phenylethylamine, a substance that occurs naturally in the brain and seems to boost mood. The D-form has been used to treat pain; the DL-form increases alertness and helps treat Parkinson's disease.

The recommended dosage ranges from 500 to 1,000 milligrams a day, but check with your doctor or health-care professional prior to supplementing. Phenylalanine should be avoided by anyone taking antidepressants; suffering from high blood pressure, the genetic illness phenylketonuria (PKU), diabetes, or migraine headaches; or being treated for melanoma, a serious form of skin cancer. The supplement could aggravate these conditions.

TYROSINE

Synthesized from phenylalanine, tyrosine is a building block of several neurotransmitters, including dopamine, norepinephrine, and epinephrine. Through its relationship to neurotransmitters, tyrosine may be beneficial for several disorders affecting the brain. Research suggests that it may help treat depression (tyrosine levels are often low in depressed patients), anxiety, dementia, stress reduction, and Parkinson's disease.

Tyrosine is available from dairy products, meat, fish, wheat, oats, bananas, and seeds. As for supplements, natural health-care practitioners suggest taking 500 milligrams to 2 grams, two to three times daily. It's best to start with the lower dosage and increase gradually to 2 grams.

Do not supplement with tyrosine if you're taking beta-blocker drugs or antidepressants or suffering from high blood pressure (tyrosine may cause blood pressure to rise even higher). If you're allergic to any foods containing tyrosine, do not supplement. Because tyrosine is so closely related to phenylalanine, the same cautions apply.

5 HYDROXY-TRYPTOPHAN (5-HTP)

5-HTP (5 hydroxy-tryptophan), a chemical cousin to tryptophan, is a naturally occurring compound shown to be effective in the treatment of depression, anxiety, stress, and other disorders. It has become very popular as a supplemental alternative to tryptophan, which is no longer available as a nutritional supplement. In 1989, thousands of Americans developed a crippling illness called eosinophilia-myalgia syndrome after taking bacterially tainted tryptophan made by a Japanese chemical company. Although some recovered rapidly after stopping the supplements, thirty-one people died and others had lingering damage. As a result of this scare, tryptophan was yanked from the market.

Commercially, 5-HTP is extracted from the bean of *Griffonia simplicifolia,* a plant native to Africa. Thus, 5-HTP is totally natural and not chemically synthesized or produced by bacterial fermentation (as was the tainted tryptophan).

Like tryptophan, 5-HTP supports serotonin production and naturally boosts its levels. Additionally, 5-HTP has been found to reduce anxiety and provide relief to patients suffering from panic disorder.

You can find 5-HTP in tablets and special drink mixes. Some formulations combine 5-HTP with St. John's wort, an herb known to naturally relieve depression. Researchers who have studied 5-HTP feel that the supplement works well at relatively low dosages—50 to 100 milligrams daily. Others have recommended a dosage of 100 to 300 milligrams taken three times a day. Supplement manufacturers may suggest other dosages, depending on how they formulate their products.

There are a few red flags associated with 5-HTP. Do not supplement with 5-HTP if you're at risk of heart disease or stroke or have high blood pressure. Nor should you take 5-HTP if you're using other medications that affect serotonin levels. These include antidepressants such as monoamine oxidase inhibitors, Prozac, or prescription weight-loss drugs. Alcohol affects the metabolism of 5-HTP so avoid drinking alcohol while supplementing.

TABLE 3.1

Supplementing with Amino Acids

Amino Acid	Mood-Boosting Actions	Dosage	Side Effects/ Cautions
GABA	Reduces anxiety.	200 mg, 4 times daily	Excess causes anxiety, shortness of breath, and tingling or numbness in the extremities.
Glutamine	Elevates levels of anxiety-reducing GABA in the brain.	500 mg to several grams daily	Avoid if you have liver or kidney disease or other preexisting medical conditions.
Phenylalanine	Elevates mood; fights depression.	500 to 1,000 mg daily	Avoid if you are taking antidepressants; suffering from high blood pressure, the genetic illness phenylketonuria (PKU), diabetes, or migraine headaches; or being treated for melanoma, a serious form of skin cancer.
Tyrosine	Treats depression, anxiety, dementia; reduces stress.	500 mg to 2 grams, 2 to 3 times daily	Avoid if you are taking beta-blocker drugs or antidepressants or suffering from high blood pressure.
5-HTP	Relieves depression, panic attacks, and anxiety.	100 to 300 mg, 3 times daily	Avoid if you are at risk of heart disease or stroke or have high blood pressure; do not take 5-HTP if you're using other medications that affect serotonin levels.

TABLE 3.2		
2 Amino Acids to Watch		
Though not yet well researched, these two amino acids show promise for their potential to sharpen mental ability.		
AMINO ACID	BENEFITS	DOSAGE
Dimethylglycine (DMG)	Sharpens mental acuity; boosts energy.	From 125 mg to more than 1,000 mg daily
Taurine	Regulates neurotransmitters in the brain; may enhance attention, cognitive performance, and feelings of well-being.	2 grams, 3 times daily

2 SURPRISE MOOD BOOSTERS YOU'VE NEVER HEARD ABOUT

Are you singing the blues a little too often these days? If so, get a grip with rhodiola rosea and skullcap—two mood-boosting herbs that are fast replacing St. John's wort and kava as the mental tonics of choice. That's because rhodiola rosea and skullcap provide even more benefits, some of which have only been recently discovered. So if you've tried other herbal antidepressants but without much relief, you'll definitely want to switch to rhodiola rosea and skullcap. Both display an astonishing power to lift your spirits and banish a bad mood, safely and effectively. Here are the basics.

RHODIOLA ROSEA

From the mountaintops of Russia and Asia comes rhodiola rosea, an herb that will make you feel on top of the world, thanks to its incredible mood-vitalizing ability. Although revered as a folk medicine for more than 3,000 years, rhodiola was first researched scientifically in 1931. Not

until the 1990s did the researchers in the Soviet Union release information to the world on the herb's numerous health benefits. As a result,
more and more people have become aware of the groundbreaking reve-
lations concerning rhodiola's value as a remedy for mental problems.
Therapeutically, the herb is used to treat mood disorders, depression,
poor mental performance, lack of concentration, stress, impaired memory, loss of physical strength, fatigue, and many diseases. The part of the
plant responsible for its medicinal value is the root of the herb.

Among the active ingredients in rhodiola are two plant chemicals
called rosavin and salidroside, which account for the herb's mood-
buoying talents. They accomplish this by jacking up levels of serotonin in
the brain. Higher concentrations of serotonin in the brain have a calming
effect on the body and help relieve depression.

Specifically, rosavin and salidroside work in two important ways.
First, they enhance the delivery of 5-HTP into the brain. As explained in
the previous section, 5-HTP is a building block of serotonin and naturally boosts its levels in the brain, an action that ameliorates the symptoms of depression.

Second, rosavin and salidroside inhibit a process that tends to degrade
serotonin in the body. Once produced, serotonin can be inactivated by
certain enzymes. Rosavin and salidroside step in and block the activity
of these enzymes. The net effect is to increase brain levels of serotonin by
30 percent, according to research. Small wonder, then, that rhodiola rosea
is such a powerful mood booster and effective treatment for depression.

Worth mentioning, too, is that this herb has other benefits to brain
health. Recent studies conducted in Russia reveal that rhodiola improved
the mental performance of students taking exams. The herb is also a
powerful antioxidant that may protect the brain from the onslaught of
disease-causing free radicals.

Rhodiola is now commercially available in capsules and sold in health-
food stores or through Internet sources. Follow the manufacturer's recommendations for dosage. In addition, look for a product in which the extract
of the herb is standardized to 1-percent salidroside and 2-percent rosavin.

Rhodiola is considered a safe herb by herbalists. In higher-than-
recommended dosages, however, rhodiola supplements have been known

to cause irritability and insomnia. Children and pregnant or lactating women should not take rhodiola. Nor should you take it with other serotonin boosters such as St. John's wort or SAM-e, since the combined effects of these supplements have not been scientifically tested. Further, anyone with an existing medical condition or prolonged illness should consult a physician prior to supplementing.

SKULLCAP

This herb's strange-sounding name comes from the resemblance of its blossoms to the human skull. It's a fitting name nonetheless because skullcap goes to work beneath the skull, acting on the brain to treat a whole constellation of conditions, including mood disorders, premenstrual tension, nervous tension, anxiety, insomnia, stress-related headaches, muscle aches, high blood pressure, and high cholesterol.

A member of the mint family, skullcap has long been used by Native American healers and European herbalists to treat conditions of the nervous system. The herb grows in Europe and in the United States from Connecticut to Florida and as far west as Texas. There is also a Chinese version of skullcap.

Skullcap goes by other names, too: mad dogweed (because it was once thought to cure rabies), blue pimpernel, and hood wort. The European and North American species of skullcap are known botanically as *Scuttellaria lateriflora*; the Chinese species is *Scuttellaria baicalensis*. The dried root of the herb yields most of the natural constituents responsible for its healing capabilities.

Although very little research has been conducted on skullcap, in practice it can modulate mood swings, take the edge off anxiety, soothe irritability, treat depression, and bring a feeling of inner peace and calm. People have also used it to control anger. Some herbalists recommend it to calm addicts who are withdrawing from narcotics or alcohol.

Although skullcap certainly sounds like a universal upper, nobody is yet sure of exactly how it works. Skullcap, however, is known to contain scutellarin, a plant chemical with mild muscle- and nerve-relaxing properties.

New evidence from Russian scientists is cropping up that the Chinese species of skullcap may be more therapeutically potent than its European and North American cousins. Preliminary research indicates that *Scuttellaria baicalensis* is an effective stress reducer. More studies are needed, however, to substantiate these findings.

For more than fifty years, skullcap was considered a sedative by the United States Pharmacopoeia (USP), the organization that sets quality standards for supplements and over-the-counter drugs. Research studies in China, Europe, and the former Soviet Union have verified the herb's sedative effects.

One reason you probably haven't heard much about skullcap is that it is often found in combination supplements formulated with other mood-balancing herbs, such as St. John's wort, valerian, chamomile, passionflower, hops, and lemon balm.

Skullcap is available in dried and liquid extracts, capsules, and teas. The usual dosage of the dried extract is 1 to 2 grams three times a day. It takes a few weeks of daily use to experience any benefit. It is rather mild, so you can take it during the day without getting drowsy.

Higher-than-recommended dosages can cause dizziness, confusion, or an irregular pulse rate. Skullcap should not be used in conjunction with prescription tranquilizers.

A report suggesting liver toxicity from skullcap has been discredited because the product in question was adulterated with germander, an herb toxic to the liver.

If you are pregnant or lactating or suffer from an existing medical condition, do not take skullcap. Safety in young children has not yet been established.

RESTORE YOUR MENTAL BALANCE WITH 12 OF THE MOST PROMISING THERAPIES

Emotional problems can strike anyone, at any time. You may feel sad, moody, anxious, lonely, or just plain overwhelmed by life. You may have trouble sleeping or eating, or you may feel like hiding from the world.

One thing is certain: You're not alone. More than 41 million Americans—nearly one in five—suffer a mental disorder at some point in their lives, according to the National Institute of Mental Health.

When you can't quite seem to shake these feelings and your mood is interfering with your life, it's wise to seek therapy—the right kind of therapy. For the very best results, the type of therapy you undergo should be tailored to your condition. Table 3.3 lists the various therapies available, how they work, as well as their pros and cons.

TABLE 3.3
Mental Health Treatment Options

THERAPY	GOALS	How It Works	BENEFITS	DRAWBACKS
Psychoanalysis	Uncover the root of a mental problem and develop coping strategies.	Talk sessions delve into a patient's past.	Effective for a wide range of mental disorders, including depression and anxiety disorders.	A long, ongoing process.
Psycho-dynamic Therapy	Help you understand the psychological forces that motivate your actions; improve coping skills and manage stress.	Focuses more on resolving specific problems, rather than on examining a patient's broad background and personality.	Effective for a wide range of mental disorders, including depression and anxiety disorders.	Can take time to achieve results.
Short-Term Dynamic Therapy	Resolve a very specific problem, such as fear of commitment to a relationship.	A few talk sessions that zero in on a single problem.	Effective for treating fears, phobias, depression, grief, and stress.	Not appropriate for long-standing mental illnesses, such as manic depression, schizophrenia, or addictions.

Therapy	Goals	How It Works	Benefits	Drawbacks
Behavioral Therapy	Change or modify unwanted behavior and replace it with more productive behavior.	Helps patient cope with and overcome difficult situations.	Teaches skills that are useful over a lifetime; effective for treating anxiety disorders and addictions.	Can take time to achieve results.
Cognitive Therapy	Change unproductive thought patterns to think more positively and realistically about the world around you.	Examines feelings and helps patient differentiate realistic from unrealistic thoughts.	Teaches skills that are useful over a lifetime; effective for treating a wide range of mental illnesses.	Can take time to achieve results.
Marital Therapy	Restore intimacy and commitment to a marriage; may focus on changing or accepting behavior.	Talk sessions that involve both spouses to examine feelings and problems in the relationship; may also involve individual sessions with each spouse.	Can dramatically enhance marriage and keep spouses together.	Often not effective if the counseling focuses on changing behavior when people are unwilling to do so.
Interpersonal Therapy	Develop and improve relationships.	Uses role-playing activities and talk sessions.	Beneficial for treating relationship problems, marital conflict, family issues, and loneliness.	Can take time to achieve results.
Pastoral Counseling	Change behavior and encourage productive living.	Provided under the auspices of a church or synagogue; through one-on-one counseling, girded in biblical principles for living.	Beneficial for a wide number of situations.	May not be effective for people who are not members of a religious faith.

(Continued)

Therapy	Goals	How It Works	Benefits	Drawbacks
Group Therapy	Learn better strategies for coping and interacting with people.	Involves meeting and interacting with a group of people under the guidance of a therapist.	Provides an environment of emotional support and social connections that makes people feel like they're not alone in their suffering; effective for treating a wide range of problems.	Can take time to achieve results.
Exposure Therapy	Overcome a specific, narrowly defined fear or phobia, such as fear of spiders, fear of flying, or any irrational fear that interferes with normal routines or relationships.	Gradual exposure to the dreaded circumstance or object in small doses at first, then bigger ones; may involve relaxation techniques such as deep breathing to alleviate anxiety.	Effective for treating fears and phobias.	Has a narrow range of application.
Cultural Analysis	Improve self-esteem; learn self-value.	Examines how societal messages of youth, beauty, thinness, etc., produce depression and low self-esteem.	Effective for treating depression, low self-esteem, and stress.	Works best for women, who are often more vulnerable to societal messages than men are.
Hypnosis	Turn negative self-thoughts into positive thoughts that change behavior.	Induces a relaxed, passive state similar to sleep but allows patient to stay awake and remain mindful of surroundings; may affect limbic system, the brain's emotional center.	Effective for treating addictions, anxiety disorders, and phobias.	Doesn't work for everyone; 25 percent of people cannot be hypnotized.

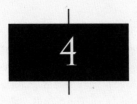

How to Improve Your Memory

Memory: It's the one thing no one wants to lose, ever. But it happens, sometimes daily. Who hasn't forgotten a password to get access to computer information or voice mail? A personal identification number at the bank? Someone's name? Where you left your glasses?

Let's face it: Memory is faulty. But happily, you can shore it up by taking steps so that memory lapses occur less often. Read on to find out how.

SNACK YOUR WAY TO BETTER RECALL: 5 RECIPES THAT ENHANCE MEMORY

Fend off fuzzy thinking and poor memory with the right between-meal snacks. Here are some examples of easy-to-fix snacks that will help you remember your PIN, the name of the client you just met, and where you put your glasses or left your car keys. Each recipe contains nutrients proven to improve memory-linked brain chemistry and protect against memory loss.

PEACHY PROTEIN SHAKE

Here's a protein-rich shake to stir up brain neurotransmitters. Made with a fortified nutritional drink, it contains a full day's worth of vitamins and minerals for total brain health. With the addition of peaches and oatmeal, this shake provides plenty of glucose, which boosts memory. Oatmeal is also loaded with a number of B vitamins that enhance brain chemistry. Quick to fix, this shake makes a delicious complete meal, for breakfast or for a snack.

8-ounce can chilled vanilla-flavored
  nutritional energy drink, such as Boost™,
  Ensure™, or similar product
1 cup frozen peaches
¼ cup raw instant oatmeal

Place all ingredients in a blender and blend until smooth. Makes 1 serving.

MEMORABLE DEVILED EGGS

Eggs are a superior source of choline, a building block for the memory-promoting neurotransmitter acetylcholine. Unless you suffer from high cholesterol, there's no reason to shun eggs.

6 eggs, hard-boiled
2 tablespoons mayonnaise or plain yogurt
1 tablespoon Dijon mustard
2 tablespoons pickle relish
¼ teaspoon salt
⅛ teaspoon pepper
Paprika

Cut eggs in half, lengthwise. Remove yolks and place in a bowl. Mash the yolks with a fork. Add mayonnaise (or yogurt), mustard, relish, salt, and pepper, and mix well. Fill egg whites with yolk mixture. Sprinkle with paprika. Makes 1 dozen. (Allow two eggs per person.)

MEMORY MIX

The nuts and seeds in this recipe supply vitamin E and protein, two nutrients that may prevent mental deterioration and memory loss. There's evidence that vitamin E in particular slows the development of Alzheimer's disease. Dried fruits such as apricots and raisins are naturally fortified with iron, a memory-boosting mineral.

½ cup dried apricots, chopped
½ cup raisins
½ cup soynuts
½ cup peanuts
½ cup pumpkin seeds

Combine all ingredients in a large plastic bag and mix well. Makes 2 to 4 servings.

BRAIN FOOD SNACKERS

Sardines are filled with brain-healthy omega-3 fatty acids, involved in strengthening memory and promoting a pleasant disposition. The crackers supply glucose and B vitamins, both essential to vitalizing memory.

1 tin sardines
6 to 8 reduced-fat Triscuits or whole-wheat
   crackers
Dijon mustard (optional)

Place pieces of the sardines on crackers and top with mustard if desired. Makes 1 to 2 servings.

REMEMBRANCE FRUIT SALAD

The fruit in this salad is rich in carbohydrates, which supplies memory-boosting glucose to your brain, as well as antioxidants, which protect brain cells from free radicals and inflammation. What's more, the wheat germ is loaded with brain-protecting vitamin E.

> *1 cup fresh strawberries, sliced*
> *1 fresh mango, peeled and cut into chunks*
> *1 banana, sliced*
> *8-ounce container nonfat, non-sugar vanilla yogurt*
> *2 to 3 tablespoons wheat germ*

Combine and toss all ingredients and serve immediately. Makes 2 to 3 servings.

FIGHT FORGETFULNESS: 8 RECOMMENDATIONS FOR OVERCOMING MENTAL BLIPS AND SLIPS

Here are some tips for improving your memory that go beyond what you eat between meals. It all comes down to this: The quality of your memory has not only to do with the state of your brain, but also with your state of mind.

BELIEVE YOU HAVE A GOOD MEMORY

What you believe about your memory influences your ability to remember, says a study at the University of Florida in Gainesville. Volunteers who were told that memory was a skill that could be improved performed better on a difficult memory task than those who were told that their memory couldn't be improved. So stop telling yourself that you're forgetful, or else forgetfulness will become a self-fulfilling prophecy. The sky's the limit when you think you can!

RELAX AND RETRACE

You can't find your favorite shirt, or you can't remember where you jotted down the password of your favorite Internet site. Don't let your frustration get the best of you. Tension and stress only make your memory fuzzy and less effective. Take a deep breath and calm down. Then retrace your steps from the last time you had the object in your hands, recreating the scene.

To prevent misplacing items in the future, make it a habit to put them back in the same place every time. Another tip is to become more aware of your actions. Tell yourself out loud: "I'm placing my keys on the desk." These cues will help you recall information when you need it.

TAKE MENTAL PICTURES

This technique comes in handy when you need to remember where you parked your car or need to navigate your way back to some location. Take mental note of your surroundings and reference points: where you parked in relation to the building, what you noticed as you parked, landmarks along the way, and so forth. The key is to pay active attention to your surroundings.

WRITE IT DOWN

If you think making lists is cheating, think again. Writing reminders makes it easier for your brain to process a larger amount of information so that it doesn't have to get clogged up with too much stuff. Alternatives to making lists include sending yourself e-mail messages, leaving reminders on your telephone answering machine, jotting things down on calendars, and keeping a diary or journal.

USE ORGANIZERS

These include address books; calendars; tickler files; special files or notebooks that list PINs, passwords, user names, account numbers, and so forth; and medication boxes. All of these memory tools help you organize information so that it is easy to find and remember.

PRACTICE

Rehearse the retrieval of information. With phone numbers, for example, memorize the number early on (the more you revert to looking it up in the phone book, the lazier your brain becomes at retrieval), then keep trying to remember it. In other words, you must work on absorbing and retaining information. This makes it easier to recollect numbers and other material in the future.

USE RECITATION

Recitation is saying aloud the information or the ideas you need to remember. If, for example, you want to remember a joke so you can retell it, recite the joke several times until you know it. When you say something out loud, you start to know it and remember it. This is because recitation transfers material into your long-term memory.

TAKE A BRAIN BREAK

Every so often during the day, give your brain time off. In other words, alternate periods of mental activity with periods of mental inactivity. This helps prevent the buildup of cortisol, the hormone secreted when you're stressed out. Chronically elevated cortisol is like poison to your nervous system because it keeps brain cells from getting enough oxygen and glucose—the nourishment they need to keep your memory sharp.

Need proof? When volunteers in a Stanford University School of Medicine study relaxed every muscle in their bodies prior to taking a three-hour memory training course, they recalled 25 percent more information than those who had not done relaxation exercises.

REMEMBER NAMES LIKE A COMPUTER:
10 PROVEN TECHNIQUES

You're introduced to someone for the first time, and just moments later the name of that person slips your mind.

Sound familiar? Probably—it happens to all of us, all of the time. In fact, forgetting names is the leading memory complaint of adults in the United States.

But it doesn't have to be if we learn and practice some simple techniques for remembering names. The benefits of doing so are worth it: no more mortifying moments, grasping to recollect names; the ability to make a great impression because you're great at remembering names; and stronger self-confidence in every social situation.

So if you're frustrated by this most common of all memory lapses and want to overcome it, read on. What follows is a look at ten proven techniques on how to remember names easily at every encounter.

When you meet someone for the first time do the following:

1. **Pay attention, concentrate, and listen to person's name as you are introduced.**

   Names often elude us because we haven't concentrated on learning the name in the first place. When you meet someone for the first time, concentrate, listen, look into the person's eyes, and focus on the name. That way, you're more likely to retain it than if you're thinking about something else at the same time— like how to get a refill on your coffee or where the restroom is.

2. **Repeat the name several times during the conversation.**

   For example, say, "I'm happy to meet you, Mary." "Where are you from, Mary?" "What type of work do you do, Mary?" "It was very nice to meet you, Mary." This verbal technique harnesses the power of repetition and thus helps imprint the person's name on your memory.

3. **Comment on the person's name, if appropriate.**

For example, say, "Are you related to the other Franklins in town?" "*Strachan*—that's an unusual name. Is it Scottish?" A variation on this technique is, "Marsha. Do you spell your name M-a-r-s-h-a or M-a-r-c-i-a?"

"If the name is unusual, ask about the origin of it to learn more about the person," advises Eileen Perrigo, coauthor with Deborah Roach Gaut of *Business and Professional Communication for the 21st Century*.

4. **Link a person's physical features to his or her name.**

This technique is rather gimmicky but is one that many memory experts highly recommend. Basically, it works like this: Say you meet a person whose name is Hazelwood, and she has hazel-colored eyes; make it a point to connect that name with the physical trait. Or suppose the person's name is Mark or Marks, and he has freckles. Remember: "Mark, the guy with freckle marks." The key is to look for a physical characteristic and hook it to the person's name.

5. **Connect the person to a famous person, past or present.**

This technique relies on the power of our visual memory to aid in recall. If you're introduced to someone named "Abe," for example, visualize Abraham Lincoln during the introduction. The next time you encounter that person, you'll think of our nation's sixteenth president, and that person's name should pop into your head.

6. **Make a name more memorable by creating an exaggerated association with it.**

This is one of the creative techniques recommended by Cynthia R. Green, Ph.D., in her book *Total Memory Workout*. Dr. Green suggests making up a story to go along with the person's name. For example, you've just met a guy named Duke Richman. Picture a duke in his castle, counting his money.

7. **Rhyme the name.**

Rhyming works like this: You meet someone and create a one-line poem in your mind for that person. For example:

"Ann's in the band. Ted can't get out of bed. Tim works out at the gym." When you rhyme a name, you stamp it on your memory.

8. **Be able to recall names in a group.**

In many social settings, you're introduced to several people at once. Remembering everyone's name is more difficult because our short-term memories can retain only five names, on average. So the key is to force those names into long-term storage as soon as possible. But how?

By using some of the same techniques discussed above: Say each person's name, ask questions about the names, and repeat each person's name. This means you'll have to spend two or more minutes conversing with each member of the group. Afterward, mentally repeat the names, and an hour later review the names in your head.

9. **Put faces with names.**

Many times, it's easier to remember a face than it is a name. If this happens to you, don't stress out because of not knowing the name. The tension will further mangle your memory and make the name harder to dredge up from your memory bank.

One technique that works for most people is going through the alphabet or a list of familiar names. For example: "Does her name begin with *A, B,* or *C?*" Or "His name is something like *Rich, Rick.*" These are memory cues that may just bring the name to mind.

10. **Practice.**

Author and memory expert Dr. Green also recommends rehearsing name-recall techniques on people whose names you don't have to remember, such as your waiter or waitress, a checkout person at the grocery store, or a salesclerk. That way, you hone your recall ability for future encounters when you need to remember names.

If you forget someone's name, relax. Just be honest and calm, recommend Deborah Roach Gaut and Eileen Perrigo in their book *Business and Professional Communication for the 21st Century.* The authors suggest responding like this: "I recall being introduced at the annual meeting, but I cannot remember your name."

Keep in mind, too, that people will forget your name. Put them at ease if you sense this is happening. Simply extend your hand and reintroduce yourself. Such commonsense etiquette overcomes awkward situations and makes everyone feel comfortable.

Part Two

QUICK AND EASY JUMP STARTS

At age sixty, seventy, eighty, or beyond, we all want to be mentally sharp. But what about right now—today—when you have to creatively solve a business problem, take a test, shift rapidly into a good mood, or have instant recall of facts or events?

Here is some powerfully good news: You can attain on-the-spot mental sharpness and fitness with a host of simple moves, some of which can be done behind your desk, in your own home, virtually anywhere, really. Others involve foods, herbs, and holistic techniques, all with ability to turbo-charge your mental capacity.

Once you begin practicing some of these moves, you'll start impressing people with your brilliance and gain a new level of self-confidence that alone will maximize your chances of success in every endeavor.

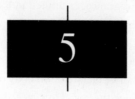

Jump-Start Your Mental Powers

If your train of thought is a choo-choo just chugging along but you want to turn it into a high-speed train, there are some quick and easy things you can do to get on the fast track. You can learn facts instantly, smash creative blocks, score well on tests, stay alert most of the day, and more. The suggestions outlined here will work for virtually anyone who needs a mental edge—and needs it now.

SNIFF YOUR WAY TO BETTER BRAINPOWER

Of all the senses, the sense of smell is the most evocative, with the power to stimulate the brain—and to do it rapidly. It's no wonder, then, that the ancient healing art of aromatherapy has been rediscovered as a way to boost brainpower.

Aromatherapy, which is one of the oldest forms of healing, employs essential oils that have been extracted from leaves, flowers, resins, seeds, fruit, grasses, wood, and other plant parts. To achieve the desired effect, the oils are diffused into the air, burned as incense to permeate the atmosphere with a pleasing fragrance, or diluted in bathwater. As you inhale, in only a millisecond the aroma is picked up by your olfactory nerve, the nerve serving the sense of smell and the only open pathway leading directly to the undersurface of your brain.

Some essential oils can be blended into body oils and used directly on the skin as part of massage therapy. However, they must first be diluted in nut or seed oils because pure essential oils are too strong and concentrated to be applied directly to the skin. When massaged into the skin, the diluted oil enters the bloodstream more quickly than if the whole herb is taken by mouth.

Although essential oils have multiple uses, certain oils can rev up your mental powers. These oils are discussed below, and ways to use them are summarized in Table 5.1 on page 136.

CINNAMON FOR PROBLEM SOLVING

Derived from a tree of the laurel family, cinnamon is no doubt the most popular spice in the world. In addition to spicing up foods, cinnamon is used as a medicine when taken internally and as an aromatic oil employed in massage therapy in a diluted form.

In aromatherapy, cinnamon oil is generally indicated for the relief of stress and exhaustion. And, according to an ongoing study at Cornell University, it may also perk up your ability to solve problems. Researchers found that subjects exposed to the aroma of cinnamon buns appeared to be more proficient at problem solving. They theorized that the smell of cinnamon evokes feelings of happiness and that happiness, in turn, promotes creativity.

JASMINE FOR ACCURACY

Native to China, India, and Iran, jasmine is an evergreen shrub whose flowers are used to produce jasmine oil, which has been dubbed "the king of essential oils."

Jasmine is among the fragrances that help you think more clearly and reduce the number of goofs you make while working. In a study conducted in Japan, researchers found that jasmine-scented air cut mistakes among workers by 33 percent.

Aromatic jasmine is also prized for its ability to decrease anxiety, depression, nervous exhaustion, and stress.

LEMON FOR PRECISION

The scent of lemon in the air may also increase precision and accuracy. That's the finding of a Japanese study in which researchers discovered that air scented with a lemon spray cut errors among workers by 54 percent.

PEPPERMINT FOR MENTAL STIMULATION

A whiff of peppermint oil is thought to invigorate the mind, so it is recommended by aromatherapists to people who need mental stimulation while performing their jobs. Indeed, some very preliminary research hints that peppermint stimulates the brain and may increase your capacity to retain facts and boost recall.

Peppermint oil can be diffused into the air, added to bathwater, or, in a diluted form, massaged into the skin to help ease tension and stress.

ROSEMARY OIL FOR MEMORY ENHANCEMENT

Diffused or inhaled rosemary oil reportedly assists in enhancing mental clarity. Only just recently has the scientific community begun to examine it as a complementary treatment for Alzheimer's disease. Supposedly, it helps oxygenate brain cells to overcome memory problems and strengthen attention span.

SAFETY PRECAUTIONS

Aromatic oils are meant for external use only. They should not be applied to the skin until diluted with a carrier oil such as grapeseed oil, almond oil, jojoba oil, or olive oil. In addition, do not ingest aromatic oils because they can be toxic if taken internally.

Anyone with a medical condition, or women who are pregnant or lactating, should not undergo aromatherapy unless under the medical supervision of a physician.

TABLE 5.1 How to Use Essential Oils	
DIFFUSION	Buy a diffuser at a health-food store or at a massage therapy clinic. Let several drops of the oil soak into the pad of the diffuser. Insert the pad into the diffuser and plug it into an electrical wall outlet. Within moments, the scent will fill your room.
MASSAGE	Dilute the essential oil according to the following: 2 to 3 drops of the essential oil to 1 teaspoon of the carrier oil. Use the oil for a full massage or spot massage on specific parts of the body.
THERAPEUTIC BATHS	Add 8 to 15 drops of the chosen essential oil to your bathwater and swish the water around for better dispersion of the oil.
INHALATION	Add 3 to 6 drops of the essential oil to a steaming bowl of water or 1 to 2 drops to a handkerchief. Breathe in deeply for about five minutes.
PERFUME	Create your own perfume by adding 20 to 25 drops of the essential oil to 1 ounce of water in a mist spray bottle. Shake well.

Air Freshener	Make your own air freshener by adding 50 to 75 drops of the essential oil to 2 ounces of water in a mist spray bottle. Shake well. Spray the air in your home or car.
Candle Incense	Place 2 drops of the essential oil into the hot melted wax of a burning candle.
Pillow	Sprinkle a few drops of the essential oil on your bed-clothes or sheets.

Sit Up for Smarts

Can't think straight? Then sit up straight.

A slouched, hunched-over position, with your head hung over, limits blood flow to your brain—a chief cause of foggy thinking and forgetfulness. (Your brain needs nearly thirty times more blood than other organs).

Anatomically, poor posture creates crimps in the two arteries that pass through the spine to your brain and reduces blood flow, much like a kink in a garden hose cuts off water supply. This hinders thinking, mental performance, and other cognitive functions.

Habitual poor posture is problematic for another reason: It can lead to mini-strokes, tiny unnoticed strokes that can damage brain tissue. Further, poor posture contributes to disabling backaches.

Thus, it's vitally important to make good posture a habit. Here are some tips:

- Imagine that there is a string connecting your skull to the bones in your ankle. Momentarily bend your knees and hunch your shoulders, then "pull" that string tight by *standing up as straight as you can*. That's good posture.
- When standing, always try to keep your back upright and your shoulders pressed back. Concentrate on tucking your stomach and buttocks in, while pulling in your chin.

- Select chairs with either straight backs or lumbar (low-back) support. Your thighs should rest parallel to the floor for even distribution of your weight.
- When seated, sit up straight, without stooping over. Keep your head and neck as straight as much as possible, too, with eyes looking forward.
- Concentrate and practice on maintaining good posture at all times.

GET SMARTER IN 12 MINUTES A DAY

There are ways to become more brilliant in only minutes a day. But before we learn them, here's some encouraging news: You may already be smarter than you think. In fact, you're smarter than your ancestors were.

The average IQ (intelligence quotient) has risen about twenty points with every generation—a phenomenon called the "Flynn Effect," after New Zealand political scientist James Flynn, who first documented the fascinating rise in IQ. In fact, today's average child is as smart as a kid considered a genius a generation ago!

Although heredity plays a strong role in determining intelligence, the steady increase in IQ has been credited to numerous environmental factors, including more education, better nutrition, better-educated parents, and technology such as smart toys and computers. Flynn and his fellow researchers also found that people with a genetic predisposition to higher intelligence tend to seek out rich learning environments and that doing so amplifies intelligence even more.

So, given that our environment factors into intelligence, are there things we can be doing that will make us smarter? You bet.

BECOME AN EXPERT

Studies conducted since the turn of the nineteenth century prove that staying in school elevates intelligence. If you're not in some type of continuing education program now, homeschool yourself. Devote twelve minutes a day to the study of a subject you're interested in so that you become an expert on that topic. This "mini-schooling" exercise will keep your mind engaged plus help you get smarter.

LEARN FACTS INSTANTLY

One of the best ways to pick up knowledge fast on just about any subject is to read a children's nonfiction book. Children's books have a knack of distilling the key information into easy-to-grasp basics. Once, I had to research and learn information about the history of banking—a voluminous topic—and so I checked out a kid's book on the subject and got everything I needed. Children's books take about ten to twelve minutes to read, so you can absorb the information quickly, even while browsing in a bookstore.

BOOST YOUR VOCABULARY

Vocabulary is routinely measured on IQ tests and used as an indicator of "smarts." Although we learn most of our vocabulary when we're younger, it's not too late to add to our personal word lists and get smarter in the process. Each day, spend twelve minutes learning one or two new words. Pluck them from the dictionary, a thesaurus, or from magazines and books. Study the definitions, memorize the spellings, and start using them in sentences and everyday conversation.

BE A MULTI-TASKER

This means learning to do two or more things at once. The easiest way to start is with your computer. Go online to research your favorite subject, but do some instant messaging (called IM'ing) with a friend at the same time. Scientists have found that teenagers who surf the Net, download information, and IM their friends simultaneously are exercising their memories (a component of intelligence), plus honing their attention skills.

LISTEN TO CLASSICAL MUSIC

Classical tunes and opera music are charged with high-frequency sounds and built with complex arrangements, both of which improve thinking and increase attention span. One study found that listening to Mozart for just ten minutes boosts brainpower. Another study demonstrated that students performed better on IQ tests after listening to Mozart.

Look Smart

Can't fit in twelve minutes a day to get smarter? That's okay. You can at least look the part. German researchers have discovered that you'll be perceived as intelligent if you are good looking, in reasonably good shape, act friendly, project confidence, have a pleasant voice, clearly articulate your ideas, dress conservatively, and wear your hair in a stylish fashion.

PASS EXAMS WITH FLYING COLORS:
12 FOODS TO AVOID BEFORE TAKING A TEST

Can you up your odds of a good test grade simply by what you put in your mouth? The answer is that the food choices you make at mealtime probably can increase alertness and recall, plus help you feel less groggy during your test. That's because the right diet supplies all the precursor and supporting nutrients you need to stay sharp.

Generally speaking, it's a good idea to eat a mixed meal of carbohydrate, protein, and some fat for breakfast or lunch to improve mental functioning. If you're taking a test in the morning or early afternoon, eat lightly at breakfast or lunch, since large meals lead to poor mental performance.

Another tip: Don't stray too far from your habitual diet. Studies show that mental performance and mood can be negatively affected if you deviate from your regular mealtime choices. So, eat what you're used to on examination day.

With this advice in mind, here's a look at twelve foods you should avoid when you're about to take a test.

CANDY BARS

Eating just a candy bar prior to taking a test pumps too much sugar into your bloodstream too rapidly. Blood sugar levels sink as quickly as they rise, causing a low blood sugar reaction, or hypoglycemia. This will make you feel tired and irritable—exactly the wrong mindset for test-takers who need to feel their best during exams. Try to eat a balance of foods that will release sugar more slowly during digestion, such as an egg, whole-grain cereal, and a piece of fresh fruit.

DOUGHNUTS

A breakfast of doughnuts and hot chocolate or coffee may be quick and convenient, but it's not the best choice for test-takers. Doughnuts are laced with sugar, which can lead to a hypoglycemic reaction, tiredness, and mental grogginess.

PANCAKES OR WAFFLES WITH SYRUP

A breakfast of pancakes or waffles with syrup is extremely high in carbohydrates, which will speed up your brain's production of serotonin. Serotonin induces sleep, which is exactly the opposite effect desired during a test when you need to be sharp and alert.

SUGARY CEREALS

Any highly sugared food should be avoided prior to taking a test because it triggers the synthesis of serotonin, which reduces alertness. In addition, sugar tends to aggravate hyperactivity in some children, reducing their attention span.

BACON AND COLD CUTS

These are heavy foods—high in saturated fats and slow to digest—and may make you feel tired during a test. By contrast, scientifically controlled studies show that diets with less saturated fat and more fiber, vitamins, and minerals improve mental performance.

RED MEAT

Even though red meat is an important source of brain-enhancing iron, it is not always the best protein choice to eat right before a test. Red meat is a heavy food that tends to digest very slowly, diverting blood to the stomach rather than to the brain where it is needed to oxygenate brain cells. A heavy meal thus makes mental tasks more difficult to perform. A better protein choice is tuna or salmon, rich in a brain-building fat called docosahexaenoic acid (DHA). This fat has been shown to reduce stress reactions in college students during final exams.

WHITE BREAD

During digestion, white bread is quickly converted into blood sugar. This drives your blood sugar up too high, giving you a quick "rush" followed by a fast "crash" into hypoglycemia. In susceptible people, hypoglycemia can bring on anxiety attacks—certainly not the mental frame of mind you want to be in during a test. What's more, white bread and other processed foods contain far fewer nutrients than natural, unrefined foods and are thus less desirable as pre-test foods. Better choices include whole grains, vegetables, and low-sugar fruits such as berries. Combine these with a protein food such as low-fat cheese to stave off a hypoglycemic reaction.

PEANUT BUTTER AND JELLY SANDWICH

This lunchtime favorite is high in carbohydrates and fat and low in protein. This is a nutrient mix that has been found in research to slow down reaction time, promote drowsiness, and muddle thinking—exactly the opposite of how you need to feel during a test.

CARBONATED BEVERAGES

Sodas and other carbonated drinks are loaded with phosphates, preservatives that can cause hyperkinesis (exaggerated muscle activity). Children diagnosed with hyperactive behavior should definitely avoid carbonated beverages to help increase their concentration and focus.

The best fluid for test-taking is water, so make sure you're well hydrated prior to and during your test. Even slight dehydration can lead to mental confusion.

MILK

A glass of milk is loaded with the amino acid tryptophan, a precursor to sleep-inducing serotonin in the brain. Tryptophan is like a natural sleeping pill. What's more, studies show that elevated levels of tryptophan increase error rate on performance tests, so you'll want to avoid milk prior to taking a test. Another high-tryptophan food is turkey.

Don't avoid high-tryptophan foods at other times, however. Research indicates that this amino acid helps you learn and retain information. So while studying for your test, fortify your brain with a turkey sandwich, washed down with a glass of milk.

ALCOHOL

Alcoholic beverages worsen mental performance, cloud thinking, and lead to mind-sapping dehydration. Best advice: Avoid alcohol for three days prior to your test to ensure mental sharpness.

COFFEE

If you're unaccustomed to caffeine, don't start drinking it on test day. Adding coffee to your diet will not improve your performance. Instead, it could make you jittery and more tense during your test. (If you are a coffee-drinker, it's a good idea to have a small cup prior to your test because caffeine makes you more alert and creative.)

Quick-Start Creativity: An Amazing Technique to Unleash Your Imagination

You're in a meeting and you have to solve a problem on the spot. Or you're up against a deadline and you need to finish an article in the next thirty minutes. With no time to let your disjointed thoughts incubate and later hatch into brilliant ideas, what do you do? Try the following revolutionary technique recommended by creativity expert Terry Persun, author of the novel *The Witness Tree* and numerous other writings.

To begin, open your eyes and become aware of specifics in your surroundings: the way the light comes through the window, how a chair is tilted, or even how the trees outside bend in the wind. Then focus in on the specifics and relate them to your present situation or problem. Let's say you're in a meeting discussing the economics behind a project, and you focus on the bright weather outside. The connection can bring instant insight into strategies for a bright future.

"Whether writing, painting, or discussing business in a meeting, this approach will bring instant creativity to the subject," Persun explains. "Similarly, if you close your eyes, your awareness is suddenly changed," he added. "One of two things will happen: You will begin to connect with your other senses and hear, feel, smell your surroundings more acutely, or you will begin to 'create' images in your head. Either way, your focus shifts quickly and you are able to connect to things outside the immediate situation. Making connections to events outside our present state of affairs brings in all kinds of creative ideas."

For people who respond better to sound than to visuals, the same method can be applied by opening or closing your ears, Persun says.

If you have more lead time to hatch ideas, be sure to read the creativity ideas featured in Chapter 19.

The Cognition Enhancer
You Can Drink Every Morning

That cup of coffee or tea you drink every morning contains one of the most amazing—and potent—mental energizers ever discovered: caffeine. Caffeine not only gets you going in the morning but also turbo-charges your alertness, boosts your mental powers, and hikes up your mood. Technically, caffeine is a drug—in fact, the most widely used drug in the world.

As a drug, caffeine is classified as a central nervous system stimulant. It works by blocking adenosine, a sedativelike neurotransmitter that slows your heart rate and blood pressure. Consequently, caffeine makes your heart beat faster, gives you that wide-awake feeling, and has some rather profound effects on behavior.

MAKES YOU MORE ALERT

After drinking a cup of coffee, you feel more alert. You can think more clearly, and you're not as tired. You're likely to feel more creative, too. These positive effects have been confirmed time after time in a number of laboratory tests, in which caffeine has been shown to radically improve performance on cognitive tests.

KEEPS YOU MENTALLY FOCUSED

If you find your mind wandering when you need to be concentrating, brew some coffee or tea right away. In a study at the University of Wales, caffeine improved subjects' performance on tasks requiring sustained attention.

HELPS YOU PROCESS INFORMATION

Whenever you're bombarded with a lot of information at once—say, during a classroom lecture or a corporate training session or meeting—make sure you're well stoked with caffeine throughout the day. That's because caffeine increases the speed at which you're able to process information, say British researchers at the University of Surrey. They gave nineteen healthy volunteers about a cup and a half of caffeinated coffee, tea, water, or a control of decaffeinated tea or plain water on three separate occasions during the day: 9 A.M., noon, and 7 P.M. When drinking caffeinated tea, the volunteers exhibited rapid increases in information processing and alertness.

ENHANCES MEMORY

In a majority of the cognitive experiments conducted with caffeine, the drug was shown to enhance memory. A good example is a study conducted at the University of Wales, showing how caffeine significantly improved volunteers' memory, mood, and powers of reasoning. In this study, caffeine (4 milligrams per each 2.2 pounds of body weight) improved a type of memory called "semantic memory," which is our permanent store of knowledge of concepts, words, and their meanings. Some scientists also define semantic memory as our general knowledge of the world. Significantly, semantic memory is a type of memory that deteriorates in Alzheimer's disease.

BOOSTS MOOD

Caffeine is a mood-altering drug with the ability to put us in a better frame of mind. In a British study, volunteers ingested a relatively low dose of caffeine (75 to 150 milligrams), roughly the amount found in a mug of brewed coffee. After having caffeine, they felt happier, with the ability to think more clearly.

Generally, researchers chalk up caffeine's mood-boosting ability to its stimulant action. As a natural stimulant, caffeine provides a psychological lift by making us feel more energetic and less fatigued. Put another way: When we're pepped up, we're less likely to feel down.

THE RIGHT DOSE

If you want the mental kick caffeine gives, how much should you drink?

With higher doses—say, 500 milligrams or more (roughly the amount in four to five cups of coffee)—mental performance begins to slide, so you'll want to keep your consumption under that dosage.

Ultimately, though, you're the best judge of how much caffeine is enough for you. Caffeine may aggravate certain health problems, such as ulcers, heart disease, high blood pressure, and anemia, to name just a few, so check with your doctor about how much you can safely tolerate.

GET A NATURAL BRAIN BUZZ: 2 HERBAL PEP PILLS TO STIMULATE YOUR SMARTS

We all have days when we can't get focused, and our thinking slogs along like a snail. At other times, we start out mentally fired up but fizzle out a few hours before the task is done.

Beyond grabbing a mugful of coffee or acquiescing to a nap, there are other ways to recharge your brain. These include supplementing with guarana or kola nut, two herbs that have been clinically proven to jump-start mental energy. But whether you should use them is the subject of controversy, since both have side effects. What follows is a brief guide to these herbs, with a look at their pros and cons.

GUARANA

Guarana is a red berry from a plant grown in the Amazon valley, and the supplement is made from the seeds of the berry. It contains seven times as much caffeine as the coffee bean and is widely sold in health-food stores as a supplement to increase physical and mental energy. It is the caffeine in guarana that stimulates alertness and boosts energy. Fifty milligrams of guarana is equal to a half cup of coffee. In contrast, though, guarana provides a longer period of stimulation because it is digested more slowly than coffee.

Another effect of guarana is that it may help maintain memory, according to a study conducted by Brazilian researchers who found that guarana-treated rats could better remember how to navigate through a maze.

But if you're sensitive to caffeine, it may be unwise to use guarana because of its stimulating effects. Also, in amounts exceeding 300 milligrams, caffeine can cause nervousness, anxiety, heart palpitations, insomnia, and irritability.

Guarana is available whole, ground, or in powder, as well as in capsules. In South America, it is found mostly in beverages.

KOLA NUT

Derived from the seed of an African tree, kola nut is considered a stimulant herb because of its high caffeine content. It is a constituent of numerous supplements marketed as natural pick-me-ups. In fact, the German Commission E has approved kola nut for treating physical and mental fatigue. One teaspoon, or 100 milligrams, of kola nut, is equal to a half cup of coffee. Kola nut also contains theobromine, a mild stimulant.

From 1891 until about 1908, the Coca-Cola Company formulated its popular cola drink with kola nuts. Today, Coke's products are made with caffeine and natural flavorings.

Many people who take kola nut notice that it reduces fatigue and helps alleviate mild depression. Some users have even reported tingles or an energy rush up their spines after supplementing with kola nut.

Kola nut is a safe herb, although one study found that higher doses (10 milligrams per kilogram, or 2.2 pounds of body weight) depressed motor activity.

Ephedra: Too Dangerous to Recommend

Also known as ma huang, Chinese ephedra, or Mormon Tea, ephedra is a plant that contains ephedrine, a stimulant that enhances the release of the neurotransmitter norepinephrine, stimulating the central nervous system, making the heart beat faster, and increasing blood pressure. Ephedra also contains pseudoephedrine, widely used as an over-the-counter nasal decongestant.

Although research into ephedrine and ephedra shows that they have positive effects on alertness, concentration, and mood, these compounds also produce adverse reactions, including high blood pressure, sleeplessness, anxiety, and nervousness. Because of these effects, people with heart conditions, high blood pressure, or diabetes should steer clear of ephedra and ephedrine.

More seriously, ephedra has been linked to heart attacks, strokes, seizures, brain hemorrhages, and some deaths. As a result, the FDA is keeping close tabs on ephedra supplements, including those spiked with caffeine-containing ingredients.

It is important to emphasize that the FDA has approved ephedrine for treating nasal congestion. The average oral dose is 25 to 50 milligrams every three to four hours, taken up to eight times in twenty-four hours. Doses exceeding those levels may produce troublesome side effects, such as tremors, rapid breathing, nervousness, and insomnia.

Dietary supplements containing ephedrine are sold as energy boosters, weight-loss agents, and bodybuilding aids. Accompanying ephedra in many of these formulations are caffeine-containing agents, such as guarana or kola nut, that promise natural highs. Products go by the following names: Herbal Ecstasy, Cloud 9, Planet X, and others. When combined with caffeine, ephedra and epinedrine can be very powerful, even dangerous at higher-than-recommended dosages, since the combination can aggravate central nervous and cardiovascular system effects such as nervousness and heart palpitations.

The 2 Most Effective
Alertness-Enhancing Drugs

You may never need them—unless your doctor says so—but there are a couple of non-amphetamine, prescription-only drugs designed to enhance alertness, increase attention span, and prevent fatigue. Generally, such drugs are prescribed for children or adults who have attention deficit disorders, but some are used to prevent the excessive daytime sleepiness suffered by adults with narcolepsy, a sleep disorder characterized by uncontrolled episodes of falling asleep, anywhere and anytime. In addition, these drugs are being used to help HIV-infected individuals fight disabling fatigue.

PROVIGIL

Approved by the FDA in 1999, Provigil (modafinil) is the first non-addictive, non-amphetamine drug for narcolepsy. In Canada, the drug is marketed as Alertec.

Until the introduction of Provigil, stimulant drugs were prescribed to treat the disorder. However, they provided only a few hours of alertness, followed by abrupt sleepiness. By contrast, Provigil induces a steadier, milder form of wakefulness.

The usual dose of Provigil, prescribed by doctors, is 200 milligrams taken as a single dose in the morning. As your doctor will advise, you should never increase the dose or take extra doses, because Provigil has the potential for abuse. It can potentially lead to dependence, although discontinuing the drug does not produce withdrawal symptoms.

According to *The PDR Family Guide to Prescription Drugs*, the most common side effects of this drug include anxiety, depression, diarrhea, difficulty sleeping, dizziness, dry mouth, headache, infection, loss of appetite, loss of muscle strength, and nausea.

RITALIN

The most popular drug treatment for children and adults with attention deficit disorders is Ritalin (methylphenidate hydrochloride), a mild central nervous stimulant. It appears to work by stabilizing the neurotransmitter dopamine, helping adults and children to focus better.

The drug is given in standard or sustained-release tablets (Ritalin-SR), taken thirty to forty-five minutes before meals. The typical adult dosage is 20 to 30 milligrams a day, divided into two or three doses. Tolerance to the drug builds, so your physician may increase your dosage. Ritalin-SR tablets keep working for eight hours and may be used in place of Ritalin tablets. Medical experts recommend that Ritalin therapy be combined with counseling to help teach people how to cope with their attention problems.

According to *The PDR Family Guide to Prescription Drugs*, the most common side effects of Ritalin are nervousness and an inability to fall or stay asleep.

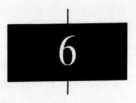

Jump-Start Your Mood

W hile it's perfectly normal for your mood to occasionally dip, a bad disposition can interfere with your ability to get things done, accomplish important goals, and interact lovingly and productively with people in your life. When you find a bad mood getting in the way of productive living, take one or more of the blues-banishing steps suggested in this chapter.

ACUPUNCTURE TO HELP YOUR MOOD

Once pooh-poohed by Western medicine, the ancient Chinese healing art of acupuncture is fast gaining respectability worldwide. In 1996, the FDA removed the "experimental" label from acupuncture needles as medical devices. And in the following year, the National Institutes of Health (NIH) concluded that acupuncture is effective enough in treating nausea to warrant further research.

Acupuncture is used primarily to relieve pain, including migraine headaches, joint problems, and neck and back pain. But it has also proven effective against an array of mental disorders, including depression, anxiety, and cognitive decline. Acupuncture is also used to treat addictions.

HOW DOES ACUPUNCTURE WORK?

In acupuncture, a licensed acupuncturist or physician inserts thin needles at specific pressure points on the body that affect physical or mental discomfort and leaves them in place for a few minutes to a half-hour. The procedure is virtually painless. Some have described the punctures as feeling like mosquito bites or tingling sensations. One or more treatments may be required. More than 1 million Americans undergo acupuncture each year.

Although numerous scientifically controlled studies show that acupuncture is effective, no one is quite sure how it works. There are some theories, however. In traditional Asian medicine, practitioners say that it balances the body's energy flow, or *qi*. Western medical experts believe that acupuncture stimulates the release of the body's natural painkilling endorphins; triggers the production of calming internal benzodiazepines (the body's internally produced tranquilizers); and elevates mood-boosting serotonin. Another theory holds that acupuncture blocks the entrance of pain signals into the brain.

HOW EFFECTIVE IS ACUPUNCTURE?

While acupuncture is now considered a legitimate pain-control technique, it is picking up steam as an effective treatment for mood disorders. If you're suffering from depression or anxiety but haven't gotten relief from conventional treatment, acupuncture from a licensed practitioner may be worth a try, considering the following evidence.

A study conducted at the University of Arizona found that acupuncture provided rates of relief from depression that were similar to those seen with the use of antidepressants. In the study, researchers divided thirty-eight clinically depressed women into three groups: a group who received acupuncture for eight weeks; a group who was told it would receive acupuncture for depression but were treated instead for loss of appetite, insomnia, and other depression-related problems; and a group placed on a waiting list for treatment.

By the end of the study, half of the patients getting acupuncture for depression were cured. Twenty-seven percent of the patients in the other group experienced symptom relief. Following the first experiment, all women received acupuncture for depression, and 70 percent experienced relief. The researchers pointed out that these rates of relief—50 to 70 percent—correspond to the rates of relief when patients receive conventional treatment such as psychotherapy or antidepressant medication.

Although the results of this rather groundbreaking study were released in 1999, this was not the first time acupuncture proved its value in treating depression. In 1987, Russian investigators studied the effects of acupuncture in treating 167 patients with manic depression (bipolar disorder) and schizophrenia. They discovered that acupuncture was highly effective in treating patients who did not respond to conventional drug treatment.

Most recently, acupuncture was found to reduce depression and anxiety in patients with mild Alzheimer's disease. This has important implications, since 70 percent of all Alzheimer's patients have anxiety, and more than half are depressed. Anxiety and depression can worsen the cognitive decline associated with the disease. Further, a Chinese study demonstrated that acupuncture improved verbal orientation and motor coordination in patients with the disease. Doctors who employ acupuncture to treat Alzheimer's patients believe that it increases sluggish blood flow and reduces inflammation—two factors thought to be a problem in Alzheimer's disease.

The take-home message here is that if you've tried other treatments for depression and mood swings, all to no avail, try acupuncture to lift your spirits.

12 HERBAL TRANQUILIZERS TO EASE YOUR MIND

A sign of our stress-filled times: From 1990 to 1998, the number of new users of prescription tranquilizers zoomed by a whopping 132 percent, according to a recent study published by the National Institute on Drug Abuse (NIDA).

Certainly, people who are seriously ill with clinical anxiety need medication. But a problem with prescription tranquilizers and other mood-stabilizing drugs is that they carry with them the risk of abuse, not to mention addiction and numerous untoward side effects.

To soothe jangled nerves and tame your tension, why not try herbal tranquilizers instead? Herbs and other natural therapies are a natural pathway to better psychological health. Their safe history of use over thousands of years is comforting when we read about the dangerous, often fatal side effects of some synthetic drugs.

Here's a rundown on twelve of the most frequently used calming herbs, along with their risks and benefits. If you take any of these, do so with the okay of your physician or psychiatrist. For a quick look at each of these herbs, see Table 6.1 on page 163.

CALIFORNIA POPPY

California poppy (*Eschscholzia californica*) is the state flower of California and a popular plant for gardeners. Except for its roots, the entire plant is used for medicinal purposes.

California poppy exerts a feeble narcotic effect and depresses the central nervous system. Plant chemicals called benzoisoquinolines are responsible for the herb's sedating effect. This plant is not to be confused with the poppy that yields opium, since it contains no narcotic derivatives.

California poppy is available as a tea or in tincture form and can be taken in combination with other calming herbs. To make tea, herbalists recommend using about 1 teaspoon per cup of hot water. If you're using a tincture, the standard dosage is 30 drops mixed in juice, taken once daily, or follow the manufacturer's directions for usage.

As yet, no safety profile has been fully established for California poppy. However, it appears to be safe when taken in recommended amounts for three to six weeks.

CATNIP

Catnip, or *Nepeta cataria* as it is known botanically, is a strong-scented herb that is a member of the mint family. The parts of the plant used medicinally are its leaves.

Catnip contains active chemical constituents (nepetalactone isomers) that act as sedatives, which are thought to be responsible for the herb's calming qualities.

Catnip is usually brewed as a minty tea, made with 1 to 2 teaspoons of the dried herb steeped in hot water. You can drink up to three cups of this tea a day. Catnip is also available as a tincture. The standard dosage is 1 teaspoon in a cup of water, taken up to three times a day. Herbalists say you should experience stress relief in about a week while taking catnip.

Catnip is considered by medical authorities to be generally safe when taken in appropriate amounts for short periods of time. Catnip may interfere with the absorption of iron and other minerals.

CHAMOMILE

Ranked as one of the top five herbs used worldwide, chamomile grows on meadows in North America, Europe, North Africa, and parts of Asia. There are several types of chamomile, but the most common is the German variety. Chamomile (*Matricaria recutita*) is a member of the daisy family. You find chamomile as tea, in standardized extracts, and as an ingredient in ointment, lotions, and perfumes.

More than 200 scientific studies have been conducted on chamomile in the last thirty years, supporting its therapeutic value. Many show that it has a mild sedative effect. Chamomile contains an active compound known as angelic acid, which gives the herb its sedative properties. It also contains a chemical called apigenin, which in animal studies demonstrates a clear antianxiety benefit.

For use as a sedative or tranquilizer, take up to 1 gram of the powdered herb daily. If using a tincture, take 40 to 60 drops, mixed in juice or water, four times a day. You can consume the tea liberally without any ill effects. Generally, you will feel the effects of chamomile within an hour.

Controversy has simmered over whether hay fever sufferers should take chamomile, since it comes from the same botanical family as ragweed. The FDA has told consumers to avoid chamomile if they're allergic to ragweed, while herbalists note that there have been only five documented cases of allergic reactions to the herb. Even so, you may want to approach chamomile cautiously if you are sensitive to ragweed.

HOPS

The ancient Romans grew hops for food, and Europeans began cultivating it more than 1,000 years ago to use for brewing beer. Today, hops (*Humulus lupulus*) is used extensively in the brewing industry to give beer its bitter aromatic flavor. A member of the mulberry family, hops has long been prized as a remedy for anxiety and insomnia. It is a distant relative of marijuana. Certain chemicals in the plant—lupulin and methylbutenol—are thought to give hops its sedating properties.

The standard dosage of hops is 0.5 gram, taken one to three times daily, or you may follow the manufacturer's recommended dosage instructions. Hops is considered safe when taken as directed for three to six weeks.

KAVA

Grown on the islands of the South Pacific, kava is a veritable dream supplement, remarkable for its ability to treat stress, anxiety, depression, insomnia, and more. Significantly, kava's benefits have been verified by extensive research.

Kava's therapeutic effects are due to at least fifteen different lipidlike compounds, collectively known by two interchangeable names, either "kavapyrones" or "kavalactones." Most of these compounds produce physical and mental relaxation but without causing addiction or harmful side effects when the herb is taken in moderate dosages. In 1990, kava was approved by the German Commission E, Germany's equivalent to our FDA, for treating anxiety, stress, and restlessness.

In a 1997 study, 101 patients suffering from anxiety were given kava over the course of a twenty-five-week double-blind study. By the eighth week, anxiety symptoms in those taking kava had subsided considerably compared to those given a placebo. The researchers noted that kava is an effective, well-tolerated alternative to drugs commonly used to treat anxiety and depression.

Kava works well in several forms: capsules, liquids, bulk, teas, standardized extracts, single-herb, and multi-herb. To relieve anxiety, the recommended dosage should generally not exceed 300 milligrams of kavalactones daily. This dosage is roughly the amount found in 3 grams of dried-root powder. You may want to start with a lower dosage at first, about 70 to 85 milligrams of kavalactones taken just before going to bed at night. Pay attention to how that dosage works, then increase it, if necessary.

Side effects from taking kava include stomach upset and allergic skin reactions. Both clear up after supplementation is discontinued. Long-term use may cause yellow discoloration of the skin, liver toxicity, allergic reactions, visual disturbances, inflammation of the eyes, and balance problems. That being so, the German Commission E recommends that kava be taken no longer than three months. If you want to stay on it for a longer period of time, you should be under medical supervision.

LEMON BALM

Grown more than 2,000 years ago in Mediterranean areas, this member of the mint family was a food for bees. Even today, beekeepers rub the leaves of this herb over beehives to encourage the insects' productivity. In fact, lemon balm's other name, Melissa, is translated from Latin as "honeybee." Lemon balm's botanical moniker is *Melissa officinalis*.

More by reputation than by scientific knowledge, lemon balm is considered a relaxant to calm anxiety, a sedative to promote sleep, and an antidepressant to combat the blues. Lemon balm contains a biologically active group of chemicals known as terpenes, which are responsible for its sedative action. Lemon balm is approved by the German Commission E as both a sedative and a remedy for nervous stomachs.

To soothe stress, herbalists recommend drinking up to three cups of lemon balm tea a day. The herb is also available as a tincture (30 to 40 drops daily, four times a day, mixed in liquid). You may feel relief within a week of regular usage. Lemon balm has no known side effects and is considered a safe and gentle herb.

LINDEN FLOWER

Linden flower (*Tilia europea*) has long had a reputation as a relaxant and mood elevator. Its flowers are used for medicinal purposes.

Very little is known about how this herb actually works. A few of its active ingredients have been isolated, and these include oils and sugarlike compounds. Animal experiments have found that linden flower reduced anxiety in mice and helped them successfully perform stressful tasks.

Linden flower is available as a tea, tincture, or dried herb. Herbalists recommend drinking three cups of the tea daily, supplementing with 20 to 40 drops of the tincture, three times a day, or taking 2 to 4 grams of the dried herb daily. The herb begins to work within a few days. Linden flower has no known side effects and is considered to be safe when taken in appropriate quantities for short periods of time.

MILKY OATS

Milky oats (*Avena sativa*) is the seed of the oat before it has ripened. It is soft and liquidlike; hence, the name "milky oats." The soft seeds are made into tinctures believed to help relieve stress and depression.

Milky oats can be used to ease withdrawal from nicotine and has a mild stress-relieving effect if taken on a regular basis. Its rich supply of B vitamins, along with a plant chemical called avenin, is probably responsible for the herb's calming action.

Tinctures (10 to 15 drops up to three times daily) are the recommended way to take milky oats because the potency changes when the
herb is dried.

Milky oats is considered a safe herb. However, high dosages (30 to
60 drops) can cause headaches.

MOTHERWORT

Motherwort is an ancient herb believed to settle a mother's womb to
aid in delivery—or so seventeenth-century herbalists claimed. Botanically, it is named *cardiaca*, a derivative of the Latin word for "heart."

Motherwort acts as a mild sedative, eases anxiety, and helps reduce
anxiety-related heart palpitations.

It is sold as a tea, in capsules of dried herb, and as a tincture. For best
results, herbalists recommend drinking two cups of the tea daily, taking
two capsules three times a day, taking 30 to 40 drops four times a day, or
supplementing with 4.5 grams a day of the dried herb. It takes about a
week to be effective, and you'll need to use it for at least a month to help
relieve anxiety.

Motherwort should not be taken during pregnancy. Additionally, the
herb may interfere with the normal thyroid function if more is taken
than the recommended dosage.

PASSIONFLOWER

Passionflower (*Passiflora incarnata*) is a perennial vine whose flowers
and fruit are made into herbal remedies for treating insomnia, anxiety,
and nervousness. In the 1500s, Roman Catholic priests dubbed the plant
"passionflower" because they believed that various parts of the plant sym-
bolized aspects of the suffering and death (Passion) of Jesus Christ.

The herb exerts a gentle sedative action and has been found in studies to relieve anxiety, counter insomnia, and reduce high blood pressure.
Laboratory studies support its use as a sedative, although the exact
chemical constituents responsible for its sedative action have not been
identified.

A compound called chrysin was recently isolated from one species of passionflower (*Passiflora coerulea*). Chrysin is not a sedative but has anti-anxiety properties. In fact, an experiment found that it was as powerful as Valium, but without the sedating side effects.

Passionflower is available as a dried herb in capsules. It is quite effective when used with other calming herbs, including kava. In fact, it is often a secondary ingredient in many kava products. The German Commission E has officially approved passionflower for nervous anxiety and recommends a dosage of 6 grams daily. With preparations containing passionflower, follow the manufacturer's directions for dosage. Many herbalists believe passionflower is safe when taken as recommended.

ST. JOHN'S WORT

Although it has been around for ages—the Greeks and Romans used it to treat infections and inflammation—St. John's wort has been a much-publicized topic in the media. In 1997, German and American researchers evaluated twenty-three studies of St. John's wort and concluded that it worked as well as prescription antidepressants for treating mild to moderate depression, a mental disorder that affects one out of every four Americans. Best of all, the herbal treatment produced fewer side effects.

St. John's wort is believed to increase serotonin levels in the brain, although no one knows exactly how. The active compound in St. John's wort is hypericin, a chemical that was first isolated from the herb in 1942 and provides a significant antidepressant effect.

Supplementing with St. John's wort relieves mild depression, elevates mood, calms anxiety, provides an increased sense of well-being, and enhances sleep.

The usual dosage is 300 milligrams of a capsulated product standardized to 3-percent hypericin, taken three times a day. It takes two to four weeks for the herb to show any effect. Unlike many prescription antidepressants, there are no withdrawal symptoms from discontinuing the use of St. John's wort nor is the herb addictive.

A side effect that has been noted with St. John's wort is weight gain.

The herb can also make your skin more sensitive to light. That means you'll be more likely to get a sunburn if you're outside. If you're fair-skinned and supplementing with St. John's wort, avoid sunlight.

The herb should not be taken in conjunction with other drugs that affect serotonin levels, such as fluoxetine (Prozac) and monoamine oxidase inhibitors (MAOIs), or with dietary supplements that influence serotonin levels such as SAM-e. Recently, doctors in the Netherlands discovered that St. John's wort interferes with the effectiveness of a common cancer drug, Camptosar. Always consult with your physician prior to taking St. John's wort.

VALERIAN

Used by Hippocrates as early as the fourth century, valerian (*Valeriana officinalis*) is a perennial herb that often grows more than 5 feet high with an attractive spray of pink or white flowers. In some areas of New England, valerian is a roadside weed. The parts of the plant used for medicinal purposes are the roots and rhizome.

Over the past thirty years, more than 200 scientific studies on valerian's constituents have been published in medical literature, particularly in Europe. As noted earlier, one study found that a combination product of hops and valerian was an effective stress reducer and sleep inducer. Overall, valerian has a gentle, tranquilizing effect.

Approximately 120 chemicals have been identified in valerian. Numerous animal studies have shown that extracts of these chemicals depress the central nervous system and thus may be antidepressants. Even so, scientists are not sure which chemicals are biologically active. As with most herbs, however, it is probably the synergistic action of many chemical components that produces valerian's sedative effect.

Herbalists suggest the following usage: capsules or tablets, 50 to 100 milligrams, taken two to three times a day to relieve stress; 300 to 900 milligrams taken one hour prior to bedtime to treat insomnia; tincture, 20 to 30 drops, mixed in liquid four times a day. (As a general rule of thumb, it's advisable to follow the manufacturer's recommended dosage.) Valerian is also available as a tea, but it has an earthy, pungent, and rather unpleasant taste.

Medical authorities consider valerian to be safe when taken in recommended quantities for no more than two to three weeks at a time. The herb is certainly a superior first-choice course of action before restoring to prescription sedatives and tranquilizers.

Very high dosages (over recommended amounts), however, can cause headaches, excitability, heart rhythm disturbances, muscular spasms, and, paradoxically, insomnia. There is some preliminary evidence that long-term overusage of valerian may cause liver damage.

TABLE 6.1
Herbal Tranquilizers at a Glance

HERB	DOSAGE	SAFETY CONSIDERATIONS*
California Poppy	*Tea:* 1 teaspoon of the whole dried herb steeped in hot water, 3 times daily; *tincture:* 30 drops mixed in juice, once daily	Safe when taken in recommended dosages for short periods of time.
Catnip	*Tea:* 1 to 2 teaspoons of the dried herb steeped in hot water, up to 3 times daily; *tincture:* 1 teaspoon in 1 cup of water, up to 3 times daily	Safe when taken in recommended dosages for short periods of time but may interfere with the absorption of iron and other minerals.
Chamomile	*Supplement:* up to 1 gram daily; *tincture:* 40 to 60 drops, mixed in juice or water, 4 times daily; *tea:* 1 tea bag steeped in hot water, taken as needed	Considered safe; individuals who are allergic to ragweed should avoid using chamomile. *(Continued)*

HERB	DOSAGE	SAFETY CONSIDERATIONS*
Hops	*Supplement:* 0.5 gram, 1 to 3 times daily	Safe when taken in recommended dosages for short periods of time.
Kava	*Supplement:* 300 mg of kavalactones daily; *dried whole herb:* 3 grams daily	Stomach upset; allergic skin reactions; possible liver toxicity in some people; stay on kava for no longer than 3 months at a time.
Lemon Balm	*Tea:* up to 3 cups daily; *tincture:* 30 to 40 drops, mixed in liquid, 4 times daily	No known side effects.
Linden Flower	*Tea:* up to 3 cups daily; *tincture:* 20 to 40 drops, mixed in liquid, 3 times daily; *whole dried herb:* 2 to 4 grams daily	Safe when taken in recommended dosages for short periods of time.
Milky Oats	*Tincture:* 10 to 15 drops daily, mixed in liquid, up to 3 times daily	Safe in recommended dosages; high doses (30 to 60 drops) daily can cause headaches.
Motherwort	*Whole dried herb:* 4.5 grams daily; *tea:* 2 cups daily; *tincture:* 30 to 40 drops, mixed in liquid, 4 times daily	Safe when taken as recommended.
Passionflower	*Supplement:* 6 grams daily	Safe when taken as recommended.

Herb	Dosage	Safety Considerations*
St. John's wort	*Supplement:* 300 mg, 3 times daily	Side effects include weight gain and greater skin sensitivity to sunlight; do not take with other drugs or herbs that affect serotonin levels; avoid if undergoing chemotherapy.
Valerian	*Supplement:* 50 to 100 mg, 2 to 3 times daily to relieve stress; 300 to 900 mg, one hour before bedtime for insomnia; *tincture:* 20 to 30 drops, mixed in liquid, 4 times daily	Safe when taken in recommended dosages for no more than two to three weeks at a time; overdoses can cause headaches, excitability, heart rhythm disturbances, muscular spasms, and insomnia.

*When taking herbs, follow the manufacturer's instructions for dosage since concentrations of the herb may vary from product to product. Do not take herbs if you are pregnant or lactating.

The Older Prescription Mood Drugs

At times, we all feel sad or bleak, but usually the feeling passes. But should your sadness become a permanent state or begin to interfere with your day-to-day activities, you may need to seek medical treatment. In such cases, your depression probably stems not from a moral failing or character flaw but from a chemical imbalance of neurotransmitters in your brain. When you are depressed, there may be a short supply of those neurotransmitters, which in turn blocks the transmission of messages between brain cells. Consequently, you feel down, sluggish, apathetic, and often hopeless.

Fortunately, you don't have to suffer in silence. Your mood disorder can be treated biologically with prescription mood drugs. Such drugs have been available for a long time, but the earlier versions had lots of side effects and are used less often today. For background, the older prescription mood drugs include the following:

- *Tricyclic antidepressants (TCAs) such as Elavil, Tofranil, and Pamelor*. These slow the rate at which certain neurotransmitters—namely serotonin, norepinephrine, and dopamine—reenter the brain. This action increases the concentration of the neurotransmitters throughout the rest of the central nervous system, alleviating feelings of depression.

  The downside of TCAs includes constipation, dizziness, and fatigue. In overdoses, some TCAs can be fatal.

- *Monoamine oxidase inhibitors (MAOIs) such as Marplan, Nardil, and Parnate*. These work by blocking the action of an enzyme called monoamine oxidase, which destroys serotonin and norepinephrine in the brain, and thus helps restore normal mood states.

  Side effects include constipation, dizziness, drowsiness, dry mouth, fatigue, digestive disorders, headache, low blood pressure, and insomnia. **Note:** *In combination with any from a long list of other drugs or even certain foods, side effects can become grave and may lead to death.*

- *Lithium*. This medication is used to treat manic (bipolar) depression and works by correcting certain imbalances in the neurotransmitters serotonin and norepinephrine. It exerts a mild antidepressive effect but is more effective for its strong antimanic effects.

  Problems associated with taking lithium include general discomfort, frequent urination, hand tremor, thirst, nausea, abdominal pain, and blackout spells. Overdosing can lead to grave side effects or death.

THE 5 NEWER AND LEAST RISKY PRESCRIPTION MOOD DRUGS

Among the newer and least risky prescription mood drugs are *selective serotonin reuptake inhibitors* (SSRIs) such as Prozac, Paxil, Celexa, and Zoloft. SSRIs act only on serotonin, a mood-regulating neurotransmitter. Serotonin levels are linked to feelings of calm and well-being. What SSRIs do is lengthen the amount of time that concentrations of serotonin stay active in the brain, elevating your mood and making you feel better. SSRIs work as well as other antidepressants. Furthermore, drug studies have shown that they are better tolerated and have fewer side effects than many of the others.

Nonetheless, *all* prescription drugs can have some side effects. Here's a rundown of the five least risky mood drugs your doctor can prescribe if you've been diagnosed with depression or another mood disorder. All but one (Wellbutrin) is an SSRI.

CELEXA

Prescribed to treat major depression, Celexa (citalopram hydrobromide) is an SSRI that boosts serotonin levels in the brain. It is normally taken once a day, in the morning or evening, with or without food. With Celexa, your depression may begin to lift in one to four weeks. Unlike some antidepressants, Celexa does not seem to impair judgment or motor skills.

According to *The PDR Family Guide to Prescription Drugs*, some of the common side effects may include abdominal pain, agitation, anxiety, diarrhea, dry mouth, ejaculation disorders, fatigue, impotence, indigestion, loss of appetite, and nausea.

PAXIL

Paxil (paroxetine hydrochloride) is prescribed primarily for serious depression but also for obsessive-compulsive disorder, panic disorder, and social phobia. For depression, the usual starting dosage is 20 milligrams, taken once a day. Your physician may increase your dosage gradually, up to a maximum of 50 milligrams daily. Paxil begins working in one to four weeks to ease depression.

According to *The PDR Family Guide to Prescription Drugs*, some of the common side effects may include constipation, decreased appetite, diarrhea, gas, dizziness, dry mouth, and nausea.

PROZAC

The most famous of the SSRIs is Prozac (fluoxetine), also among the top-selling drugs of all time. In addition to depression, it is also prescribed for obsessive-compulsive disorder and bulimia. Under the brand name Sarafem, it is used to treat premenstrual dysphoric disorder (PMDD), a premenstrual condition characterized by debilitating depression and anxiety.

Prozac is usually taken once or twice a day, as prescribed by your doctor. The usual starting dosage is 20 milligrams a day; however, your physician may increase the dosage after several weeks if no improvement occurs. Generally, the drug begins working in about four weeks. There is a newer version of Prozac that is taken just once a week.

According to *The PDR Family Guide to Prescription Drugs*, the most common side effects of Prozac include abnormal dreams, abnormal ejaculation, agitation, amnesia, nausea, weakness, dizziness, insomnia, sweating, tremors, suppressed appetite, and nervousness.

WELLBUTRIN

Wellbutrin (bupropion hydrochloride) is a relatively new antidepressant designed to treat depression and attention deficit disorder. Under the trade name Zyban, it is prescribed to help people quit smoking. Wellbutrin is neither an SSRI nor a TCA, but in a different chemical class. It works by increasing levels of the neurotransmitters dopamine and norepinephrine in the brain, thus relieving the symptoms of depression.

The normal dosage is three equal doses spaced six hours between doses, for a total of 300 milligrams a day. Your doctor may start you at a low dosage, and gradually increase it. Usually, you'll start feeling better in one to four weeks after taking Wellbutrin.

According to *The PDR Family Guide to Prescription Drugs*, common side effects include abdominal pain, agitation, anxiety, constipation, dizziness, dry mouth, sweating, headache, loss of appetite, and weight loss.

ZOLOFT

Zoloft (sertraline) is prescribed mainly for depression. It is also prescribed for panic disorder and posttraumatic stress disorder. An advantage of Zoloft is that it appears to have the least effects on cognitive function.

Available in capsules or oral concentrate (to be mixed with liquid), Zoloft is usually taken once a day (50 milligrams), either in the morning or evening. You will begin to feel better in several days to a few weeks. Your doctor may increase your dosage, depending on how you respond to the drug.

According to *The PDR Family Guide to Prescription Drugs*, some common side effects include agitation, anxiety, constipation, decreased sex drive, diarrhea, ejaculation problems, dizziness, dry mouth, fatigue, gas, headache, decreased appetite, sweating, nausea, and indigestion.

INSTANT CALM: LEARN HOW IN 30 SECONDS

It could be snarled traffic, a looming deadline, a computer glitch, or an argument with your boss. Whatever the provocation that's stressing you out, you must disable it before it disables you.

Fortunately, there's a super-fast way to regain your calm and become immediately refreshed, something so simple and easy to learn that you can do it right where you are.

Want to give it a try?

Good. Follow these steps:

1. Sit comfortably, with your feet flat on the floor and your shoulders relaxed. Close your eyes.
2. Breathe in deeply through your nose to a count of five. This action activates nerve receptors in the lower lungs that calm your body.
3. Pause for five counts. Then breathe out through your mouth to a count of five. As you exhale, feel your body releasing all inner tensions. Repeat this breathing sequence once more, or until you feel less anxious. Breathing in this manner not only de-stresses you but also helps oxygenate your blood, refreshing and reenergizing your body.
4. While breathing in and out, keep the muscles of your body relaxed. Pay attention to your breathing. If you concentrate on your breathing, you can't think about the troublesome circumstances around you.
5. After you've finished, open your eyes and sit quietly for a while.

If you practice this breathing exercise every day, you can cut your tension level in half, according to research. Other studies show that regular practice of controlled breathing lowers blood pressure (which is elevated by stress) and reduces the risk of cardiovascular disease.

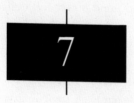

Jump-Start Your Memory

There will be times when you need to learn and recall things fast—such as remembering the right answers for an exam or memorizing someone's phone number. Remembering information is easier if you use certain tricks, hints, or cues. You can also help your recall by the way you initially learn information. What follows is a look at tips for jump-starting your memory.

OXYGEN AND YOUR BRAIN: 4 WAYS TO TAKE A BREATHER AND ENHANCE YOUR MEMORY

One of the quickest ways to jolt your memory is to get a good whiff of oxygen. That's because your brain thrives on oxygen, a gas necessary for life. You take in oxygen from the atmosphere through your mouth, nose, and breathing passages into your lungs. The job of the lungs is to supply oxygen to the body—including your brain—and remove from it carbon dioxide, a byproduct of oxygen consumption.

If your memory and mind power feel dulled, you probably need a good dose of fresh air. Here's what to do.

GO OUTSIDE AND TAKE A BRISK STROLL

Walking, particularly outdoors, steps up oxygen supply to your brain. University of California researchers observed that regular walking reduced mental declines by 13 percent. Also, with physical and mental exercise, the rate of brain cell production may double, according to an animal study conducted at Princeton University.

MAINTAIN A REGULAR AEROBIC EXERCISE PROGRAM

While it's beneficial mentally to take short walking breaks, it's an even better move to engage in a regular aerobic exercise program at least three to five times a week for thirty to forty-five minutes each time. This strengthens your lungs and improves your body's use of oxygen intake from the atmosphere.

TRY AN OXYGEN BAR

One place to get a hit of memory-boosting oxygen is at an oxygen bar, an establishment where you can sit back, fill your lungs with pure oxygen inhaled through a tube, and get a revitalizing buzz. You can have your oxygen straight or scented with herbs and other flavors. The experience costs about a dollar a minute, and most patrons purchase enough for a twenty-minute whiff of the gas. Devotees of recreational oxygen claim that it can:

- boost alertness.
- enhance memory.
- fight fatigue.
- ease headaches.

- cure hangovers.
- relieve stress.

There may be some truth to these claims. A few studies have demonstrated that supplemental oxygen administered to older adults with memory deficits can boost memory and recall. In one study, German researchers observed an increase in short-term memory capacity by 19 to 23 percent after oxygen therapy.

TAKE OXYGEN-BOOSTING SUPPLEMENTS

Another way to keep your brain oxygenated is to consider supplementing with ginseng and ginkgo biloba, two herbs that increase the level of oxygen to the brain.

MUSIC: AN OVERLOOKED WAY TO BOOST YOUR RECALL FAST

If you've ever tuned in to the oldies, you know that music has the power to conjure up memories of the past. After all, music has a deep personal and intimate meaning for most people.

Clinicians have harnessed this power to help patients with dementia strengthen their failing memories. At Royal Holloway University in London, investigators played background music while interviewing older adults with mild-to-moderate dementia. Patients' recall of past events was much better when music was played, compared to no background sound.

In a recent issue of the medical journal *Lancet*, Elizabeth Valentine, one of the lead investigators, was quoted as saying: "Music should be played when physicians are interviewing or attempting to get information from patients with dementia and should also be tried in combination with other treatments for dementia management."

That said, start listening to more of your favorite music, pursue music-accompanied physical activities such as aerobic dance, or get involved in group singing or music lessons.

MEMORIZATION MADE EASY:
6 REMARKABLE MNEMONIC TECHNIQUES

Derived from the name of the Greek goddess of memory (Mnemosyne), mnemonics is a technique of enhancing quick recall through the use of memory and learning aids. It is very effective for retaining lengthy and difficult information. There are a variety of mnemonic techniques. Here are six of the most popular.

ACRONYMS

A tried-and-true memory device, acronyms are created by using each first letter from a group of words to form a new word. You commonly find acronyms in many fields. Some examples are MADD (Mothers Against Drunk Driving), NBA (National Basketball Association), ALCOA (Aluminum Company of America), and SCUBA (Self-Contained Underwater Breathing Apparatus).

Acronyms are useful when you need to remember words in a particular order. Let's suppose you need to remember the major anatomical parts of the eye for a class: (1) pupil, (2) cornea, (3) iris, (4) retina, and (5) optic nerve. Take the first letter of each part you're trying to remember: PCIRO. Next, rearrange them so that they sound like a word: PRICO. The acronym will trigger your recall.

Acronyms are also useful for everyday memory tasks. If you have to pick up some items at the grocery store, for example, turn the list into an acronym like CAMP (cereal, apples, milk, and potatoes).

ASSOCIATIONS

This technique links words and ideas in order to help learn information. For best results, the association should be unusual or ridiculous. Let's suppose you need to memorize state capitals. The capital of Virginia is Richmond. If you want to remember that, you might associate Richmond with "rich man" and Virginia with "virgin." Then you could create the sentence "A rich man marries a virgin" to help trigger recall of Richmond as the capital of Virginia.

Similarly, when remembering a locker or safe combination, try to link the numbers to dates that are meaningful to you, such as a birthday or anniversary.

CHUNKING

Chunking is used mostly to remember numbers. Basically, it involves breaking a long string of numbers, such as a telephone number or Social Security number, into smaller, easier-to-remember "chunks." To remember the telephone number 555-0040, for example, you'd break it up into 555 (triple fives), 00 (double zeros), and 40 to help learn the number. When you chunk information in this manner, it takes up less space in your memory, making it easier to recall.

METHOD OF LOCI

Developed by Roman orators to memorize long speeches, the method of loci involves selecting rooms in a building (such as your house) or identifying landmarks along a path and using each room or landmark to remember your material. Basically, you mentally associate each piece of information you need to remember with one of these rooms or landmarks. For example, you might choose the bed in your bedroom, the closet in your hallway, and the bathtub in your bathroom as loci. Any time you want to remember one or a list of things, form a visual picture of the thing you want to remember, then mentally place it on or in one of the loci.

RHYME

This technique employs a rhyming verse to aid memorization. One of the most familiar is "30 days has September, April, June, and November" to remember the number of days in the months of the year.

SENTENCES

Using this method, you create sentences in which the first letter of each word is the one you want to remember. Some familiar examples include *Every Good Boy Does Fine*—for E, G, B, D, F—the notes on the lines of the treble clef in music; or *My Very Educated Mother Just Served Us Nine Pickles* for remembering the planets in order of distance from the sun.

Part Three

PREVENTING PROBLEMS

Your brain can get out of order like any other part of your body. Sometimes, this can make you lose your ability to think normally, feel good, or remember clearly.

You'll be surprised and delighted to know, however, that a lot of what goes wrong with the brain, though distressing, is eminently preventable or highly treatable—mostly by adopting healthier lifestyle habits. So if you want to help your brain, start by getting to know the brain depleters, the mood depressors, and the memory losers—and what to do about them.

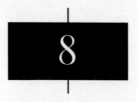

Stop the Brain Depleters

Three of the main contributors to "brain drain"—technically known as permanent or temporary loss of faculties—are alcohol abuse, poor nutrition, and mental laziness. Are there ways to stop these brain depleters?

Absolutely. By bringing a few things in your life under control, brain drain in most cases can be reversed, even prevented.

ALCOHOL'S SURPRISING SHORT-TERM EFFECTS ON THE BRAIN

After enjoying a few drinks you're relaxed, perhaps a bit euphoric and less inhibited. As the familiar saying goes: You're feeling no pain.

But your brain may feel otherwise. That's because alcohol is essentially a toxin, and your body treats it as such. In fact, were alcohol discovered today, it might be banned because of its potentially lethal impact! Even in moderate, one- to two-drink doses, alcohol has some surprising short-term effects on the brain.

ALCOHOL IMPAIRS NORMAL THOUGHT PROCESSES AND BODILY CONTROL

Alcohol requires no digestion and rushes to your brain within a minute. Its first stop is your frontal lobe, the reasoning part of your brain. As alcohol molecules diffuse into the cells of this lobe, they interfere with your judgment. With a few more cocktails, the speech and vision centers of your brain become dulled. Still more booze works on the cells of the brain responsible for large-muscle control. That's when you start staggering or weaving. Poor judgment, dulled senses, disturbed motor skills, and reduced coordination all occur because alcohol prevents blood from carrying oxygen to brain cells. When oxygen is in short supply, brain cells are impaired or can die.

With continued drinking, you can pass out. Passing out—believe it or not—may save your life. It stops you from consuming a higher dose, which can anesthetize the deepest brain centers that control breathing and heartbeat, leading to death.

ALCOHOL ACTS AS A DEPRESSANT

The description of alcohol as a "depressant" technically means that it slows down the activity of your central nervous system, of which your brain is a part. The reason is that alcohol replaces the water normally found around nerve cells. The movement of electrically charged atoms, which send messages along nerve fibers, is thus impaired. As a result, messages dawdle as they travel along nerve fibers. We're slower to react, and our speech becomes slurred.

ALCOHOL SHRINKS THE BRAIN

Brain cells are very sensitive to alcohol and can actually self-destruct when you're "under the influence." The destruction of cells causes the brain to shrivel—even if you are a moderate drinker (one to two drinks a day). The trouble is, the more alcohol you consume, the more your brain shrinks. Brain shrinkage impairs your memory and interferes with your ability to learn. Alcoholics pay the heaviest price: In someone with an alcohol addiction, the brain shrinks by as much as 30 percent. This shrinkage can be permanent unless the alcoholic abstains from drinking altogether.

ALCOHOL BLOCKS PRODUCTION OF THE BRAIN'S ANTIDIURETIC HORMONE

It's no secret that drinking alcoholic beverages means frequent trips to the restroom. That's because alcohol steps up your body's urine output by depressing your brain's production of antidiuretic hormone. Your body loses precious water as a result, and you're at risk of becoming dehydrated—unless you alternate alcoholic beverages with water or non-alcoholic choices to keep your body watered. Incidentally, alcohol-related dehydration drains water from your brain cells. When these cells re-acquire water the morning after, they swell, causing nerve pain, which is one of several factors that produces a hangover.

ALCOHOL INTERFERES WITH NORMAL SLEEP PATTERNS

A drink or two is sedating and can make you feel sleepy. However, after you hit the pillow, the alcohol in your system prevents you from entering a deep, restorative stage of sleep known as rapid eye movement (REM) sleep. During REM sleep, your eyes dart around rapidly as you dream. The big deal about REM sleep is that it helps your body recover from mental stress. But when you're under the influence of alcohol,

REM sleep is disturbed. Deprived of REM sleep, you're likely to lose mental focus and alertness.

ALCOHOL ALTERS THE ACTION OF
KEY BRAIN CHEMICALS

Another big problem with alcohol is the way it alters the action of glutamate, which is among the chemicals that transmit messages in the brain. Glutamate is involved in memory and learning. Scientists have discovered that even very tiny amounts of alcohol block the action of glutamate—an interference that can affect memory and quite possibly be responsible for a short-lived condition known as the "alcoholic blackout."

Another brain chemical affected by alcohol is GABA, technically known as gamma-aminobutyric acid. GABA is the brain's natural tranquilizer. A few alcoholic beverages can enhance GABA's tranquilizing effects, thus mildly sedating your brain.

Alcohol also overstimulates the release of serotonin, a feel-good brain chemical. Although this stimulation contributes to the temporary "high" you feel when intoxicated, a flood of serotonin also produces mental grogginess.

ALCOHOL WORSENS PHYSICAL AND MENTAL
PERFORMANCE EVEN WHEN IT'S GONE

Don't swallow the myth that hangovers are harmless. If you have one the day after a bender, even after alcohol has exited your bloodstream, you'll experience poor judgment, impaired vision, poor skill at judging distances, and loss of manual dexterity, according to an analysis of nearly fifty scientific studies on the effects of alcohol on performance.

DANGER ZONE: THESE 6 NUTRITIONAL SUPPLEMENTS COULD BE HAZARDOUS TO YOUR BRAIN

Americans pop supplements by the handful. In fact, a survey by the Centers for Disease Control and Prevention shows that more than 60 percent of the general population takes supplements daily.

Although supplements are great nutritional insurance in pill form, there are some you should *never* take, namely, supplements made from bovine (cow) parts. That's because they may put you in harm's way of getting mad cow disease, a brain-wasting illness.

That's the expert opinion of a Food and Drug Administration (FDA) advisory panel, which expressed concern in January 2001 that some dietary supplements are made with brain or spinal-cord tissue, or other glandular tissue, that may come from cattle, including European cattle.

Mad cow disease, or bovine spongiform encephalopathy (BSE), infects cattle and eats away at their brain tissue. The human form of mad cow disease, Creutzfeldt-Jakob disease, has caused the deaths of more than fifty people in Great Britain. Scientific research strongly suggests that humans get the disease by eating infected cow parts. Eating tissue from a cow's brain and spinal cord pose the greatest danger; pituitary and adrenal glands, the spleen, and lymph nodes are medium risk, says the FDA.

Even though there has been no evidence of mad cow disease in the United States, the panel urges consumers to avoid supplements made with bovine parts. What's more, in July 2000, a Maryland doctor wrote a letter to the *New England Journal of Medicine,* stating that he had found one dietary supplement containing ingredients from seventeen bovine organs.

Although it's important to read the labels of supplements before you buy them, these labels don't state the country of origin of the cow parts used in the formulation. So until there is tighter regulation of nutritional supplements containing cow tissues, it's best to avoid them altogether. See Table 8.1 for a rundown of six potentially risky supplements.

	TABLE 8.1		
	Potentially Risky Supplements		
SUPPLEMENT	USES	BOVINE PART(S) USED	COMMENTS
Bone Meal	A calcium supplement used to prevent and treat osteoporosis	Bovine bone and bone marrow	Bovine bone and marrow are considered low-risk parts; nonetheless, some supplements are made from the bone and marrow of livestock raised in Europe.
Chondroitin sulfate	Treatment of arthritis	Cartilage obtained from beef trachea	The risk of contracting mad cow disease from beef trachea is low because the proteins thought to cause the disease are mainly found in bovine brain and nervous tissue, and are not prevalent in cartilage.
Colostrum	Immune protection; muscle growth	A pre-milk fluid harvested from a cow within twelve hours of giving birth to a calf	Colostrum is low risk because it does not contain high-risk bovine parts. Colostrum gathered from organically grown cattle or certified by the manufacturer to be free of mad cow disease is the safest choice.

Supplement	Uses	Bovine Part(s) Used	Comments
Creatine monohydrate	Muscle growth and energy enhancement in bodybuilders, athletes, and exercisers	Sarcosine, a protein found in nature (including various bovine tissues), and used to manufacture creatine monohydrate	If the sarcosine used to make creatine originates from bovine tissues, there is risk of contamination. For this reason, authorities in France have banned the sale of products containing creatine.
Glandulars	Promotion of glandular health; treatment of stress-related diseases	Bovine brain, adrenal and pituitary glands, thymus gland, spleen, liver, and other bovine organs	These supplements are high risk due to their high content of bovine parts, particularly brain and glandular tissue.
Vitamin B$_{12}$	Prevention and treatment of vitamin B$_{12}$ deficiencies	Bovine liver	This supplement carries a modest risk because it is made from a bovine organ.

WHY SOME WEIGHT-LOSS DIETS
MAKE YOU DUMB

When you go on a diet to lose weight, you may shed more than just pounds. You may shed some of your "smarts," particularly if you are on a crash diet. Research reveals that dieters:

- become easily distracted from tasks at hand.
- lose alertness.
- process information more slowly.
- have slower reaction times.
- score lower on memory tests.
- have trouble recalling simple lists.

In addition to those problems, there are other serious psychological repercussions to cutting back on your eating, specifically on behavior. In a famous World War II study, normal-weight men were asked to restrict their food intake for six months to lose 25 percent of their body weight so that researchers could study the effects of semi-starvation on the body. Their goal was to use the findings to learn how to treat the starving survivors of concentration camps in Europe.

In six months, the men lost an average of 50 pounds. The psychological reactions that emerged were startling. The men became increasingly obsessed with food. They collected recipes, pinned up pictures of food on their walls, even pursued food-related careers such as becoming a chef. Emotionally, the men turned irritable, upset, and combative. One subject was quoted as saying: "We lost our semblance of humanity and became similar to beasts."

What's more, the subjects turned apathetic and lost interest in sex. There's more: Once the men were allowed to resume normal eating, they tended to binge on food. In other words, food restriction turned normal eaters into binge eaters.

Other scientists have studied the psychological effects of food deprivation, too, and the findings are strikingly similar. Food-deprived people—restrictive dieters included—tend to experience mental processing problems, decreased intelligence, and behavioral disorders such as anxiety, low self-esteem, and irritability.

Why these cognitive and psychological side effects occur remains a mystery. But there are some theories. One theory holds that dieting disrupts the synthesis of neurotransmitters, thus altering brain chemistry. Also, dieting depletes bodily stores of iron, a key nutrient for optimal mental functioning. A USDA study, for example, demonstrated that iron deficiency in dieting women shortened their attention spans.

Thus, in ways that haven't been fully spelled out, mental performance and behavior are related to your nutritional status. If you must lose weight, it's best to take the prudent approach—a safe, gradual loss of no more than 2 pounds a week, without severe caloric deprivation. That way, you'll lose mostly fat—plus stay smart in the process.

PURSUE LIFELONG LEARNING: 15 ACTIONS TO KEEP YOUR MIND SMART AND SUPPLE

The scientific evidence is cascading in: Use your brain or lose it. Stimulating the brain with ongoing intellectual activity keeps your brain cells healthy, according to research. And one of the best ways to stimulate your brain is by becoming a lifelong learner.

If you're a lifelong learner, your brain is getting sharper and stronger. Researchers believe that when you try to learn new things, you promote the growth of new dendrites, the branches of brain cells that help transmit messages. A higher number of dendrites helps maintain short-term and long-term memory as well as overall brain fitness. What's more, many researchers theorize that keeping the brain active may help prevent or postpone Alzheimer's disease later in life.

With that in mind, here are fifteen ways you can keep your brain cells active and alive, plus get smarter in the process.

1. Read textbooks, habitually. Challenging yourself to learn more about history, science, literature, economics, politics, or any other challenging subject on a regular basis not only leaves you with more facts but it also increases your ability to learn.

2. Enroll in a continuing education class in crafts, photography, conversational German, nutrition, computers, Shakespeare,

English as a second language, a personal development course, or whatever strikes your fancy.

3. Return to college to obtain your degree. If you already have a degree, earn another one.

4. Attend a home-improvement workshop.

5. Enroll in a cooking class.

6. Sign up for a work-related conference or training seminar to help you get ahead in your career.

7. If your profession offers them, accumulate Continuing Education Units (CEUs), which provide opportunities to study and expand your knowledge in your field.

8. Take courses in your field to earn professional certifications and advance your current job.

9. Join a Bible study class, Sunday school class, or religious studies group.

10. Become a member of a book group.

11. Take a distance education or correspondence course. Check out the following Web sites to locate colleges, universities, and training companies that offer either full degrees, individual courses, or certificates: www.eCollege.com, www.edupoint.com, and www.petersons.com/dlearn.

12. Teach yourself a new computer program once every couple of months.

13. Audit college classes on a regular basis.

14. Take an educational vacation such as those provided through Elderhostel, a learning program for adults aged thirty-five and older. It has programs on more than 2,300 campuses in the United States and abroad.

15. Teach others. There's an old saying that goes like this: "When you teach, you learn twice." Apply or volunteer for a job to teach a subject on which you're an expert.

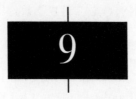

Stop the Mood Depressors

You'd be surprised at the list of conditions that can cause a depressed mood: chemical imbalances in the brain, heredity, stress, a traumatic life event, diseases, nutritional deficiencies, lack of exercise, low blood sugar, the time of year, relationship problems, financial difficulties, and grief, to name just a few.

Fortunately, though, these depressors can be controlled, even stopped. For example, certain medications and herbs act as antidepressants, treating chemical imbalances in your brain and restoring them to normal. In addition, depression can be stopped by pursuing stress-reducing behaviors or by talking through your problems and changing the way you think. In the sections below, you'll learn how to recognize depression and stop the mood depressors before they take their toll on your physical and mental health.

The 5 Major Types of Depression: Know the Signs

Sadness. Hopelessness. A sense that life's not worth living. These are just a few signs of "depression," a mental illness that affects one of every four Americans and is on the rise in the United States. Depression is a very common mental disorder—in fact, it has been dubbed "the common cold" of psychiatric problems—but it is the most treatable, provided the sufferer seeks treatment. Depression is also preventable.

Preventing depression is vital not only to preserve mental health but also to ward off some serious physical problems. For example, depression is a risk factor for heart disease. It speeds up the loss of bone mass that leads to the crippling disease of osteoporosis. Depression compromises immunity, making you more vulnerable to disease. Depression also shrinks parts of the brain, causing cognitive decline. And, tragically, 15 percent of all depressed people kill themselves.

So far, there are no hormonal or blood tests to diagnose depression; laboratory tests are used only to rule out potential medical causes. A diagnosis is made by a doctor or psychiatrist based on the symptoms you report. Thus, it is important to recognize the signs of depression in order to initiate treatment as soon as possible. There are various types of depression, each discussed below, and many share some of the same symptoms.

MAJOR DEPRESSIVE DISORDER

Affecting approximately 15 million Americans at one point during their lives, this form of depression goes beyond merely having the blues. Patients are emotionally incapacitated, unable to find pleasure in anything, hold down a job, or interact with other people.

If at least five of the following symptoms are present for at least two weeks, you may be suffering from major depressive disorder:

- depressed moods on most days.
- loss of interest in pleasurable activities such as sex.

- significant increase or decrease in appetite.
- sleep problems, either insomnia or excessive sleepiness.
- change in physical demeanor, either agitation or a dragged-out feeling.
- loss of energy.
- feelings of inappropriate guilt and worthlessness.
- inability to concentrate.
- suicidal thoughts or behavior.
- no apparent trigger or precipitating event (such as alcohol, drugs, or grief).

Although extremely serious because of its association with suicide, major depressive disorder tends to run its course, even without treatment, and usually subsides in six months. It can recur, however. Treatment generally involves psychotherapy and antidepressants.

CHRONIC DEPRESSION (DYSTHYMIA)

This type of depression is a milder form of the illness but one that lasts much longer—at least two years. Sufferers generally feel sad most of the time; however, the disorder doesn't interfere with their normal, everyday tasks. Nearly 10 million Americans may suffer from chronic depression each year.

Chronic depression has many of the same symptoms as major depressive disorder with the exception of agitation, a dragged-out feeling, suicidal thoughts or behavior, and loss of interest in pleasurable activities.

Treatment includes antidepressants and therapies such as individual psychotherapy, group therapy, or family therapy.

BIPOLAR DISORDER (MANIC DEPRESSIVE ILLNESS)

Afflicting about 1 percent of the population, this form of depression is characterized by extreme and unpredictable mood swings. Periods of depression alternate with feelings of excitability and hyperactivity (mania). Other symptoms include:

- inappropriate elation.
- insomnia.
- increased, hard-to-understand speech.
- disconnected thoughts.
- exaggerated belief in one's own ability.
- increased sex drive.
- increased energy.
- poor judgment.
- inappropriate social behavior—usually impulsive and sometimes dangerous.
- depressive symptoms (see above).
- thoughts of death and suicide.

Bipolar disorder is usually chronic. Tranquilizers, antidepressants, and psychotherapy are used to treat bipolar depression. In severe cases, hospitalization may be warranted.

PREMENSTRUAL DYSPHORIC DISORDER (PMDD)

It's not uncommon for women to experience psychological and physical symptoms associated with their menstrual cycle, symptoms collectively known as premenstrual syndrome, or PMS. But for 3 to 5 percent of women with PMS, symptoms are so severe that they interfere with normal living. Dubbed premenstrual dysphoric disorder (PMDD), this condition is characterized by debilitating depression and anxiety. Depressive symptoms are similar to those for chronic depressive disorder. If five or more of those symptoms are present, a diagnosis of PMDD is made.

By far the best treatment for PMDD appears to be fluoxetine (Prozac). That's the conclusion of a three-month clinical trial comparing four treatments: vitamin B_6 (300 milligrams daily); alprazolam (Xanax) (0.75 milligrams daily); propranolol (Inderal) (20 milligrams daily, increased to 40 milligrams daily during the menstrual period); and fluoxetine (Prozac) (10 milligrams daily). Fluoxetine reduced symptoms the most—by nearly 66 percent. The researchers noted that the drug "presented the best results for treating premenstrual syndrome."

SITUATIONAL DEPRESSION

Suppose you lose your job, your spouse leaves you, or a loved one passes away. Distressing environmental factors like these can trigger the blues, known technically as situational depression. Its symptoms include:

- a sense of hopelessness.
- grief.
- shattered self-esteem.
- anxiety or worry.
- irritability.
- a retreat from social relationships.

Situational depression is often a side effect of certain life choices, too. Alcohol, for example, acts as a depressant, although it may temporarily boost your mood. It also interferes with the dreaming periods of sleep, known as rapid-eye-movement (REM) sleep. This leads to fatigue and, with it, depression. Prolonged dieting triggers depression, too, particularly if you do not eat enough carbohydrate-rich foods, known to boost mood.

Normally, situational depression resolves itself as the disappointment or loss fades and you begin to get on with your life. Yet, if the depression persists without resolution, you may need counseling to explore solutions to life problems, resolve feelings of hopelessness or low self-esteem, or overcome self-defeating ways of thinking.

16 DEPRESSION-DEFEATING MOVES YOU CAN MAKE NOW

Given the very serious problems stemming from depression, what can you do to prevent it from clouding your life?

Plenty! Here's a sixteen-point plan for preventing depression.

NOURISH YOUR BODY WITH
VITAMINS AND MINERALS

A better-balanced diet will do wonders for your mental health. A number of vitamin and mineral deficiencies have been linked to symptoms of depression. Deficiencies of iron, thiamine, selenium, magnesium, and carbohydrates, for example, produce depressive symptoms, low moods, anxiety, and fatigue.

CONSIDER OMEGA-3 FATTY ACIDS
FOR BIPOLAR DEPRESSION

As long you have the blessing of your doctor, look into omega-3 fatty acid supplements, which have been studied for their ability to combat bipolar disorder. Research-backed recommended supplements include:

- Fish oil, especially an omega-3 fatty acid formula containing 440 milligrams of EPA and 240 milligrams of DHA per capsule. Take seven capsules twice a day.
- Flaxseed oil (1 tablespoon daily).

REDUCE SUGAR INTAKE

The rapid spike in energy supplied by sugar is quickly followed by a drop in blood sugar (hypoglycemia), which can lead to depression and fatigue. Cut back on sugar in your diet by avoiding sweets, desserts, and other processed foods.

AVOID RAPID WEIGHT-LOSS DIETS

Crash diets—in which caloric intake is slashed to under 1,000 calories or less a day—starve your body and mind of vital nutrients, such as proteins, carbohydrates, essential fats, vitamins, and minerals. These are your "armed forces" for good physical and mental health. When in short supply, these nutrients cannot adequately provide the raw material to fuel your brain or manufacture the neurotransmitters necessary for proper mental functioning.

STAY ACTIVE

The more you make exercise a habit, the better your mood and the lower your stress level. But you've got to make a commitment to it. Researchers in Australia studied three groups of people: long-term exercisers, short-term exercisers, and non-exercisers. The long-term exercisers had a more positive outlook on life and were less depressed and stressed out than those in the other two groups, based on the results of questionnaires filled out by the participants.

QUIT SMOKING

Smokers are more likely than non-smokers to be depressed, according to research. A recent study, for example, found that teenagers who smoked cigarettes were nearly four times as likely to develop depression as their non-smoking peers.

Scientists aren't exactly sure why smokers are more depressed than non-smokers, but there is a theory. Nicotine and other tobacco byproducts alter brain chemistry, probably interfering with the uptake of serotonin, the feel-good neurotransmitter. This theory is bolstered by evidence that antidepressant drugs that increase serotonin uptake are helpful in getting adults to kick the smoking habit.

SEE THE LIGHT

If you want to maintain a sunny disposition, get outdoors as much as you can, brighten up your house in the winter with more light or light coats of paint, sit near windows, or take your winter vacations in the tropics or other sunny climates. Exposure to sunlight increases levels of feel-good serotonin in the brain.

CHALLENGE YOUR THINKING

Scientists have learned that most depression is caused by the way we respond to events and experiences. For example, some people take things personally, even when the situation is not personal. Or they look at life in terms of black and white, with no shades of gray. With either response, there can be a negative interpretation that can bring on depression.

In addition, try not to engage in all-or-nothing thinking. When faced with a situation, realize that there may be a variety of choices rather than a single right choice that you must make. Life can be ambiguous at times, with many possible paths to follow.

GET INVOLVED

Moods can worsen if you're lonely, isolated, unhappy with your surroundings, or around people who "bring you down." You may have to change your lifestyle or make new social contacts. Volunteering is a good way to reduce social isolation and meet new people. Pick a cause you want to support, and volunteer your time and talents to help make a difference. You won't be sorry, and you'll be better off both physically and mentally.

LIVEN UP YOUR LOVEMAKING

Intimate, fulfilling sex with a committed partner releases endorphins to produce a natural euphoria and increase levels of immune cells that protect the body. In women, regular sexual activity also jacks up levels of estrogen, a natural antidepressant. In addition, satisfying sex leads to better communication and strengthens relationships—two important hedges against depression.

BE CREATIVE

Tap into your talent, whether it's painting a picture, tending a garden, or writing a poem. Creative pursuits will give you a sense of accomplishment in addition to rescuing you from the doldrums.

REDUCE YOUR USAGE
OF PRESCRIPTION DRUGS

Some of the regular medications you're taking—or thinking about taking—might be drugs that help your physical health but also give you the blues. Examples include blood pressure medication (reserpine, methyldopa, clonidine, and beta-blockers); antiarrhythmic drugs such as digitalis; cortisone; glaucoma medication such as timolol; antihistamines; and oral contraceptives. If you suspect that your medication is bringing on depression, discuss the issue with your physician. See if there's an alternative medication he or she can prescribe that is free of depressive side effects or find out if your dosage can be reduced.

NURTURE YOUR SOUL

There is a documented scientific link between faith and mental health. People who are religious or come from a religious family have a lower risk of depression, suicide, drug abuse, alcoholism, and depression. Having faith gives you peace and hope—two feelings that reduce depression, stress, and anxiety. The key is to reconnect with the faith of your youth, join a house of worship, and reconnect with God.

SLEEP WELL

Do you pull frequent all-nighters, whether to cram for tests, socialize into the wee hours, have trouble falling asleep, then drag yourself out of bed early in the morning for school or work?

If so, such behavior—technically known as sleep deprivation—could be making you feel down in the dumps. One of the side effects of sleep deprivation, including insomnia, is depression. Lack of sleep causes the body to churn out too much cortisol, a stress hormone. Excesses of cortisol can lead to memory impairment, high blood pressure, weakened immunity, and depression. So avoid depression by getting a better night's sleep, every night.

PREVENT RELAPSES

If you've suffered depression in the past, you'll want to prevent its recurrence. Scientifically controlled studies show that the combination of medication and psychotherapy is more effective in preventing relapses than either treatment alone, particularly among older patients.

GET REGULAR CHECKUPS

If you haven't been to a doctor in a while, make an appointment now for a thorough medical checkup. There are many physical conditions that can produce depressive symptoms, including thyroid malfunctions, menopause, diabetes, and anemia.

2 BLOCKBUSTER ANTIDEPRESSANTS FROM NATURE'S PHARMACY

The following two mood enhancers are very effective but less well known than other natural remedies for depression.

HOLY BASIL

Doctors in India consider holy basil (*Ocimum sanctum*), or Gai Pad Bai Gaprow, an important treatment for depression. It is not the same basil you use in cooking but a different plant altogether.

Indian researchers have recently discovered that holy basil is as effective as the antidepressant desipramine. In mice, it helps heal various types of ulcers, including those induced by stress.

Herbalists recommend taking a 500-milligram capsule one to two times a day. If you're using a tincture, try 5 to 10 drops on your tongue, up to ten times a day or as needed. You can find it in health-food stores, some specialty culinary stores, and on the Internet. No side effects have yet been associated with this herb.

S-ADENOSYL-L-METHIONINE (SAM-E)

Since becoming available over the counter in the United States in 1998, SAM-e has been a popular and well-researched natural antidepressant— one that works rapidly, usually within one week. That's a real plus because prescription antidepressants often take weeks before any relief from depression becomes noticable.

SAM-e is derived from the amino acid methionine and participates in the production of brain chemicals. Specifically, it appears to elevate levels of dopamine, which is involved in mood regulation, among other functions. It is also involved in the formation of myelin, the sheath that envelops neurons.

Studies show that SAM-e may be one of the most effective natural antidepressants available. The suggested dosage for treating depression ranges from 400 to 1,600 milligrams a day. Most manufacturers recommend up to 800 milligrams daily. For better absorption and use by the body, take it on an empty stomach with water.

With the exception of minor gastrointestinal upset, there are virtually no side effects associated with taking SAM-e. At dosages above 400 milligrams daily, however, you may experience dry mouth, restlessness, and abdominal discomfort.

5 WAYS TO CHASE AWAY WINTERTIME BLUES

Do you get the "winter blahs" or feel down in the dumps on gloomy days? Granted, we all do, every now and then. But if your mood goes beyond a mere "blue funk," especially during the winter months, you could be suffering from seasonal affective disorder (SAD), a form of depression that strikes 10 to 25 million Americans, usually in the fall and winter.

This extreme form of the wintertime blahs is thought to stem from abnormalities in the brain's neurotransmitters. Low levels of light in the winter disturb the balance of neurotransmitters being released, particularly serotonin. Although serotonin levels normally dip during the winter, people prone to SAD are not able to handle the slack and thus become depressed more easily.

Other symptoms include:

- depressive feelings during a specific season of the year (usually winter).
- headaches.
- irritability.
- low energy.
- food cravings.
- crying spells.

If you've been diagnosed with SAD, follow the five recommendations below.

UNDERGO BRIGHT-LIGHT THERAPY

SAD sufferers respond well to light. Scientists think that certain parts of the brain are stimulated by sunlight. If you have SAD, try getting outdoors as much as you can, brightening up your house in the winter with more light or light coats of paint, sitting near windows, or taking your winter vacations in the tropics or other sunny climates.

If you can't get enough time in the sun, consider a light box, which is highly recommended by mental health therapists to treat SAD. Constructed with fluorescent or incandescent lights in front of a reflector, these devices emit light that is fifty times as bright as ordinary room light. Ask your therapist about purchasing a light box, and try to spend thirty minutes a day under it.

DISCUSS ANTIDEPRESSANT THERAPY
WITH YOUR DOCTOR

If light therapy doesn't work, you may have to take a selective serotonin reuptake inhibitor (SSRI), which acts only on serotonin. Since

SSRIs lengthen the amount of time that concentrations of serotonin stay active in the brain, these medications can elevate your mood and make you feel better.

As mentioned earlier, the best known of these drugs is fluoxetine (Prozac). Another SSRI is sertraline (Zoloft). Studies indicate that SAD can be effectively treated with either antidepressant. In many cases, a combination of antidepressant therapy and bright-light therapy will chase away wintertime blues.

TRY ST. JOHN'S WORT

A number of studies show that St. John's wort combats SAD. At a dosage of 300 milligrams, taken three times a day, it may work as well as Prozac (fluoxetine). Like its prescription-drug counterparts, St. John's wort increases serotonin levels in the brain.

SUPPLEMENT WITH THE HORMONE MELATONIN

Your body produces less melatonin in the day (light suppresses its release) and more at night. This helps you fall asleep at bedtime. More melatonin is secreted during winter, too, when the days are shorter. This can negatively affect mood and cause sleepiness among SAD sufferers, who may already have higher-than-normal levels of melatonin. Another theory holds that people with SAD release too much melatonin at the wrong time.

A few researchers have experimented with the hormone melatonin to see whether tiny doses can reset the body's internal clock and help restore the normal release of this hormone. In one study, small amounts of melatonin (0.125 milligrams twice a day) appeared to reduce wintertime depression.

WORK OUT

In addition to the approaches described here, exercise is emerging as an important adjunct to treatment. A Russian study found that exercise (one hour daily of stationary cycling) significantly improved the dispositions of women with SAD—and did so in just one week. One reason for the positive outcome may be that exercise releases natural mood-elevating chemicals called endorphins.

STRESS AND YOUR MOOD

Blowing a sales call, missing a deadline, failing a test, getting laid off, working too hard, losing a loved one—these are just a few of the things in life that trigger stress and, with it, mood disorders such as depression.

In fact, stress-related events bring on 50 percent of all depression. What's more, stress early in life leads to depression later in life.

When you're persistently under stress, your adrenal glands churn out cortisol and adrenaline, two emergency hormones. Normally, these hormones help us handle stress. But if that stress is chronic, these hormones stick around. Cortisol, in particular, isn't metabolized well.

Studies show that depressed people have higher-than-normal levels of cortisol in their bodies, and recent research suggests that high cortisol levels may trigger depression. Further, stress can cause huge disruptions in brain chemistry—disruptions that lay low for many years, only to rear up later as depression. In other words, you get through the stress-producing problem and go on with your life but show up in a therapist's office many years later to be treated for depression. This sequence of events has been observed in victims of child abuse and other forms of trauma.

Clearly, stress is hazardous to your mood and mental health. How well you cope with stress makes a huge difference in your well-being.

From Here to Serenity:
29 Tips for Stress-Free Living

1. Fortify yourself nutritionally.
2. Cut down on stress-inducing substances such as caffeine as well as depressants such as alcohol.
3. Exercise. It jogs the mind by increasing blood flow to the brain, which in turn leads to a better memory.
4. Take yoga classes. Yoga requires concentration, which calms the mind.
5. Pursue spiritual activities such as prayer and meditation.
6. Get a massage.
7. Practice deep breathing.
8. Pamper yourself at a day spa.
9. Listen to soothing music.
10. Talk out problems with a friend.
11. Pursue your favorite hobby.
12. Take a vacation.
13. Laugh a little or a lot.
14. Smile.
15. Try cognitive therapy.
16. Get more rest.
17. Take control of your time by making "to-do" lists, but don't get upset if you fail to complete everything on your list.
18. Don't bring your work home.
19. Redecorate your house to make it a more relaxing, soothing, and healthier environment.
20. Get a grip on your budget with better financial management.
21. Stop trying to keep up with the Joneses; income and material possessions aren't worth it if they bring you hassles over happiness.
22. Stop crying over spilt milk or wishing for something you may never get; instead, set realistic, achievable goals for yourself.
23. Take mini-time-outs to read or relax.
24. Get enough rest.

(Continued)

25. Organize your home or office to reduce clutter.
26. View and label stressful situations as challenges rather than "problems."
27. Take the advice capsulized in the title of a popular book, *Don't Sweat the Small Stuff*.
28. Stop trying to be perfect.
29. Think positively.

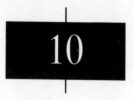

Stop the Memory Losers

If someone tells you your memory is terrible, don't believe it! Your brain has a remarkable ability to remember things—thousands of words, myriad facts, details of encounters, any number of complex tasks—if only you take good care of it. One of the best ways to do that is to shun the memory losers, those things—from diseases to toxins to medicines to stress—that can turn your mind to mush.

THE 4 MAIN DEMENTIAS: WHAT YOU NEED TO KNOW TO HALT MEMORY LOSS

Dementia is a condition in which you gradually lose the ability to remember, think, reason, interact socially, and care for yourself. It is not a disease, but rather a cluster of symptoms triggered by diseases or conditions that adversely affect the brain. Some of these triggers can be treated and are referred to as "reversible" dementia; others cannot be cured and are termed "irreversible" dementia. Irreversible dementia causes permanent brain damage.

There are four main types of dementia: Alzheimer's disease, which accounts for 60 percent of all dementia; multi-infarct dementia, 25 percent; reversible dementia, 14 percent; and miscellaneous causes, such as Parkinson's disease, 1 percent.

ALZHEIMER'S DISEASE

Named after Dr. Alois Alzheimer who discovered the disease in 1906, Alzheimer's is a disease in which you lose your mind, literally. It gradually impairs your memory, behavior, thinking, personality, judgment, language, movement, and coordination. Irreversible, it is the most feared of all dementia, and about 4 million Americans have it.

In Alzheimer's disease, a protein called beta amyloid peptide builds up outside of the brain cells, forming brain-cell-killing plaques, and inside brain cells, causing fibrous tangles. These changes adversely affect the way brain cells operate, primarily by decreasing the number of synapses, the tiny gaps between brain cells that are the units of communication between these cells. Also, in Alzheimer's disease, the brain's supply of acetylcholine, a neurotransmitter involved in memory formation, gradually diminishes.

The exact cause of these brain-damaging changes has not yet been pinned down; however, scientists and medical experts believe it arises from a combination of factors, including environmental toxins, viruses, free-radical activity, head trauma, and heredity.

Environmental Toxins

Among environmental toxins, exposure to aluminum has been studied the most. In one investigation, autopsied brains of Alzheimer's patients were found to contain thirty times the level of aluminum than that found in healthy brains of people the same age.

Other environmental agents that may be implicated in Alzheimer's disease include pesticides, solvents, and mercury dental fillings. (For a more detailed explanation of brain toxins, see "Top Defense Against Dementia: Avoid These 4 Memory-Damaging Toxins" on page 210.

Viruses

Evidence is piling up that many viruses, including HIV and herpes, may enter the brain and cause Alzheimer's disease but without producing the overt symptoms of infection. In 2000, British researchers discovered that the combined presence of herpes simplex 1 (the kind that causes cold sores) and an Alzheimer's gene known as ApoE-e4 increased the likelihood of Alzheimer's disease. In the study, the herpes virus was detected in 74 percent of Alzheimer's-affected brains. Also, the ApoE-e4 gene was four times more common in cold-sore sufferers than among patients without any sores.

Free Radicals

Oxidative stress—a condition that arises when free radicals outnumber antioxidants—may also be involved in Alzheimer's disease. Oxidative stress further aggravates brain cell damage caused by plaques in the brain that are characteristic of Alzheimer's disease.

Supplementing your diet with antioxidants, particularly vitamins E and C, may thus help minimize free-radical formation and retard the onset of Alzheimer's disease. Smoking increases oxidative stress and is a risk factor for Alzheimer's disease. A Japanese study published in 2000 found that moderate to heavy smoking more than doubles the risk of developing the disease.

Head Trauma

If you've had a history of head trauma, including concussions or head injury, you may be at an increased risk of Alzheimer's disease. Boxers, for example, have a higher incidence of the disease.

To a certain extent, however, you can control this risk factor. Take precautions, such as wearing seat belts and helmets and avoiding contact sports that may involve head injuries.

Heredity

Genetic factors are also involved in Alzheimer's disease, and several Alzheimer's genes have been identified. However, you can have the gene and not get the disease; and you can develop the disease without having the gene.

Currently, no cure exists for Alzheimer's disease, although there are some drugs and herbs that improve its symptoms (see Part 5). The two major risk factors for the disease—age and family history—are beyond our control. Even so, the other factors mentioned above can be controlled and may reduce risk.

MULTI-INFARCT DEMENTIA

This common form of dementia is caused by a series of strokes (bleeding or lack of blood supply in the brain) that leave pockets of dead brain cells (infarcts). The accumulated effect of these strokes leads to gradual loss of memory; personality changes; depression; sudden, involuntary laughing or crying; partial paralysis of one side of the body; and other symptoms. Another term for multi-infarct dementia is "vascular dementia." It can coexist with Alzheimer's disease.

Although irreversible, multi-infarct dementia is largely preventable by taking measures to reduce your risk of stroke, as well as your risk of high blood pressure and atherosclerosis (the narrowing and thickening of arteries), two conditions that can lead to stroke. Anti-stroke measures include controlling your weight, cholesterol levels, and salt intake; getting regular exercise; quitting smoking; avoiding or decreasing the frequency of situations known to cause stress in your life; and getting regular medical checkups. (For more on stroke prevention, see Chapter 15.)

REVERSIBLE DEMENTIA

Treatable, reversible dementia is caused by a number of factors, including the following:

- *Nutritional deficiencies*. Virtually any shortfall of nutrients, particularly the B vitamins, will cause dementia, particularly in the elderly. Adhering to a nutrient-rich diet and taking nutritional supplements will "cure" the dementia.
- *Depression*. Severe cases of depression can lead to dementia. Happily, treatment with antidepressants can chase away the blues and, with them, the dementia.
- *Treatable diseases*. Dementia is a worrisome side effect of some diseases. An underactive thyroid, for example, produces slowed physical and mental functioning. Treating the disease with daily replacement of thyroid hormone rectifies these and other symptoms. Brain tumors and viral infections can also cause dementia.
- *Drug interactions*. Among elderly people, a common cause of reversible dementia is medication. In fact, the elderly take seven different medications each day, on average. Dementia may occur as a result of unintentional overdoses, reactions to a single drug, or as a consequence of interactions among several drugs.
- *Alcohol dependence*. Alcohol is essentially a toxin that, if abused, can damage the brain and induce dementia. Treatment for alcohol dependence is very straightforward: abstinence.

MISCELLANEOUS CAUSES OF
IRREVERSIBLE DEMENTIA

Other causes of dementia include certain incurable brain and nervous system disorders, including the following:

- *Parkinson's disease*. First described by Englishman James Parkinson in 1817, this disorder is a progressive degeneration of nerve cells in the part of the brain that controls muscle movements. The disease results in the loss of dopamine in the brain. Dopamine is a neurotransmitter that transports signals from one cell to another in the brain to help control voluntary movements such as walking, talking, and writing. Dementia is evident during the very late stages of the disease.

- *Pick's disease*. This is a rare disorder in which only some cells in parts of the brain shrink, die, or become abnormal and swollen. In Pick's disease, there are slow, progressive changes in behavior and speech. Dementia occurs in the late stages of the disease. The disease was first described by Arnold Pick in 1892.

- *Lewy body dementia*. This disorder, which can coexist with Alzheimer's disease or Parkinson's disease, is a progressive form of dementia characterized by abnormal structures in brain cells called "Lewy bodies." Unlike Alzheimer's disease, this dementia tends to progress more rapidly.

- *Huntington's disease*. Often striking in midlife, this disease stems from a disorder within the cerebrum that causes nerve cells to wither away. It is an inherited disease that develops slowly, beginning with personality changes and unusual twisting movements of the body and progressing to dementia. The disease is named after American physician George Huntington, who first documented the disorder in 1872.

- *Creutzfeldt-Jakob disease*. A rare and fatal brain disorder, this disease is a progressive form of dementia in which brain cells have a spongy appearance due to cell death. There are four types: a sporadic form, where the cause is unknown; an inherited form; a transmissible form, thought to occur through organ transplants and the contamination of surgical instruments; and mad cow disease, caused by exposure to contaminated meat.

TOP DEFENSE AGAINST DEMENTIA: AVOID THESE 4 MEMORY-DAMAGING TOXINS

Exposure to certain environmental toxins is a prime suspect in triggering dementia, including Alzheimer's disease, Parkinson's disease, and other cognitive problems, according to a growing body of scientific studies into brain diseases. Specifically, there are four toxins you should shun in order to protect your memory and other brain functions. They are discussed below.

ALUMINUM

For years, researchers have been mystified by the high levels of aluminum found in the brains of Alzheimer's patients. It is not clear whether exposure to aluminum causes the disease or if the deposits are a side effect of Alzheimer's. A study by the University of Toronto, however, found that high levels of aluminum in drinking water increased the odds of developing Alzheimer's disease. Residents with the disease were 1.2 to 3.6 times more likely to have lived in areas where the drinking water was high in aluminum.

Aluminum, which can be absorbed by the body, is used in water purification and in drinking water. It is also used in the manufacturing of many products as well as in the processing of food, cosmetics, and medicines.

A review article on aluminum and the brain published in a 2000 issue of *Neurotoxicity* pointed out that aluminum is a neurotoxicant (a brain toxin) in humans and animals. One of the ways it poisons the brain is by promoting the formation and accumulation of beta amyloid peptides, proteins that are responsible for the destruction of brain cells in Alzheimer's disease. The article goes on to recommend that avoiding aluminum, when practical, is a wise move.

If you're concerned about exposure to aluminum, do the following:

- Avoid cooking foods (especially acidic ones such as tomatoes) in aluminum pans.
- Stop drinking soda from aluminum cans. According to medical experts, one aluminum can may deposit up to 4 milligrams of aluminum inside your body, an amount that exceeds the maximum safe limit.
- Purchase a water filter that removes aluminum and other metals from your drinking water.
- Reduce your use of food products, cosmetics, and over-the-counter (OTC) medicines that contain aluminum. A number of these products are listed in Table 10.1.

TABLE 10.1		
Aluminum-Containing Products		
FOOD PRODUCT*	COSMETIC*	OTC MEDICATION*
Nondairy creamers	Douches	Antacids
Food mixes	Antidandruff shampoos	Buffered aspirin
Processed cheese	Deodorants	Antidiarrheal medications
Frozen dough	Antiperspirants, including aerosol antiperspirants	
Baking powder		
Salad dressings		

*Read product labels to check for the presence of aluminum.

LEAD

Scientists have known for a long time that lead damages the central nervous system, including the brain, and harms other body tissues. In fact, people who have worked in jobs with high levels of lead exposure are 3.4 times more likely to develop Alzheimer's disease, according to researchers at Case Western Reserve University in Cleveland, Ohio. Presented at the 2000 meeting of the American Academy of Neurology, this finding emerged from a study of the work histories of 185 people with Alzheimer's disease and 303 people without it. Workers involved in casting or smelting lead, welding, sandblasting, paint removal, or working with lead products were at the highest risk.

Exposure to lead has also been linked to attention deficits, learning problems, and intellectual impairment in children, according to a growing number of studies. Young children are at a greater risk for lead poisoning because they absorb four times as much lead as adults do.

Fortunately, less lead has been finding its way into our bodies, thanks to bans on lead-based paint, the availability of lead-free gas, a reduction in lead used to solder food cans, and limits on allowable levels of lead in drinking water.

But, by far, lead still poses the biggest toxic problem to your health. Fortunately, you can further protect yourself and your family from lead contamination. Here are some important guidelines:

- Purchase a water filter that reduces the lead in your drinking water.
- Avoid purchasing lead-glazed ceramic products, particularly those made in foreign countries. Lead can leach from these containers into your foods.
- Keep your home clean. Lead is found in soil, so if you work in your yard, or if your child plays outside in the dirt, be sure to wash and keep areas inside your home free from dirt.
- Check to learn whether your home paint contains lead. If your home was built as recently as 1978, it may contain lead paint. The problem with this is that children can accidentally ingest minute amounts of paint, or the lead can generate harmful lead dust. Contact your local or state health department to test your home for lead paint and, if needed, have a contractor who specializes in lead paint removal to take off the paint.
- Be cautious when refinishing old furniture that has previously been painted. The paint may contain lead. If you suspect that it does, purchase a lead-paint testing kit at your local hardware store or home-improvement center. Should the paint test positive for lead, contact the local arm of the U.S. Environmental Protection Agency (EPA) for further instructions.
- Follow a lead-reducing diet. A diet with adequate amounts of calcium and iron helps reduce the amount of lead absorbed by the body. Foods high in calcium include dairy products; those rich in iron include lean red meats and poultry.

MERCURY

Mercury contamination is responsible for a wide range of emotional problems, including excitability, lack of concentration, loss of memory, and depression. It can also lead to permanent brain damage.

In the brain, mercury causes special scaffoldlike structures in developing brain cells to break down, and the cells stop functioning normally. This degenerative process was recently observed and videotaped by scientists at the University of Calgary, using brain cells from snails, whose brain cell structure resembles that of humans. Some of the degenerated brain cells clumped or tangled together, a characteristic seen in the brains of Alzheimer's patients.

Found naturally in the environment, mercury is a shiny white metal used in thermometers and some electrical switches. We're exposed to metallic mercury in two major ways. First, it can be released into our bodies from dental fillings. When these fillings are inserted, they emit small amounts of mercury vapor that can be absorbed into the brain, where they can damage neurons.

To be on the safe side, talk to your dentist about having your mercury fillings removed and replaced. Or consider seeing a holistic dentist. Holistic dentists are licensed dentists who use an interdisciplinary approach in their practice, often employing such methods as homeopathy, nutrition, and acupuncture to achieve a healing effect. In addition, holistic dentists emphasize wellness and preventive care and avoid such treatments as mercury fillings.

The second major way we're exposed to mercury is by eating contaminated fish. Here's how: Mercury is capable of evaporating to form colorless, odorless vapors. After being released into the atmosphere, mercury is deposited in bodies of water, where it is converted by bacteria into a more dangerous form called methylmercury. Fish absorb methylmercury as they feed on aquatic organisms. It binds very tightly to the proteins in fish tissue, and, unfortunately, cooking does not reduce the mercury content in fish.

Certain species of fish are higher in this toxin than others, according to tests conducted by the FDA, *Consumer Reports*, and some environmental groups. Table 10.2 lists fish that have tested for high, moderate, and lower levels of methylmercury.

TABLE 10.2 Fish Consumption Advisory		
FISH WITH HIGH LEVELS OF MERCURY	FISH WITH MODERATE LEVELS OF MERCURY	FISH WITH LOWER LEVELS OF MERCURY
Bass	Canned tuna, chunk light	Cod
Canned tuna, white meat		
Freshwater fish from contaminated waters*	Shrimp, boiled	Haddock
King mackerel		Pollack
Orange roughy		
Pike		
Shark		
Swordfish		
Tilefish		

*Waterways in the following states have been found to have widespread mercury contamination, according to the Environmental Working Group: Connecticut, Florida, Indiana, Maine, Massachusetts, Michigan, Minnesota, New Hampshire, New Jersey, Vermont, and Wisconsin.

How to Limit Your Exposure to Mercury-Contaminated Fish

Although fish is an important source of high-quality, brain-building nutrients, FDA seafood specialists recommend the following precautions to avoid the danger of mercury poisoning:

- For the general population, fish that has been tested for high levels of mercury should be eaten no more than twice a week.

- If you're pregnant, lactating, or of child-bearing age, you should limit your consumption of high-mercury fish to no more than once a month. Tuna, a fish with moderate levels of mercury, should be limited to no more than one 6-ounce can a week. Fish with lower levels of mercury can be consumed up to 14 ounces a week.

- Young children (with a weight up to 45 pounds) should eat even less fish—no more than one tuna sandwich (with just 2 tablespoons of tuna), or the equivalent, a week.

- When purchasing fish, select a smaller fish within the species. It is typically younger and probably hasn't been exposed to toxins for as long as an older, larger fish has.

- Buy farm-raised fish, if available. These are raised under controlled conditions with less exposure to toxins and bacteria.

- Don't eat the skin or the fatty portion of fish because this is where toxins tend to congregate.

- Avoid eating the same species of fish all the time to minimize possible exposure to the pollutants over and over again. In other words, plan your diet to include a variety of fish.

PESTICIDES

If you handle garden pesticides or in-home pesticides, you may be at risk of developing Parkinson's disease. That's the finding of a study presented at the annual meeting of the American Academy of Neurology in 2000. Investigators from Stanford University interviewed 496 people who had been diagnosed with Parkinson's disease about their past use of pesticides. The use of garden pesticides was tied to a 50-percent increase in the risk of the disease, and the use of in-home insecticides was linked to a 70-percent chance. The study was the first to look into home and garden pesticides as a Parkinson's disease risk.

More recently, scientists at the University of California demonstrated that several pesticides—including rotenone, paraquat, and dieldrin—

accelerated the rate of formation of the protein alpha synuclein in the brain. Abnormalities in the formation of this protein have been linked to the development of Parkinson's disease. For a closer look at these pesticides, see Table 10.3.

TABLE 10.3 Pesticides to Avoid		
PESTICIDE	SOURCES	CAUTIONS
Rotenone	Pet shampoos, flea and tick powders	Causes Parkinson's disease–like symptoms in rats.
Paraquat	Weed killers	Use in the United States is restricted to certified applicators.
Dieldrin	Found residually in soil, although levels are slowly decreasing	Banned by the Environmental Protection Agency (EPA) in 1987.

The link between pesticides and brain disease isn't clear-cut, but if you want to hedge your bets, use alternative approaches to health-damaging pesticides. For example:

- Try "biopesticides." These are pesticides derived from natural materials such as animals, plants, bacteria, and certain minerals. Examples include synthetic pyrethroids and neem oil.
- Vacuum pests from plants. If you have a problem with mites or other common pests among your houseplants or in your garden, you're better off removing them with a handheld vacuum cleaner than with a pesticide.
- Spray aphids and other bugs with a diluted soapy solution.

- Use "biological control agents" such as ladybugs. They are natural predators that eat the offending pests.
- Try pheromones, a sex attractant released by the female of the insect species. Made by various companies, these natural chemicals are extracted from the pest or made in the laboratory and are designed to lure pests into traps.
- Use insect hormones. Introduced at the right time, these chemicals disrupt the insect's growth and development cycle, halting its reproductive capacity.

CAUTION: DO TOO MUCH OF THIS AND YOUR BRAIN MAY TURN TO MUSH

If you spend long hours watching television, you could be a candidate for memory-destroying Alzheimer's disease, according to a study from the Cleveland Clinic released in 2001 and published in the *Proceedings of the National Academy of Sciences*.

Clinic researchers surveyed about 550 people in their seventies about their hobbies and leisure activities during early (age twenty to thirty-nine) and middle (age forty to sixty) adulthood. Of the respondents, 193 were Alzheimer's patients, and the rest (the control group) were not. The information from the Alzheimer's patients was gathered from their friends and families; the control group was questioned directly.

The activities were categorized into passive (watching television or listening to music); intellectual (reading, doing crossword puzzles, playing musical instruments, doing board games, or knitting); and physical (swimming, walking, riding bicycles, playing sports, and so forth).

The research suggested that adults with pastimes that challenge and stimulate the brain, such as reading, playing chess or bridge, or knitting, were two and half times less likely than others to develop Alzheimer's disease. Other safeguards against the disease were physical exercise, as well as certain passive activities such as listening to music, talking on the phone, and socializing.

But watching too much television (around four hours a day, on average) was linked to a higher risk of developing Alzheimer's disease, the study found. The researchers believe that being glued to television puts the viewer in a semi-conscious state in which the brain is not active. By contrast, brain-stimulating activities build up a greater supply of neuron connections. If Alzheimer's disease did strike, it would take longer for the disease process to destroy enough brain cells before symptoms would appear.

These findings send an important message: We need to engage in activities that keep our brains active—and to do so for a lifetime.

7 Memory Manglers and How to Outsmart Them

If your memory seems cloudy and your thinking feels fuzzy, certain memory manglers may be the reason. Many conditions—from coronary bypass surgery to worry—can make you feel like your mind is turning to mush. Here's a look at seven factors that can mangle your memory—and what to do about them.

DEPRESSION

When you've got a bad case of the blahs, neurotransmitters involved in memory—dopamine, norepinephrine, and acetylcholine—get out of whack and you can't remember a thing, or so it seems. Fortunately, though, some depression is only temporary and so are the memory problems that go with it. Protracted depression is treatable and can be outsmarted with therapy, antidepressant medication, exercise, or natural remedies such as St. John's wort or SAM-e. Resolving depression is a great way to protect your memory, as well as to stay emotionally fit. (For more information on how to overcome depression, see "16 Depression-Defeating Moves You Can Make Now" in Chapter 9.)

EMOTION SUPPRESSION

Hiding your emotions can harm your memory, says a Stanford University study. In this experiment, participants viewed slides of injured accident victims and were told personal information about each one. A third of the participants were told to hide their emotions; another third to regard the information with emotional detachment; and the rest received no special instructions. Those who concealed their emotions recalled fewer details about the victims than the other participants. The researchers believe that defusing emotions helps people pay close attention to events and situations.

If you have a hard time saying what's on your mind, consider therapy or an assertiveness training course. Both will help you get your feelings out in the open.

JET LAG

Published in the journal *Nature Neuroscience* in 2001, a British study found that chronic jet lag significantly impaired short-term memory and cognition (thinking skills) in a group of flight attendants. Jet lag is a condition experienced by many travelers who travel over time zones. Its symptoms include fatigue, disorientation, and insomnia.

The researchers believe that their findings have implications not only for airline workers but also for shift workers and parents of small children—anyone who experiences disruptions in their circadium rhythms, the cycle of sleeping and waking and of light and darkness.

Fortunately, you can outsmart jet lag in a number of ways. Here are eleven tips:

1. Prior to your trip, get some extra rest. Try to sleep and wake up as close as possible to the times in your destination city.
2. Drink lots of fluids (particularly water) before and during the flight.
3. Avoid caffeine and alcohol; they interfere with normal sleep.

4. Avoid antihistamines and tranquilizers; these induce drowsiness and can interfere with your sleep cycle.

5. Eat high-protein, low-fat meals during the traveling portion of your trip. These tend to keep you more alert—in contrast to high-carbohydrate foods, which produce drowsiness.

6. Stretch and move around the plane every so often.

7. Acclimate yourself to the schedule of the new time zone as soon as you arrive.

8. Expose yourself to natural light as soon as you land, if possible. Light suppresses the production of melatonin, a sleep-inducing hormone normally secreted in the evening.

9. Pop some supplemental melatonin to help keep your circadium rhythms in line with the new time zone. If traveling east, take ½ milligram at 3 P.M. on the day of departure to fool your brain into thinking that night is coming earlier. Take another dose at 3 P.M. the following day. If traveling west, take ½ milligram on the morning of your departure. Supplement with 3 milligrams in the evening to sleep through the night in the new time zone.

10. Instead of supplemental melatonin, try a dietary supplement called NADH, shown in research to help travelers stay alert while traveling across time zones. Take the supplement one hour prior to arrival at your destination. For correct dosage, follow label recommendations.

11. As you head home, try to shift your sleeping time to match that of your home time zone.

CORONARY BYPASS SURGERY

Although it has saved the lives of millions of people, coronary bypass surgery can induce memory loss and stroke in patients. A Duke University study found that more than one-third of coronary bypass patients had lost some degree of mental sharpness by five years after the procedure.

Doctors have been aware of bypass-induced memory loss for a long time but have been unable to zero in on the cause. One theory holds that the use of a heart-lung machine during surgery may have something to do with the problem. Another theory is that clots are forced during bypass surgery from the aorta into cerebral vessels, ultimately leading to stroke, which causes memory problems and other cognitive impairments.

If you are scheduled to undergo bypass surgery, discuss these potential side effects with your surgeon to learn whether they can be minimized. Unquestionably, the best way to outsmart this side effect is by avoiding bypass surgery altogether. Take care of your heart health through proper diet, exercise, and regular checkups.

ILLNESSES

It's no secret that Alzheimer's disease brings on memory failure, but did you also know that memory loss is a symptom of many other illnesses? The following diseases can temporarily impair your ability to remember: viral or bacterial infections, diabetes, hypertension, Parkinson's disease, chronic fatigue syndrome, alcoholism, thyroid problems, thiaminee deficiency, vitamin B_{12} deficiency, and multiple sclerosis. If you're under a doctor's care for a medical condition and find your memory becoming more fuzzy than usual, talk to your physician right away. He or she should be able to pinpoint whether your problem is due to your illness or to some other cause.

Further, if you're diagnosed with a medical condition, follow your doctor's orders, along with a healthy lifestyle, to outsmart potential memory loss. That way, you're more likely to prevent long-term complications that could further impair your memory.

Also, if you're having memory lapses for no apparent reason, have a complete physical examination to rule out medical causes.

WORRY

Are you a worrywart? You know, turning everything into a worst-case scenario—and doing it a lot?

Memory lapses occur most frequently when we're in a state of chronic worry. Worrying reduces your attention span. Reduced attention also zaps your memory.

Psychologists say that it's perfectly normal to spend as many as ninety minutes a day worrying. After all, a little healthy worrying is good. If you're a parent, for example, it's reasonable to be concerned over the safety of your children. Healthy worrying—let's call it "concern"— prompts you to take action. It's only when you worry all the time and can't stop that you may have a serious problem.

To outsmart excessive worrying, ask yourself: When worrying, do I resolve my worry through action or stop dead in my tracks? If worry serves no useful purpose, you need to nip it in the bud.

MARIJUANA

Regular marijuana users have reduced blood flow to a part of their brains involved in memory and other mental abilities, say University of Iowa researchers. The brain region in question is the posterior cerebellum, which is associated with memory, language, and sense of time. The researchers found that long-term use of marijuana has a noticeable effect on memory and brain function, contradicting accepted beliefs that smoking marijuana is not harmful to the brain.

Outsmart this illegal memory mangler by abstaining from marijuana use. If you're having trouble breaking free, see an addiction counselor.

5 TYPES OF DRUGS THAT CAN DESTROY YOUR MEMORY

A surprising culprit behind your forgetfulness may be a medicine you're taking. A worrisome side effect of some medications is that they can impair your memory by acting on brain chemistry or interfering with the function of your central nervous system. If you experience memory problems while taking a medicine, talk to your doctor about prescribing another treatment, if feasible, but do not stop taking a prescribed medication without consulting your doctor first.

Drugs known to cause memory problems include those discussed below.

ANTIHISTAMINES

They're the pills and capsules you take to halt the wheezing and sneezing of allergies and are available over the counter and in prescription form. While they nip allergies in the bud, they unfortunately can interfere with the ability to recall information.

Two antihistamines that may cause disorientation and mental confusion are Phenergan (promethazine hydrochloride) and Tussionex (hydrocodone polistirex).

BENZODIAZEPINES

This is a class of drugs used to treat anxiety. They relax you by slowing your brain function. Some of the more familiar antianxiety drugs that can cause memory loss include Ativan (lorazepam), Klonopin (clonazepam), Tranxene (clorazepate dipotassium), Valium (diazepam), and Xanax (alprazolam).

BETA-BLOCKERS

These medications are prescribed for the treatment of a wide range of heart problems, including high blood pressure. They lower blood pressure by reducing the force and speed of the heart. Because they can cross the blood-brain barrier, beta-blockers act directly on the central nervous system, often producing side effects such as memory loss, confusion, disorientation, anxiety, depression, and hallucinations. The following beta-blockers have been known to induce memory impairment: Inderal (propranolol hydrochloride), Inderide (a combination of propranolol hydrochloride and hydrochlorothiazide), and Lopressor (metoprolol tartrate).

OPIATES

This class of drugs includes painkillers such as morphine and codeine. They interfere with memory centers in your brain.

SLEEPING PILLS

These medications are prescribed for people who have trouble falling asleep and are intended for short-term use. Among the listed side effects of some of these drugs is amnesia, or memory blackouts. The following medications may induce this side effect: Halcion (triazolam), ProSom (estazolam), Restoril (temazepam), and Sonata (zaleplon).

BE KIND TO YOUR MIND:
STRESS AND MEMORY

Picture two scenarios. *Scenario one*: You're fleeing from a suspicious-looking stranger in an alleyway. Your heart pounds. Adrenaline rushes throughout your body as you run for your life. *Scenario two*: You're at work, enduring yet another frustrating day of criticism and lack of support from your boss. Which scenario would you rather be in?

Probably neither. But, for your brain's sake, the first scenario is the better bet.

Surprised? Here's the deal: Fleeing from a mugger provokes a short-lived stress response called the "fight or flight" mode—a reaction your body is wired to handle. Life-saving responses kick in: Heart rate accelerates. Digestive activity decreases so that extra blood and glucose can be diverted to your muscles for energy. Your pupils dilate so that you can see more clearly.

Adrenaline and other stress hormones such as cortisol surge. They activate the hippocampus, a brain region responsible for memory formation, so that you'll remember the stressor should you ever encounter it again in the future. In short, your body prepares you to defend yourself against danger. Once the threat is gone, your body returns to its normal state.

But if stress is chronic—like working for a bad boss, day in and day out—stress hormones stick around and become toxic to brain cells. The good deeds they do are reversed: Cortisol, in particular, damages short-term memory in the hippocampus. Prolonged elevation of stress hormones shrinks the hippocampus, a finding observed in a number of studies.

Researchers studied a group of thirty-eight women, twenty with a history of sexual abuse. Using magnetic resonance imaging (MRI) to peer into their brains, the researchers discovered that in those women who had been sexually abused as children, the hippocampus was smaller than normal. They speculate that this shrinkage may be caused by prolonged exposure to cortisol and other stress hormones.

Furthermore, studies on stress in children have found that long-term family conflict interferes with the development of the hippocampus. And a study of Vietnam combat veterans showed that traumatized veterans averaged an 8 percent smaller hippocampi in their right brains.

In other studies, a shrunken hippocampus has been linked to memory loss and other cognitive impairments. Thus, stress can make you not only frazzled but forgetful, too. In fact, day-to-day stressors, such as marital conflict, job pressures, and financial worries, seem to inflict the same degree of brain and memory damage seen in victims of abuse and trauma.

At McGill University in Montreal, researchers studied a group of elderly women for four years. They discovered that women whose stress hormones had increased over the experimental period had hippocampi that were 14 percent smaller than their counterparts who were not so stressed!

Given the evidence of what stress can do to your brain and memory, is there anything you can do to prevent or reverse the process? Quite possibly. Studies with animals indicate that several therapeutic agents may be able to reverse the stress-induced shrinkage of the hippocampus. Promising new treatments include the following:

- DHEA (dehydroepiandrosterone), a supplemental hormone available over the counter.
- Dilantin (phenytoin), an anticonvulsant.

- Selective serotonin reuptake inhibitors (SSRI), which are anti-depressants. (Prozac is an SSRI.)
- Tianeptine (Stablon), an antidepressant used in Europe that combats anxiety and depression.

4 Memory-Building Herbs You Can Grow in Your Own Garden

Stimulating your memory can be as easy as stepping outside, harvesting a few herbs from your very own garden, and brewing a pot of tea with them. Among these are lemon balm, rosemary, sage, and stevia—all known to have their own unique memory-building properties. Another plus: They're easy to grow, no matter how brown your thumb.

LEMON BALM

Lemon balm (*Melissa officinalis*) is a member of the mint family believed to stimulate memory, probably because it contains choline, a nutrient necessary for optimal brain functioning.

The herb is a hardy plant that grows throughout the world. For your home garden, buy a small pot of lemon balm from a nursery and plant it in rich soil with full sun and regular watering. Lemon balm is a perennial that can grow up to 3 feet high.

You can brew a tasty tea of lemon balm by making an "infusion," a method of preparing whole herbs that is similar to brewing tea.

Follow these steps to make an infusion:

1. Boil water, then remove it from the heat.
2. Add several teaspoons of the fresh, chopped leaves of the herb.
3. Let the mixture sit for ten to twenty minutes (or until it has cooled off) to extract the active ingredients.
4. Strain off the plant material and drink the beverage cool or lukewarm, or gently reheat it.

ROSEMARY

In ancient writings, rosemary is mentioned in connection with remembrance (it has been nicknamed the "remembrance herb"). The ancient Greeks and Romans would toss sprigs of rosemary into graves to express their desire to remember the departed. The herb was also used medicinally by the Greeks to strengthen memory.

There is some scientific validity to the legendary claims about rosemary's effectiveness in boosting memory. The herb is rich in antioxidants that actively protect brain cells from attack by free radicals. Rosemary is also full of compounds that prevent the breakdown of acetylcholine, a neurotransmitter involved in memory formation.

As a perennial herb, rosemary is easy to grow, particularly in climates near the ocean. It prefers soil that has been prepared with compost and sand. When growing rosemary, don't overwater it, or else a fungus may appear on the plant. Rosemary grows best in full sun.

If you live in a cooler climate, bring the rosemary indoors and place it next to your sunniest window. Let it dry out between waterings.

You can easily propagate rosemary from cuttings placed in a small container of water. Roots will appear on the cuttings in about four weeks. Dip the cutting in a hormone rooting powder and plant it in a pot or in your garden.

You can prepare a tea of rosemary using a few teaspoons of the fresh leaves steeped in a cup of boiling water.

SAGE

Sage (*Salvia officinalis*) is best known as a culinary herb for seasoning poultry or sausage, as well as for spicing up dressing at Thanksgiving. But it has medicinal properties, too, and its use dates back to ancient times. In fact, Hippocrates believed that the oils in sage could cure illnesses of the brain, and herbalists down through the ages have claimed that it can restore a weak memory.

Interestingly, modern-day researchers have discovered that sage contains two constituents that block an enzyme that degrades acetylcholine, thus preserving a neurotransmitter that becomes depleted in patients with Alzheimer's disease. (The current drugs used to treat this disease work in much the same way.) Sage is also loaded with cell-protecting antioxidants.

It's best to purchase your sage plants because the seeds are difficult to germinate. A hardy perennial, sage requires little water and prefers full sun. Usually, every three years you can divide the plant and replant the sections.

To make sage tea, steep 2 teaspoons of fresh leaves in a cup of boiling water for five to ten minutes. **A note of caution:** Go easy on sage tea. Don't drink it habitually or for prolonged periods because the herb contains a toxin called thujone, which in large amounts can cause convulsions.

It is safe to drink one to three cups a day in a pattern of one week on, one week off, for no longer than four to six weeks. Do not drink sage tea if you are pregnant or nursing.

STEVIA

Known as the sweet-leaf plant, this herb (*Stevia rebaudiana*) is native to Paraguay but grows well in herb gardens, particularly those in southern climates. The reason stevia is important for brain health and memory fitness is that it is an excellent substitute for aspartame, an artificial sweetener that has been linked to memory problems. In a study at Texas Christian University, investigators found that students who regularly drank diet sodas containing aspartame were more likely to report long-term memory lapses, such as whether or not they had completed certain tasks.

Thus, all-natural stevia is a healthier alternative to artificial sweeteners. Its leaves yield a sugarlike derivative called steviocide, which is 250 to 300 times sweeter than sugar and is noncaloric.

Stevia has been used in Japan as a sweetener for more than twenty years. Although you can grow it in your garden, it is available as tea, powdered leaves, liquid extract, and purified steviocide. The herb is considered a dietary supplement in the United States by Food and Drug Administration (FDA) definition.

To grow stevia, plant it in full sun and make sure it has plenty of water. A cold snap will temporarily damage the herb, unless you bring it indoors. Even so, the herb is capable of growing back after winter.

The best use of stevia leaves is for sweetening cold or iced tea. When preparing any type of tea, simply add stevia leaves to the boiling water and let the concoction steep for five to ten minutes. Several leaves will sweeten a cup of tea; several sprigs of the plant will sweeten a pot of tea. Stevia is also available commercially in powdered form at health-food stores and markets.

Put Senility in Reverse with Phosphatidylserine (PS)

Between the ages of twenty-five and forty-five, our ability to learn and remember begins to fade by as much as one-third, depending on how well we've taken care of our brains. Good lifestyle habits—including diet, exercise, stress reduction, avoidance of environmental pollutants, and mental stimulation—go a long way to halt age-related mental deterioration.

So does a rather new nutritional supplement called phosphatidylserine (PS), which has the power to rebuild brain function and put mental decline in reverse. Researched for more than two decades, PS is a natural substance that is highly concentrated in brain cells, where it supports many cellular functions. Specifically, it facilitates the action of neurotransmitters, elevates brain energy, corrects hormonal imbalances, and coordinates activities between the brain and the adrenal glands to help the body handle stress. PS is also believed to work synergistically with nerve growth factors to help repair, restore, and even regrow damaged nerve networks in aging brains, according to studies with animals.

Technically, PS is a phospholipid, a phosphorus-containing fat that forms the structure of cell membranes. Thus, it is also an essential building block of cells.

PS is backed by an impressive body of research that demonstrates its value as a memory booster. Stanford and Vanderbilt researchers found that volunteers who supplemented with PS for a month significantly improved their ability to recall phone numbers and match names to faces. In another study, PS partially restored learning and recall ability in subjects suffering from age-related cognitive decline. Also, patients with advanced dementia improved their sociability, paid greater attention to personal welfare, and better cooperated with their caregivers after taking PS.

In addition to its ability to help recover lost memory power, other research with PS shows that it:

- improves mood.
- relieves anxiety and depression.
- reduces cortisol production in the body. (Cortisol is a stress hormone that, when chronically elevated, can damage tissues and organs, including the brain.)
- reinforces treatment with Ritalin to further improve attention span, behavior, and learning performance in attention-deficit children.

PS has proven so effective as a brain and memory restorer that many experts recommend its use in supplement regimens to support brain health. PS has virtually no side effects and does not interact adversely with prescription medications.

When purchasing PS, make sure you buy a product made from soy and not from bovine brains. PS supplements were originally manufactured from cattle sources, but a few years ago soy-based supplements were introduced and found to be as effective in boosting memory as the animal-derived variety.

For memory loss, supplement with 300 milligrams of PS daily; for maintenance of brain health, supplement with 100 milligrams of PS daily.

Bring Back a Fading Memory with Memory-Boosting Zinc

Worried about losing your memory? Then make sure you're getting enough zinc in your diet. Present in every nook and cranny of the body, zinc plays a role in nearly all biologically important functions. A short supply can lead to memory impairment as well as decreased alertness.

Case in point: Researchers at the University of Texas tested thirty-four women (ages eighteen to thirty-four) who were marginally deficient in zinc and observed that their recall ability was within normal ranges. But when given 30 milligrams of zinc daily, the women performed up to 20-percent higher on standard tests for memory. These findings suggest that boosting zinc intake may stimulate memory.

Zinc is also an antioxidant. It helps make superoxide dismutase, an antioxidant enzyme that inactivates certain free radicals.

As with most nutrients, it's much better if you get zinc from food. Zinc is plentiful in seafood and animal foods but is also present in whole grains, peas, corn, and carrots. But to ensure that you get enough of the brain-enhancing nutrient, take a mineral supplement that has 100 percent of the daily reference intake (DRI) for zinc (11 milligrams for men and 8 milligrams for women).

Part Four

UNDERSTANDING WHY

Ever wonder why some people are so smart even as they get older? Why others are so happy? Why certain people seem to control the mood of a room? What do those dizzy spells and headaches mean? Why you're so forgetful at times?

Such questions have challenged human beings for ages. For the most part, the answers lie in the tantalizing mystery of the brain.

In this part of the book, you'll explore intelligence and how you can boost both yours and your children's. You'll delve into some new and fascinating information about mood—for example, that it doesn't always stem from faulty brain chemistry or events in your life. Other factors are at work, too, such as infectious diseases and infectious people.

You'll also discover what memory is, how it works, where it occurs in the brain, and you'll find out how to distinguish between ordinary memory lapses and Alzheimer's disease. You'll learn about all sorts of state-of-the-art brain tests that can pinpoint with amazing accuracy what might be going on in your head. Finally, you'll see that the aging brain isn't just getting older, it's getting wiser, too.

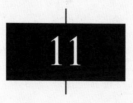

The Mind Connections

Whatever makes your brain maintain intellectual vigor throughout your lifetime is a "mind connection." Listening to music, learning to play a musical instrument, mastering a foreign language, staying socially plugged in, and other fun activities—these all build new connections in your brain and keep it active throughout your lifetime. In this chapter, you'll learn a host of secrets for keeping your mind physically and intellectually fit.

What's Your IQ?

Intelligence is the measurement of your ability to think through problems and come up with successful solutions. The question is: Do you lose it as you get older?

(Continued)

Not really. The latest word on intelligence comes from a growing body of evidence suggesting that if you stay mentally active over your lifetime, you'll retain your intelligence and may even boost it, particularly in the areas of information and vocabulary.

You can easily find out what your IQ is in a mere five or twelve minutes. Simply log on to www.brain.com and access the site's 5-Minute IQ Test or 12-Minute IQ Test. You'll be required to give your e-mail address so your scores can be sent to you.

Both IQ tests are "speeded" intelligence tests, meaning that you have an allotted amount of time in which to complete them. Speeded intelligence tests are being used more and more by clinicians as diagnostic tools to help identify brain disorders.

- The 5-Minute IQ Test measures mental quickness, also known as "fluid intelligence." During the test, you'll be asked to select the most appropriate word to complete short sentences. The test measures mostly vocabulary, verbal processing speed and accuracy, and correlates well with standardized IQ tests.

- The 12-Minute IQ Test is a conventional type of IQ test. Like standardized IQ tests, it measures "crystallized intelligence," which refers to the knowledge you've acquired through education and experience, as well as your ability to apply it. The fifty-question test assesses your verbal, math, and spatial reasoning, plus your problem-solving skills.

Both tests were developed in the United States and incorporate commonly used words and phrases found in American English. If you're not a native speaker of American English or grew up in a household where English was not spoken, your score may not be an accurate reflection of your true IQ. According to Brain.com, neither test is to be used as a medical or diagnostic tool.

RAISE SMART KIDS: 30 RECOMMENDATIONS

It's every parent's fondest desire: to have a child who's among the best and the brightest. What does it take to have a bright child? Are some children just born geniuses, or can intelligence be shaped?

While genetics does play a role in a child's brain growth and mental development, research shows that numerous other factors have a tremendous influence on your child's intellectual capacity and performance. With that in mind, here are thirty things you can do to raise a smarter child, starting in the womb and beyond.

AVOID ALCOHOL WHEN PREGNANT

Raising smart kids starts when they're in the womb. If you're pregnant or planning a pregnancy, abstain from drinking alcohol. Children exposed to alcohol before they are born are slower at information processing, have difficulty with problem solving, have trouble figuring math problems, and generally have difficulties performing in school, according to a growing body of research. Alcohol exposure during pregnancy can lead to fetal alcohol syndrome (FAS), which causes deficits in growth, physical structure, and central nervous system functioning.

QUIT SMOKING

Kids whose moms smoked at conception have lower IQs, according to researchers at the University of Bergen in Norway. Published in the *Archives of Disease in Childhood* in 2001, their report noted that maternal smoking tends to result in smaller-than-normal infants, a condition associated with lower intelligence. The researchers found that children, tested at age five, who were smaller than normal scored three to four points lower than those with an average birth weight.

HAVE YOUR THYROID LEVELS CHECKED

An underactive thyroid gland, medically termed hypothyroidism, could compromise your baby's intellectual development, according to the study from the Foundation for Blood Research in Scarborough, Maine. Investigators also discovered that, compared to mothers without the deficiency, women with undiagnosed hypothyroidism were four times as likely to have babies with lower-than-average IQ scores.

One out of fifty pregnant women has hypothyroidism, so it's a good idea to be screened prenatally for the disorder. Hypothyroidism is easily treated with synthetic thyroxin, a hormone that is normally produced by the thyroid gland.

"WOO" YOUR INFANT

In the first few months of life, the beginning of learning takes place as an infant learns to distinguish Mommy and Daddy from other people. To facilitate this learning, child-development experts recommend that you let your baby play with your nose or other part of your face, as well as with rattles and other toys.

PROVIDE A STIMULATING ENVIRONMENT FOR YOUR BABY

Throughout your child's formative years, trillions of connections (synapses) are formed between brain cells. The more synapses a child has, the faster information can be processed.

Crucial to learning, synapses are developed through stimulation: light, color, smell, and sound, for example. Because of this, many experts believe that by stimulating a baby's senses, you can boost his or her IQ.

Playing classical music, showing your baby colorful pictures or objects, and providing toys that can be touched and moved are ways that can encourage stimulation and supposedly develop a baby's brain. However, simply interacting with your baby through playing games like peek-a-boo or singing to your child also provides stimulation that fosters intellectual growth.

TOUCH AND CUDDLE

There's an amazing emotional component to brain development in infants. Case in point: Investigators at Baylor College of Medicine in Houston discovered that children who were rarely played with or touched as babies develop brains 20- to 30-percent smaller than normal for their age. By contrast, babies who were cuddled frequently have 25 percent more brain connections than understimulated infants, according to other research. A mother's touch triggers the release of hormones in a baby's brain that helps it grow.

Clearly, this research indicates an emotional component in brain development. The take-home message is touch, play with, and love your baby.

BREAST-FEED YOUR BABY

Research indicates that children gain three to eight IQ points by age three if they were breast-fed as infants. One study found that breast-fed babies have a 38-percent greater likelihood of completing their high school education than formula-fed babies.

Why? Scientists believe that breast milk contains immune factors that protect children from diseases which diminish energy and tissue repair, factors that affect nervous system functioning, and healthy fats. Some researchers speculate that DHA, found naturally in breast milk, may also have an intelligence-boosting effect on babies. Studies confirm that breast-fed infants have higher levels of DHA in their brains than do formula-fed babies.

SING TO YOUR BABY

Singing to your infant has been shown in research to stimulate the brain to start building strong language circuits.

ENGAGE TODDLERS IN
CHALLENGING INTERACTIONS

As they approach the toddler stage, children begin learning more about the world around them and how to use ideas. To encourage learning at this level, engage your child in more complex interactions. If your child wants a cookie, for example, have him guide you to the pantry and point to what he wants. As you see your child start to use toys in more creative ways—such as having dolls socialize or interact—get involved in the interaction by being a "guest" at a tea party, for example, with your child and the other dolls. This helps bolster creativity and communication skills.

BE A TALKATIVE MOM

Engage your kids in conversation. It helps develop their brainpower. Evidence for this comes from research showing that kids who aren't getting enough stimulation at home lag behind academically. At the University of Kansas, investigators discovered that mothers on welfare were less likely to converse with their toddlers. On average, a child in a welfare home heard 616 words an hour compared to 2,153 words in families where the heads of households were professionals.

Speech by a young child's mother helps build vocabulary, and vocabulary is a common component of IQ tests. In one study, psychologists at the University of Chicago taped moms interacting with their children, who were between the ages of sixteen and twenty-six months, a time when kids' language skills are developing very quickly. The tapings were conducted every two to four months. The toddlers who had the most talkative mothers had the largest vocabularies by the time they reached twenty-six months.

Baby Talk

Don't wait until your child becomes a toddler to strike up a conversation. Talk to your infant—and use "baby talk." Experts say baby talk—the singsong inflections we use around babies—holds an infant's interest much better than adult speech does. In fact, it helps babies learn the rules of language.

READ TO YOUR CHILDREN

Reading to your child helps foster a love of books and language and provides a wonderful time of bonding—all of which optimize a child's intellectual potential.

CHOOSE A STIMULATING
DAY-CARE ENVIRONMENT

Research shows that the quality of infant and toddler day-care programs can drastically affect IQ. So if your child must go to day care, make sure the program provides an enriching, stimulating environment with gamelike learning activities built into the day. These activities should help improve language, cognitive performance, and motor skills. In addition, look for a day-care program in which there is a small adult-to-children ratio, such as one to three for toddlers and one to six for preschoolers, so that your child gets enough attention.

Also worth mentioning: A recent study funded by the National Institute on Child Health and Human Development found that while children taken to day-care centers tended to be more disobedient than kids cared for at home, day-care children are more likely to develop better language skills and stronger short-term memory.

REDUCE STRESS IN YOUR HOUSEHOLD

Chronic stress can have a devastating effect on learning by elevating levels of cortisol, a stress hormone. Cortisol disrupts learning and may retard the growth of brain cells. Furthermore, research on stress in children has found that long-term family conflict interferes with the development of the hippocampus, the part of the brain that deals with learning and memory.

CREATE A NURTURING ENVIRONMENT

One of the most important ways to foster intelligence in your kids is to spend time with them—playing with them, conversing with them, loving them. Children who grow up in a secure, trusting, and loving relationship with their parents tend to be smarter, better adjusted, and more intelligent. When children feel valued, they want to become the best they can at whatever they set out to do.

EXPOSE CHILDREN TO A WIDE VARIETY OF THINGS IN THE WORLD

Along with a nurturing environment, create a stimulating one for your kids—lots of music playing, and things that children can touch, smell, taste, and see. In addition, take them on sightseeing trips to local museums, county fairs, concerts, parks, and other attractions. All of these activities help develop smarter, more well-rounded children, say child-development experts.

SHARE YOUR INTERESTS WITH YOUR CHILDREN

One of the best ways to foster talent and intelligence in your kids is to present and model your interests to them. Children are more likely to develop an interest in a hobby, musical instrument, academic subject, sport, or other activity if they see their parents do it and genuinely enjoy it.

In a study at the University of Chicago conducted in the 1980s, researchers interviewed 120 highly talented men and women and their parents to pinpoint how they became so gifted. The subjects in the study ran the gamut from Olympic swimmers to concert pianists to neurologists. Interestingly, the parents had all shared their interests with their children, practically from the day they were born. This all goes to show that talent isn't something we are necessarily born with or beat into us by pushy parents but more often is a result of a loving environment in which various activities are modeled in a positive way.

FOSTER CREATIVITY

Look for cues as to what interests your children. If they spend a lot of time drawing or coloring, give them additional materials to help them do this. Or, if they like music, give them lessons. Another idea: Grab your video camera, script a movie with your kids' ideas, and cast them in roles.

In short, provide your kids with the resources—materials, exposure to art shows or concerts, summer workshops—that will give them opportunities to develop. Equally important: Listen and pay attention to your children when they're singing, coloring, and creating, and never criticize or critique their efforts.

BE AN INVOLVED DAD

A growing body of evidence indicates that fathers are crucial to a child's development, contrary to popular sentiment emphasizing a less significant role in their children's lives. Family researchers have found that the way fathers play with their kids involves more games and teamwork, healthy competition, risk-taking, and independence—all of which foster academic achievement. Furthermore, studies indicate that children who have healthy relationships with their fathers do better academically as well as in their chosen professions.

FEED YOUR CHILDREN WELL

Strive to prepare menus made from natural, wholesome foods, particularly meals free of preservatives, dyes, and colorings. In an intriguing analysis of 1 million kids enrolled in the New York City school system, there was a 14-percent improvement in IQ scores after additives, preservatives, dyes, artificial flavorings, and colorings were removed from their lunches. So one factor that improves IQ scores among kids is better nutrition.

AVOID DELAYED SCHOOLING

In a study of the intellectual capacity of children of Indian descent in South Africa, investigators found that for each year of delayed schooling, the children experienced a decrease in five IQ points. Similar findings have been reported among American children.

BE INVOLVED IN YOUR CHILDREN'S SCHOOL

Know your kids' teachers and be aware and supportive of what's going on at school and in the classroom. Involvement sends a message to your kids that education is important and that you care about them.

HELP YOUR CHILDREN WITH THEIR HOMEWORK

Helping your children with their homework shows that you care about their academic performance and want them to excel. But doing homework for them makes your kids intellectually lazy. So don't do it for them.

ENCOURAGE YOUR CHILDREN TO EXERCISE

Physically active kids do better in school, according to nearly fifty years of educational research. Sports and exercise build self-esteem, which translates into greater confidence in academic ability; promotes the development of more brain connections (synapses), which are critical to learning and memory; and increases the number of capillaries in the brain for an increased supply of blood, oxygen, and nutrients.

INVOLVE CHILDREN IN DECISION MAKING

Get older children involved in such decisions as where to go on vacation. Ask them to come up with the advantages and disadvantages of various choices so that they experience decision making firsthand. This type of interaction helps kids learn how to problem-solve and better equips them for life.

ENROLL YOUR CHILDREN IN CHOIR
OR MUSIC LESSONS

You can increase your preschooler's intelligence by enrolling him or her in group singing activities (such as choir) or in keyboard instruction. That's the finding of a study conducted at the University of California at Irvine in which preschoolers who participated in such programs dramatically enhanced their ability to perform complicated math and science exercises.

Other studies demonstrate that training in music at an early age exercises higher-brain functions such as complex reasoning; stimulates the formation of connections (synapses); and promotes the growth of branches (dendrites) in the brain. Learning musical skills also helps kids develop in other intellectual areas such as math, language, and spatial reasoning.

BE OPEN TO YEAR-ROUND SCHOOLING

If the school system in your community is considering year-round school, don't pooh-pooh the idea. Increasingly, researchers have found that IQ in kids is negatively affected by summer vacations: IQ scores decline with each passing month over the summer. The decline is worse for kids who are less academically inclined. The bottom line is schooling increases IQ.

LOOK INTO HOMESCHOOLING

The fastest-growing alternative to public education is homeschooling, in which parents teach their kids at home using specially designed curricula. As a group, homeschooled children score significantly higher on standardized tests than students in public or private schools, according to a growing body of studies.

If you are considering homeschooling, talk to parents who homeschool and find out what materials have worked best for them; contact local and national homeschooling organizations to identify programs and resources to help you; conduct an Internet search for information on materials, teaching methods, and other activities; and talk to librarians about books, programs, and resources that are helpful to homeschooling families.

ENCOURAGE FURTHER SCHOOLING

Set an expectation that your kids will go to college. For each year of schooling completed, a child gains 3.5 IQ points. What's more, people who have completed more school tend to generate more earning power. For example, college grads currently earn $812,000 more than high school dropouts over a lifetime; people with professional degrees earn $1,600,000 more than college graduates.

GET SMART YOURSELF

Better-educated parents tend to produce smarter kids with higher IQs—so consider going back to school yourself. Not only may it boost your child's academic performance but it also sets a good example.

LET KIDS BE KIDS

Kids used to go to school, come home, play, do a little homework, and go to bed. Now they're shuttled off to ballet, soccer, music lessons, and so forth, or they may have to stay at school longer in an after-care program waiting to be picked up by Mom or Dad. Kids these days are as busy as grown-ups. While such activities have their value, they can create pressure—and the mind-numbing stress that goes along with it.

Child-development experts recommend that parents strive for balance between activities and quality family time. Spending time with kids helps develop social skills such as sharing and interacting with other children. When kids master these skills, they learn reading, writing, and other academic skills much more readily. Give your kids some down time so they don't get overstimulated. Fussing, wriggling out of your arms, throwing a tantrum, or refusing to participate in an activity are signs that your child needs a break.

Your Brain on Music:
5 Reasons Why Your Mind Needs
a Dose of Musical Medicine

There's an incredibly easy and fun way to boost your mindpower—something that many of us are already doing and loving: listening to music.

Exposure to music has a rather astounding effect on intelligence. In a groundbreaking study at the University of California at Irvine, researchers had thirty-six undergraduate students listen to ten minutes of a piano sonata by Mozart, then take a standard intelligence test. After listening to Mozart, the students scored eight to nine points higher on the spatial IQ section, which tests the ability to recognize objects visually, form mental images of them, and decipher variations among them. They did not score as high when the test was preceded by a period of silence or mental relaxation.

The outcome of this experiment has since become known as the "Mozart Effect." The same researchers have tested it in Alzheimer's patients, with impressive improvements in thinking and reasoning.

Listening to classical compositions, such as Mozart's, is believed to excite and enhance firing patterns in the brain that are used to process and execute complex tasks that require advanced reasoning, such as math and engineering.

But music does more to the mind than just make it smarter. What follows is a closer look into five other reasons your brain needs a dose of musical medicine.

MUSIC EXERCISES YOUR BRAIN

It's not just listening to music that's good for your brain. Playing a musical instrument gives your brain a terrific workout, too, because it involves vision, hearing, touch, motor coordination, and symbol interpretation—faculties and skills that activate different brain systems.

MUSIC BUILDS YOUR BRAIN

Imaging studies of the brains of musicians have revealed that musical experience enlarges an area on the left side of the brain that is associated with processing sounds. So if you are a musician or plan to learn to play an instrument, you'll build your brain.

MUSIC INCREASES BLOOD FLOW
TO YOUR BRAIN

Research has demonstrated that rhythmical music, in particular, boosts blood flow to both hemispheres of the brain. Increased blood flow aids in concentration, memory, and other mental tasks.

MUSIC HELPS YOU SLEEP BETTER

If you're having trouble sleeping, try listening to classical music prior to tucking in. When twenty-five elderly patients with sleep problems listened to classical music right before bedtime, all but one reported improved sleep during the night, according to a 1994 study published in the *Journal of Holistic Nursing*. Improved sleep helps ward off numerous mind-numbing problems: lack of alertness, depression, and stress, to name just a few.

MUSIC IMPROVES MOBILITY IN
PARKINSON'S DISEASE AND STROKE

Listening to rhythmic music improves motor coordination of Parkinson's patients and those recovering from stroke, helping them walk up to 50-percent faster. That's the finding of a study in which patients walked faster, more steadily, and with better balance when they synchronized their movement with music that had a strong rhythm. Thus, music therapy can be an important component of physical rehabilitation to stimulate and regulate movement.

WHY YOU SHOULD MASTER
A FOREIGN LANGUAGE

Something rather amazing happens to your brain if you learn a foreign language as an adult: A new brain region is created.

Scientists have long known that people who learn a new language when they're teenagers or adults have two brain regions for generating complex speech, one for each language. By contrast, infants who learn two languages simultaneously have a single brain region for both languages.

The evidence for two language regions was first observed in bilingual epileptics who, during seizures, lost their ability to speak in one language but not the other. Similarly, stroke victims may lose their ability to speak a foreign language but still be able to speak in their native tongue.

As reported in a study published in *Nature* in 1997, scientists at Memorial Sloan-Kettering Cancer Center in New York City used magnetic resonance imaging (MRI) to peer into the brains of twelve bilingual people, half of whom had learned two languages as babies. The other half had learned a second language around age eleven. The subjects were asked to think about their day's activity, first using one language, then the other, while undergoing MRI scanning. The scan pinpointed where the thinking occurred by ascertaining changes in blood flow.

What the scientists observed was fascinating: Subjects who had acquired a second language during adolescence had two distinct regions in a part of the brain known as Broca's area. Those who were bilingual since infancy had a single area.

Named after its discoverer, French surgeon Pierre Paul Broca, Broca's area is a part of the brain involved in speech as well as in some grammatical aspects of language. Sentences are first created in an area of the brain called Wernicke's area (so named after a German neurologist, Carl Wernicke, who identified it), then sent as a signal to Broca's area, which tells your tongue and vocal cords to make the sounds.

Scientists believe that babies are able to distinguish sounds from several languages and that the neuron connections in their brains become hard-wired, or fixed, for the languages they hear during their first year of life. In people who have been bilingual from birth, the two languages seem to be crystallized and comingled in Broca's area. Thus, the complex speech sounds of both languages are naturally embedded in the brain.

Let's assume you're not bilingual but want to master French. To do so, you must learn all sorts of new skills in order to produce the complex speech patterns of the new language. Your Broca's area is wired for American English only. But as you learn French, an auxiliary Broca's area forms in your brain—a phenomenon observed in the Sloan-Kettering study. So, in a sense, learning a second language as an adult is a terrific brain-builder.

That's certainly a good reason for learning another language, but there are others:

- You'll get the best out of visiting a foreign country if you know the language.
- Communicating with another person in his or her native language is a good way to break down barriers.
- You'll learn more about grammar, which you may have forgotten, and this will improve your written and spoken communication.
- Knowing another language helps cement business deals if you're conducting business internationally.
- Fluency in another language increases your job prospects.

8 Unusual Ways to Master a New Language

1. Live in the country where the language is spoken. If your employer has offices overseas, ask for a transfer to a foreign country. Or volunteer to serve in a foreign country or become an exchange student.
2. Watch foreign films or television shows.
3. Keep a diary or journal in the language you're learning. That way, you'll use the language every day.

4. Recite poetry in the language you're learning.
5. Read children's books written in foreign languages.
6. Listen to—and sing—songs in the foreign language you're learning. Research indicates that foreign-language music helps you better learn and reinforce the words, grammar, and language structure of the new language.
7. Find a foreign pen pal through www.epals.com.
8. Participate in language chat rooms that let you converse in real time with people from other countries.

His Brain/Her Brain: New Discoveries About How Men and Women Really Think

The anatomical differences between men and women are not only the obvious physical differences we see but also what we don't see: in the brain.

The differences mainly involve the corpus callosum, a band of tissue connecting the right and left hemispheres of the brain. In men, the corpus callosum is less dense, a phenomenon that initially occurs while a male baby is developing in the womb, when the male hormone testosterone is produced. Testosterone mildly damages nerve fibers in the corpus callosum, leaving male infants with less nerve tissue. In female infants, that nerve tissue is left intact.

Further, the male corpus callosum tends to shrink with age. It does not shrink in women, however. And some areas of women's brains contain more neurons than corresponding areas of men's brains, even though, overall, men have more neurons than women. These differences have been detected mostly in studies using the donated brains of cancer victims as well as in imaging studies of babies as they develop in their mothers' wombs.

But what do these physical differences actually mean?

For one thing, they may explain why men have trouble expressing emotions. The corpus callosum is involved in communication between the two halves of the brain. A man's smaller corpus callosum may mean that information flows less fluidly from the right side to the verbal left side, which controls emotional expression. So when your husband or boyfriend doesn't express his love often enough, it may be due to brain anatomy rather than to problems in your relationship.

Research into the brain anatomy of men and women is part of a growing body of studies suggesting that the mental divide between the sexes may be rooted more in fundamental biology than in social conditioning. Here's a look at what other brain-sex studies have discovered.

MEN USE HALF THEIR BRAINS AT TIMES

For some types of mental activity, men use only a portion of their brains, while women use both left and right hemispheres. This was observed in a Yale study in which investigators electronically monitored men's and women's brains as the subjects were asked to match nonsense words such as "jete" and "lete."

During the test, a half-inch portion of the men's brains, near the left temple, was active, while in women, mental activity was spread throughout the brain. Because both sexes performed equally well on the test, the experiment suggests that male and female brains work at a similar capacity but process information differently.

Basically, women seem to draw on both sides of their brains when they read rhyme or do verbal tasks, while men use left-brain regions exclusively. In practical terms, this may explain why girls usually speak sooner than boys and learn to read more easily. In addition, women regain their speech abilities faster than men after suffering strokes that damage the left side of the brain, hinting that women can better use other regions of the brain to compensate.

WOMEN POSSESS BETTER VERBAL SKILLS

Women have the edge over men when it comes to verbal skills. Research shows that girls have significantly superior writing skills and higher reading comprehension scores than boys. As adults, women are better at certain language puzzles.

MEN ARE BETTER AT THINKING IN THREE DIMENSIONS

Men have an advantage over women in visual-spatial abilities (the ability to mentally picture and manipulate three-dimensional objects) and mathematical reasoning. This observation is supported by a growing catalog of studies showing that only 20 percent of American girls in elementary school attain the average level of performance of boys in spatial ability.

As adults, men are better at mathematical reasoning and playing games involving projectiles (like darts). In men, the right side of the brain appears to be dominant, which may explain their well-developed spatial and reasoning abilities.

In addition, men are more skilled at mentally rotating objects to solve a problem (a skill indicating that you have a good sense of direction).

Does this mean that women are more prone to getting lost?

Not at all. Read on.

WOMEN HAVE BETTER MEMORIES

Women usually perform better than men on tests of recall and generally have better memories. Because of this memory advantage, women are better at remembering the placement of objects and the location of landmarks, enabling them to better locate destinations.

MEN ARE MORE VISUAL

A man's visual cortex is larger than a woman's, which means that men respond more quickly to things they see. This may also explain why a man is attracted more to a woman's looks—at least initially—than to her personality.

WOMEN ARE MORE COORDINATED

That's because a man has fewer connections in his cerebral cortex, a brain center associated with movement and coordination.

MALE AND FEMALE BRAINS AGE DIFFERENTLY

With age, men lose brain cells at rates up to three times faster than women. However, men have more brain cells to lose, so the biological significance of this phenomenon is not yet known.

WHAT THIS ALL MEANS

The actual physical differences between the male and the female brain do not mean that either sex is unequal or inferior but that each processes information differently.

So the next time you're frustrated over poor communication with your spouse, boyfriend, girlfriend, or opposite-sex coworker or boss, remember: Men and women are wired to think differently, and this results in major differences in perceptions, thought, emotional expressions, and behavior.

DIAGNOSING BRAIN DISORDERS: 7 TESTS PERFORMED IN YOUR DOCTOR'S OFFICE

Suddenly and without warning, you start experiencing some worrisome symptoms: poor balance, frequent dizziness, unusual headaches, blackouts, memory loss, or disorientation. Such symptoms point to a brain disorder, but how do you know for sure?

Only your physician can properly diagnose a brain disorder. For starters, he or she will require information obtained from your medical history and the symptoms you report. Next, your physician will conduct a neurological examination. This examination is usually the first test given if you complain of headaches, blurred vision, tingling sensations, blackouts, memory loss, and other symptoms that may point to a brain disorder. It involves a series of simple tests and is usually conducted by your physician in his or her office.

During this exam, your physician will check several nervous system functions, including the following:

1. *Tendon reflexes*. To evaluate nerve functions, spinal cord connections, and nerve conditions, your physician will stimulate your reflexes by tapping your knee or ankle lightly with a special rubber-tipped hammer.
2. *Babinski reflex*. Your physician will lightly stroke the bottom of your foot. If this produces an involuntary movement of your big toe, there may be an abnormality in the neuron circuits that originate in the brain.
3. *Muscle strength*. Your physician will test your muscles for any weakness, which can be a sign of a neurological disorder.
4. *Muscle tone*. Your physician will look for spasms, rigidity, or flaccidity, all of which could indicate problems in nerves that stimulate various muscle groups.
5. *Sensory function*. Your physician will evaluate your ability to experience nerve-conducted sensations such as pain, heat, touch, and vibration by asking you what you feel when touched by various types of objects. Your taste, smell, and hearing will be evaluated as well.
6. *Balance and coordination*. Your physician will check your gait, posture, coordination, and sense of balance by asking you to stand, walk, or move your body in a particular way.
7. *Mental state and memory*. You may be asked questions that help your physician evaluate your thinking, judgment, attention span, and memory. (See Table 11.1.)

If abnormalities are detected, your physician may order further tests such as blood tests or imaging tests (in which x-ray or other technologies are used to view the brain) that can provide a more definitive diagnosis.

TABLE 11.1

What's Your Mental State?

To check for signs of cognitive problems, your doctor will test your mental state and memory by probing in the following areas.

AREAS TESTED	PURPOSE OF TEST	WHAT YOUR DOCTOR WILL ASK	WHAT ABNORMAL RESULTS MAY MEAN
Orientation	To evaluate your sense of time, place, and person.	Questions pertaining to time, date, and season; where you live; the type of building you're in; the city and state where you live; your name, age, and occupation.	Alcohol or drug intoxication; low blood sugar; concussion; nutritional imbalances; fever; environmental illness (such as heat stroke); brain disease.
Attention Span	To check for attention-deficit problems, confusion, depression, and other mental problems.	Your doctor will test your ability to complete a thought by observing your conversation or asking you to follow a series of instructions.	Attention-deficit disorder; confusion; depression; or other mental disorders.
Memory, recent	To assess your memory of people, places, and events that have occurred recently.	Questions pertaining to people you've met recently, places you've visited, and recent activities.	Brain disease if long-term memory remains intact.
Memory, long-term	To assess your memory of people, places, and events that happened earlier in your life.	Questions about your childhood, school, or historical events.	Alzheimer's disease; dementia.

Areas Tested	Purpose of Test	What Your Doctor Will Ask	What Abnormal Results May Mean
Word Comprehension	To test your knowledge of everyday items.	Your doctor will point to everyday items in the room and ask you to identify them.	Alzheimer's disease; dementia; brain injury; stroke.
Judgment	To evaluate your judgment and ability to apply alternative solutions to a problem or situation.	Questions that ask you what you would do in a given situation, such as: "What would you do if you found someone's wallet on the ground?"	Brain disease; emotional dysfunction; schizophrenia; mental retardation.

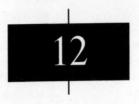

What Makes Your Mood?

Have you ever felt like an emotional basket case for no apparent reason, even when everything in your life is humming along perfectly? Can you blame it on a full moon, or is something else going on?

Don't worry, you're not crazy. There are a couple of common but unwitting perpetrators that can make you feel down in the mouth. In this chapter, you will learn how to deal with them, plus find out how to join the ranks of the most content and fulfilled people on Earth.

THE CONNECTION BETWEEN INFECTION AND MENTAL ILLNESS: HOW TO PROTECT YOURSELF

Mental illness is caused by a variety of factors: abnormalities in genes, brain chemistry imbalances, or things that happen in your life (environmental factors). Add to that list an unlikely source: infections.

The bacteria and viruses that invade our bodies and cause the flu, sore throats, and other ailments can inflict damage on our brains as well. This invasion of the brain snatchers can result in a host of mental illnesses including schizophrenia, obsessive-compulsive disorder, anxiety, and dementia.

What follows is a brief overview of bacteria and viruses that have emerged as culprits in various types of psychological illnesses—and what you can do to fend them off.

CHLAMYDIA PNEUMONIA

Chlamydia pneumonia is among the pathogens that cause pneumonia and other respiratory diseases. It has also been implicated in Alzheimer's disease. Scientists have found this pathogen in specific areas of the brain affected by Alzheimer's disease, where it sets off an inflammatory response that injures brain cells; however, more research into a possible association is needed. Fortunately, chlamydia pneumonia responds very well to treatment with antibiotics, which halt the inflammatory response and rid the body of the infection.

CREUTZFELDT-JAKOB DISEASE

Otherwise known as "mad cow disease," Creutzfeldt-Jakob disease is caused by a "prion," or infectious protein, which acts in the same manner as a virus. It is transmitted by eating contaminated meat, through organ transplants, and through the contamination of surgical instruments. The disease causes brain-cell death and leads to dementia. There is no known cure for Creutzfeldt-Jakob disease.

HUMAN IMMUNODEFICIENCY VIRUS (HIV)

This virus causes AIDS (acquired immune deficiency syndrome). Transmitted through sexual intercourse, shared needles among intravenous drug users, or from infected mother to unborn child, HIV infects immune cells called macrophages. Macrophages are "search and destroy" cells that are on the lookout for foreign invaders, particularly bacteria and tumor cells that can harm the body.

HIV attaches itself to macrophages and travels into the brain, where it starts churning out cytokines that decimate brain cells. The result can be anxiety, confusion, and psychosis. There is no cure for HIV infection or AIDS, although the infection can be treated with a combination of various types of drugs.

INFLUENZA

Scientists believe that a mother-to-be, infected with the influenza ("flu") virus, may transmit the bug to her unborn child, increasing the risk of later development of schizophrenia in that child. The evidence for this comes from studies of flu outbreaks in various countries, followed a generation later by a rise in schizophrenia.

Apparently the virus works its way into the fetal brain at a key point in its development, damaging neural connections. The damage does not manifest itself until the brain reaches full maturity in early adulthood. The result is shrinkage of the cortex, thalamus, and basal ganglia—all parts of the brain affected in schizophrenia.

STREPTOCOCCAL BACTERIA

The same bacteria that cause strep throat—streptococcal bacteria— may also lead to obsessive-compulsive disorder (OCD), particularly in susceptible people. These bacteria attack the body in a rather strange way. Upon invasion, they mobilize the body's antibody force but hide themselves inside proteins that resemble the body's own proteins, thereby dodging attack.

In certain people, especially children who have underdeveloped immune systems, the antibodies mistakenly attack the body's own tissue, including cells in the basal ganglia, a group of small structures within the brain concerned with voluntary movement. The basal ganglia are also involved in emotions and thinking.

TREPONEMA PALLIDUM

This bacterium causes syphilis, a three-stage bacterial disease transmitted by sexual contact or through infected blood. The final stage of the disease can produce depression, dementia, mania, and delusions.

After entering the body through sexual intercourse or from an infected mother to her unborn child, treponema pallidum travels through the lymph system—a secondary circulatory system in the body—until it reaches the brain. There, it inflames nerve cells and erodes the myelin sheath, a tube that envelops nerves. Without this sheath, nerve cells neither heal nor regenerate themselves if damaged. Consequently, they cease to function.

A diagnosis of syphilis can be confirmed by blood tests. If caught early and treated appropriately (with antibiotics), syphilis can be completely cured. But, if left untreated, the disease leads to death.

WHAT YOU CAN DO

Thankfully, not everyone who gets a bug will suffer mental illness, because our immune systems protects us from most infections. The most vulnerable, however, are those with weakened immune systems, children, people in poor health, and, quite possibly, individuals with a genetic susceptibility.

The best way to protect yourself from infectious brain snatchers is to follow standard commonsense advice and to fortify your body with some special immune-boosting supplements. Here's what you can do:

- Stick to a nutritious diet that emphasizes natural foods and antioxidant supplements. How sick you get as a result of a bacterial or viral infection depends partly on your overall health and immune strength.
- Eat cultured foods such as yogurt and sauerkraut. These supply beneficial bacteria that protect your body against disease-causing bacteria and boost immune functioning.

- Get plenty of sleep.
- Reduce stress.
- Understand that having multiple sex partners increases your risk of infection.
- Wash your hands properly to reduce your chances of contracting an infection and spreading it to others.
- Have a flu shot, which is recommended for people age sixty-five or older, anyone with a chronic heart or lung conditions, and those living in institutions. Flu shots have a 60- to 70-percent success rate in preventing infection.
- If you're pregnant, take special precautions to avoid infection.

Bugs

Another avenue of protection is to take special immune-boosting supplements to enhance your immune system. These include:

1. Alkylglycerols, found in shark liver oil extract, beef up the immune system by activating macrophages. *Suggested daily dosage for immune support and disease prevention:* two to three 250-milligram capsules.
2. Astralagus is an Asian herb that stimulates germ-fighting white blood cells. *Suggested daily dosage:* 35 drops of the liquid extract in teas or soups, or follow dosage recommendations on the label.
3. Garlic has antibacterial and antiviral properties. *Suggested daily dosage:* two to three capsules.
4. Maitake mushroom extract fights viral infections. Other mushrooms with immune-boosting power include shitake and reishi. *Suggested daily dosage:* Follow label directions.
5. N-acetyl cysteine (NAC), a form of the amino acid cysteine, increases bodily levels of glutathione, an antioxidant vital for a healthy immune system. In addition, research shows that NAC can reduce the severity of flu symptoms. *Suggested daily dosage for preventing infections:* one 300-milligram capsule.

6. Probiotics such as acidophilus help restore and maintain healthy, disease-fighting bacteria in the intestines. *Suggested daily dosage:* Follow label directions.

7. Prebiotics are a type of starch that arrives in your colon undigested and nourishes health-building bacteria such as *Lactobacillus* and *Bifidobacteria. Suggested daily dosage:* ¾ teaspoon (3 grams) in powder or capsules.

8 Ways to Cope with Toxic People

Just as germs can infect your mood, so can people—your coworkers, relatives, even some of the people you hang out with on a regular basis. They're people who are rude, insensitive, negative, abusive, depressed, good put-down artists, or all of the above.

Some researchers who study depression and other mood states believe that certain people can be "mood transmitters" or "mood receivers." When you're in the same room with a mood transmitter, that person, if depressed or anxious, can subconsciously transmit those negative mood states to you. Consequently, you "catch" a case of the blues just as if you had caught a cold. Your susceptibility to catching depression in this manner is heightened if you're a "mood receiver," someone who is easily influenced by the changing moods of people around you.

Given the potential seriousness of toxic people on your mood, how can you inoculate yourself? Here are eight tips:

1. Counter their gloom with a genuine upbeat attitude.

2. When someone puts you down, adopt a feel-sorry-for-them mindset: Remember that he is insecure, trying to make himself feel good by putting you down. Or maybe she's clinically depressed and not totally responsible for her behavior.

3. Let a "woe-is-me" person rant on until he or she runs out of things to say. If she asks why you've been silent, tell her: "I've been waiting for *my* turn."

4. Forgive. Forgiveness releases you from the bonds of negative emotions.

(Continued)

5. Be firm. If someone bullies you, tell the person you don't allow people to treat you that way.
6. Rather than dwelling on a person's negativity, see if you can uncover something that is there to like.
7. Avoid toxic people if all else fails.
8. Study up on toxic people. Several authors have written about this phenomenon. Three of the best reads are *Thank You for Being Such a Pain: Spiritual Guidance for Dealing with Difficult People* by Mark Rosen (Crown Publishers, 1999); *Toxic People: 10 Ways of Dealing with People Who Make Your Life Miserable* by Lillian Glass (St. Martin's Press, 1997); and *Contagious Emotions: Staying Well When Your Loved One Is Depressed* by Ronald M. Podell (Pocket Books, 1993).

GET RELIGION: 5 ASTOUNDING REASONS WHY THE FAITHFUL ARE LESS DEPRESSED AND MORE FULFILLED

A rather remarkable hedge against depression is religion. At least fifty scientific studies have found that religious commitment—defined as participation in and endorsement of a set of beliefs associated with an organized community of faith—works wonders in averting depression, curing it, and preventing its most tragic outcome, suicide. Here's a look at five scientific facts.

1. **People of faith are less likely to get depressed.**

   A string of scientific evidence suggests that if you're a person of faith and committed to your religious beliefs, you'll have a lower risk of depression. The reason, according to researchers, is that having faith fills you with peace and hope—feelings that reduce stress, anxiety, and depression—and links you to a community of people who will love and support you, an atmosphere that is good for your body and soul.

2. **People with no religious affiliation appear to be at an elevated risk for depression, compared to those who are affiliated with a religion.**

People without a religious affiliation (about 8 percent of the U.S. population) are more prone to depression, according to several studies. When researchers at Duke University, for example, assessed 850 medically ill men, aged sixty-five and older, they discovered that those who had no religious connection had a greater number of depressive symptoms than men who identified themselves as Protestants, Catholics, or nondenominational Christians.

3. **People of faith are less likely to commit suicide.**

The most severe and tragic outcome of depression is suicide. In fact, 15 percent of all depressed people kill themselves, according to studies.

A bright silver lining in this heart-wrenching statistic is religious commitment. Research has consistently found that having religious faith protects against depression-related suicide. One study of suicide victims found that people who did not attend church were four times more likely to kill themselves than regular churchgoers. And several studies have documented a link between increases in suicide rates nationwide and a corresponding national decline in church attendance.

4. **People of faith bounce back more quickly from depression.**

Few events in life are as depressing as being diagnosed with a serious or life-threatening illness. Religion, however, can help you cope with a health problem and get over the depression that accompanies it.

Case in point: A Duke University study of eighty-seven patients, all aged sixty and older, found that depressed medical patients to whom religion was important recovered much faster from depression than those who were less religious. Harold G. Koenig, M.D., one of the lead researchers of this study, shed light on this finding in an article he wrote for the *Harvard Mental Health Letter:* "The reports of patients suggest that it [religious faith] gives suffering a meaning and purpose or promotes a sense of control that stimulates recovery."

5. **People of faith are less likely to abuse alcohol.**

Today, alcohol is the most abused drug in the United States. Ten percent of users are addicted, and 10 to 20 percent are abusers or problem drinkers. A major problem with alcohol is that it is a depressant that can make your mood plummet.

Several studies have found that religious commitment is linked to a lower incidence of alcohol and drug abuse. When surveying a group of alcoholics about their religious backgrounds, Duke researchers learned that 89 percent of the alcoholics had lost interest in religion during their teenage years.

In another study, Dr. Koenig and his research team investigated the relationship between religion and alcohol dependence among 3,000 North Carolina residents aged eighteen and older and discovered that recent and lifetime alcohol problems were less frequent among weekly churchgoers and among people who considered themselves born-again Christians.

WHAT THIS MEANS TO YOU

If you're already among the faithful, count your blessings: Your beliefs and commitment are helping you handle the inevitable ups and downs of life and are protecting you against depression. Continue to pray—individually and with others; attend religious services; and read the Bible or other sacred texts that are important in the context of your religion.

On the other hand, if you've parted from religious beliefs and practices, it may be time to embark on a soul-searching journey. Consider reconnecting with the faith of your youth or finding a faith that gives you everlasting hope and security.

Menopause: 5 Strategies
for Managing Mood Swings

If your moods start to teeter-totter for no apparent reason, you could be entering menopause, a natural stage in life that marks the end of your reproductive years.

These troubling changes in your emotional climate are tied to the sudden dropoff in estrogen, a decline that affects the normal ebb and flow of neurotransmitters. Happily, though, these mood swings are short-lived. As your body adjusts to its lower levels of estrogen, they dissipate. In other words, you're not doomed to a lifetime of depression, anxiety, and irritability. Life events such as retirement and loss of youth and attractiveness may also be involved in causing mood swings during this period of your life.

Whatever the cause, you can restore your mental and emotional balance and start feeling better in no time—and do so naturally. Here's a look at five natural mood-stabilizing strategies that really work.

1. Boost your intake of natural carbohydrates.

    Eating natural unrefined carbohydrates such as whole grains, legumes, potatoes, and yams throughout the day helps elevate levels of mood-enhancing serotonin in your brain. When combined with protein, they also help stabilize blood sugar to keep your mood on a more even keel. Therefore, populate your diet with ample carbohydrates when you need a natural mood boost.

2. Try mood-lifting herbs.

    Several herbs are notable for their proven ability to help manage the emotional changes brought on by menopause. They include St. John's wort (300 milligrams of a standardized extract, three times daily); kava (60 to 120 milligrams of kavalactones, or follow the label directions); and black cohosh (as a dry powdered extract, 250 milligrams, three times daily).

3. Consider homeopathic mood busters.

    Numerous homeopathic remedies may help mend your mood and

(Continued)

control your emotional ups and down. Try one of the following: ignatia, lilium tigrinum, natrum nuriaticum, and pulsatilla. Homeopathy dosage directions vary, so it's best to consult the instructions printed on the label.

4. See the light.

Some researchers believe that there may be a connection between a woman's mood swings and a serotonin deficiency. An easy way to raise levels of serotonin is by stepping outside on a sunny day. Sunlight reaches the brain through your eyes and stimulates the release of serotonin. For best results, get fifteen to thirty minutes of sun exposure each day.

5. Move your body.

Working out three days a week or more with a combination of aerobic exercise and weight training helps banish the menopausal blues. That's the consensus of a body of research showing that women who exercise regularly have consistently more positive moods and fewer swings than non-exercising women. Exercise makes you feel better about yourself, increases feel-good endorphins, and improves your sleep at night (poor sleep has been implicated in menopausal mood changes).

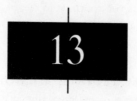

The Workings of Memory

It's a fact of life: Your memory will let you down on occasion. You'll forget where you parked your car, left your glasses, or put the last book you were reading. Does that mean you have Alzheimer's disease? Or are you just absentminded? Read on to find out.

THE MANY TYPES OF MEMORY AND WHY THEY'RE IMPORTANT

Memory—the ability to retain and recall information and experiences—is an indispensable part of life and survival. You need it to remember who you are, how to walk and talk, and how to avoid danger. Without memory, living would be impossible. Memory makes us who we are.

We all have various types of memories, classified by scientists into the categories discussed below.

SENSORY MEMORY

Sensory memory lets you continue to see, hear, or feel an experience for a short time after it stops.

IMMEDIATE MEMORY

This is a fleeting type of memory that takes a quick snapshot of an experience or stimulus. Unless that image is transferred to short-term memory, it is rapidly lost. Immediate memory lasts less than a minute.

SHORT-TERM MEMORY

Short-term memory stores information for only a brief time. Also called "working memory," it is the part of your brain used to follow conversations or remember a telephone number you've just looked up.

The capacity of short-term memory is limited, however. Research shows that it can hold up to only nine pieces of information. After about thirty minutes, facts in your short-term memory are replaced by new ones. The old facts either drop out of your memory completely or are transferred to long-term memory.

Short-term memory is also easily disrupted. You've probably experienced this when you forgot what you were looking for or couldn't recall something on a mental shopping list. This usually happens because you got distracted.

LONG-TERM MEMORY

Long-term memory stores most of everything you know. For example: your vocabulary; the names of your friends and loved ones; your favorite movies; how to read, write, and add; how to perform work-related skills; and how to find your way to the grocery store. Unlike short-term memory, long-term memory is less vulnerable to distractions in the environment. And information stays in your long-term memory for months, years, or even for the rest of your life.

Scientists further classify long-term memory into the following:

- *Priming memory* helps you recognize objects and words.
- *Semantic memory* holds facts, principles, and rules that make up your general knowledge of the world—gained through books, televisions, and various common experiences like knowing that a burner is hot when the stove is turned on. Some types of semantic memory are referred to as "explicit or declarative memory," in which you have to actively recall information such as events and facts. These memories are stored up rapidly in your head and can be recalled quickly. Semantic memory usually does not decline with age.
- *Procedural memory* stores such information as how to operate a computer, type a letter, or do arithmetic. Some procedural memory, described as "implicit memory," involves skills and habits that are performed practically automatically, without much active thinking on your part. An example would be driving your car or riding a bike. You don't consciously remember how to do them; you just get in your car or mount your bike and go. The memories of the emotions associated with an event are another type of implicit memory. Procedural memory does not normally decline with age.
- *Episodic memory* involves specific personal experiences from the past and the ability to recall those experiences. Unlike semantic and procedural memory, episodic memory can fade with age.
- *Remote memory* includes our knowledge of how to speak and read. It is so deeply fixed in our brains that we don't ordinarily lose it.

How Your Brain Records and Constructs Memories

The formation of memories involves four interrelated processes: encoding, consolidation, storage, and retrieval. These are described below.

ENCODING

In encoding, your brain takes the things you learn and experience and turns them into new pathways of nerve connections, called memory traces or engrams. For a memory trace to be formed, you have to pay attention and focus on the event, experience, or material to be remembered.

CONSOLIDATION

Occurring over several weeks or more, consolidation is a process by which a memory trace becomes permanent. During this time, your memory is malleable and susceptible to modification and distortion. It is important to point out that the consolidation of memories is not like the process of videotaping an event by recording, and later replaying, the exact images. Rather, memories are always undergoing revision and editing as we revamp them to suit our present situation and thinking. For example, a woman who is divorced may look back on her former husband and believe that she never really loved him, when in fact their courtship was one of bliss.

STORAGE

With storage, your brain keeps the memory trace over time. Memories are not, as was previously thought, stored in file folders organized in specific regions of the brain. Rather, memories are cached everywhere throughout the brain.

RETRIEVAL

Retrieval brings the memory out of storage into consciousness. A memory is retrieved each time a memory trace is activated, usually by "cues" or reminders in your environment. We tend to remember recent experiences more clearly and past experiences more vaguely. Also, we tend to remember what we consider unusual or important.

WHY WE FORGET

Scientists are not yet sure exactly what physiological processes are involved in activating memory traces, but they do know that the master controller of memory is the hippocampus, the seahorse-shaped area deep inside the brain, where memories are first created. Acting as a sorter, the hippocampus stores the memories temporarily, then parcels them out (probably during sleep) to permanent storage sites throughout the brain. This can take minutes or hours.

But during the process, memories can be lost unless the nerve connections responsible for the memory are reinforced so that the memory can exist independent of the hippocampus.

Here's an example: When you teach yourself a new skill, such as playing the piano, and practice it over and over again, you are strengthening certain nerve connections so that the skill will be stored permanently. One reason we forget things is that some connections break down through lack of use.

Another reason we're forgetful is because the brain never encoded the memory in the first place. For example, you may not have registered where you parked your car when you went grocery shopping. That simply means your brain didn't lay down the memory.

Ever wonder why the name of that person approaching you is on the "tip of your tongue"? Chalk it up to a delay in information processing. The sound of a name or word is stored in the brain in a different place than its context or meaning. You may know that his name begins with "T" (sound) and that you met him at a party (context), but if the links between the two are weak, you will have trouble remembering the name although you know the face. Proper names and seldom-used words are prone to this tip-of-the-tongue phenomenon.

And don't worry about being absentminded—like the time you forgot to return a library book or pick up shampoo at the drugstore. Being absentminded mostly means that your brain is concentrating on higher-priority matters. If we remembered every detail with the same degree of concentration, our brains would get overloaded with unimportant information and lose focus on priorities.

WHY WE REMEMBER SIGNIFICANT EMOTIONAL EVENTS

On the other hand, some memories are so vivid that they become virtually indelible. For example, most people can recall exactly where they were and what they were doing when President John F. Kennedy was assassinated in November 1963. Similarly, in later years, you may be able to recall where you were when terrorists attacked the World Trade Center in New York City and the Pentagon in Washington, D.C., on September 11, 2001.

Other memories (particularly those involving a traumatic event) are intrusive—and haunting—and can lead to posttraumatic stress disorder (PTSD), characterized by flashbacks of the trauma, hallucinations, anxiety, and other mental problems.

Why do memories of a significant emotional event such as an assassination or a trauma become forever etched on our brains? During such an experience, the brain takes advantage of two powerful stress hormones, adrenaline and noradrenaline, which flood the body in times of stress and strong emotion, to carve the memory into the brain—forever. This process is actually a life-saving defense mechanism: We need to be able to recall danger or threats in order to take precautions should we ever encounter them again.

Also involved with strong emotional events is the amygdala, an almond-shaped structure in the brain. The amygdala is involved in mood and emotions, particularly the acquisition and expression of fear and anxiety. It also helps you vividly recall emotionally charged events from your past.

Scientists are still unlocking the many mysteries of memory. But with each new discovery, they expand their knowledge of how memory works—knowledge that will lead to better treatments for repairing memory when it malfunctions.

How Sharp Is Your Memory?
Take This Quiz to Find Out

If you're like most people, your memory slips from time to time. You may even have wondered if you're losing your memory permanently or if the early stages of dementia are setting in. How do you know? What are the differences between normal forgetfulness and memory loss that's a cause for concern?

Only your physician can tell for sure, but here's a memory self-test that may give you an inkling of just how sharp your memory is. It was developed by the Memory Assessment Clinic in Bethesda, Maryland.

MEMORY QUIZ

Step 1. Read through the following list of 14 foods once, concentrating on each word.

ONIONS	SHRIMP	PASTA
PLUMS	TONIC WATER	HAM
EGGS	MAYONNAISE	BROWNIES
BLACKBERRIES	BASIL	OATMEAL
HAZELNUTS	MANGOES	

Step 2. Turn away from the list and write down as many of the foods as you can remember.

(Continued)

Step 3. Match your list to the foods listed above.

Scoring

You have a sharp memory if you scored accordingly:

- Ages 18 to 39: You remembered 10 items.
- Ages 40 to 59: You remembered 9 items.
- Ages 60 to 69: You remembered 8 items.
- Age 70 or older: You remembered 7 items.

Assessing Your Memory Performance

If you scored below what is considered normal for your age group, you may want to undergo further testing at your physician's office or at a memory clinic. The major tests used to diagnose other memory problems, dementia, or Alzheimer's disease are discussed below.

A Test to Determine Dementia

Called the Abbreviated Mental Test, this test is used to detect the possibility of dementia, particularly in elderly individuals. An individual under evaluation will be asked to answer the following questions posed by a health-care professional:

1. What is your age?
2. Without looking at your watch or clock, what time is it to the nearest hour?
3. What is your address?
4. What month is it?
5. What year is it?
6. Where do you live—or where are you right now?
7. What is your date of birth?
8. When did World War I start?
9. Name a current world leader.
10. Count backward from 20 to 1.

SCORING
- 8 to 10 correct answers: Normal
- 7 correct answers: Possible dementia
- Less than 7 correct answers: Usually suggests dementia

IS IT AGE-RELATED MEMORY LOSS, OR IS IT ALZHEIMER'S? THE 7-MINUTE SCREEN

Designed to be part of a yearly physical checkup, this screening test can help distinguish between age-related memory loss and dementia such as Alzheimer's disease. In fact, results of a study testing the usefulness of this test found that it is more than 90-percent accurate in differentiating between people with memory loss due to normal aging and those with symptoms characteristic of Alzheimer's disease. The test is useful for identifying patients who should be evaluated for Alzheimer's disease.

The seven-minute test was developed by Paul Solomon, M.D., of the Memory Clinic at Southwestern Vermont Medical Center. It involves the following four components:

- *The Benton Temporal Orientation Test.* This portion of the test assesses the participant's knowledge of month, date, year, day of the week, and time of day.
- *Clock Drawing.* The participant is asked to draw a clock with all the numbers on it, then draw the hands so that they are set at twenty to four, or to some other time.
- *Memory Test.* This test requires the participant to verbally recall sixteen pictures, presented four at a time on flash cards. When the participant is asked to recall each set of pictures, the tester (test administrator) will offer a cue or hint. Healthy individuals benefit from the hint, while people with Alzheimer's disease do not.

- *Verbal Fluency*. The participant is asked to state as many words as possible within a specified category (such as fruits) in a one-minute period.

During the test, the tester keeps score in a special test booklet. After all four tests are completed, the scores are entered into a customized calculator to produce a summary of results for the physician.

Patients in the early stages of Alzheimer's disease generally have trouble performing well in the four test categories. Those who test positive should have a full diagnostic and neurological examination.

Is It Forgetfulness, or Is It Alzheimer's Disease?
10 Signs You Shouldn't Ignore

What's the difference between Alzheimer's disease and plain old forgetfulness? To find out, read through the following checklist of common symptoms developed by the Alzheimer's Association. If they seem to apply to you, check with your doctor. Only he or she can make a final diagnosis.

☐ MEMORY LOSS

One of the most common early warning signs is forgetting recently learned information. While forgetting names, appointments, or telephone numbers is normal, people with Alzheimer's disease forget this information more often and have trouble remembering it later.

They also have trouble remembering what common items are. For example, someone with normal forgetfulness might forget where he left his keys, but someone with early Alzheimer's disease will look at the keys and say, "What are these?"

☐ DIFFICULTY PERFORMING FAMILIAR TASKS

People with Alzheimer's disease have trouble completing everyday routine tasks that most people can do without thinking, such as cooking a meal, getting dressed, and participating in a familiar hobby.

☐ Problems with Language

Although it's normal to mentally grope for the right word every now and then, people with Alzheimer's disease tend to forget familiar words or substitute a wrong or vague word instead. As a result, their speech or writing is difficult to understand.

☐ Disorientation to Time and Space

People with Alzheimer's disease can get lost on their own street, forget their location and how they got there, and not know how to find their way home.

☐ Poor or Decreased Judgment

No one has perfect judgment, but those with Alzheimer's disease may dress inappropriately for the weather, give away large amounts of money to strangers, or make other decisions that seem foolish or odd.

☐ Problems with Abstract Thinking

Many people have problems balancing their checkbooks or making a budget. Those with Alzheimer's disease, however, forget completely what the numbers mean and what should be done with them.

☐ Misplacing Things

Everyone misplaces a pair of glasses, car keys, or other item. With Alzheimer's disease, the person puts items in strange places: keys in the refrigerator or glasses under the bed, for example.

☐ Changes in Mood or Behavior

Anyone can feel down in the dumps from time to time. Someone with Alzheimer's disease exhibits rapid mood swings for no apparent reason.

☐ Changes in Personality

With age, people's personalities change a little. But in those with Alzheimer's disease, personality can become radically different. The person may become very confused, suspicious, fearful, or dependent on others.

(Continued)

☐ Loss of Initiative

From time to time, anyone can get bored with housework, business activities, or social events. But a person with Alzheimer's disease loses all desire to participate in such activities and may passively watch television all day, sleep more than usual, or avoid social activities.

Memory Problems and More: The Mini-Mental State Examination (MMSE)

The MMSE is a more comprehensive mental status test. It is the most widely used such test in the United States and the most comprehensive of the short tests. It is used to help diagnose memory problems, cognitive decline, dementia, or Alzheimer's disease. On average, this test takes about thirty minutes to complete.

In this test, patients are asked to do the following:

- Give the year, season, month, and day of the week.
- State their present location: state, country, town, building, floor, or room.
- Name three unrelated objects, repeat them, and remember them for later in the test.
- Count backward from 100, subtracting seven each time and stopping after five answers; or spell the word "world" backward.
- Recall the three objects mentioned earlier.
- Point to an object in the room and identify it.
- Repeat the phrase "No ifs, ands, or buts."
- Follow a three-stage command: Take a sheet of paper, fold it in half, and place it on the floor.
- Read the sentence "Close your eyes" and do as it instructs.

- Write a complete sentence on a piece of paper.
- Copy a picture of two intersecting pentagons.

Patients are scored on the accuracy of their responses.

5 Myths About the Aging Brain

You've probably heard that your mental powers go south after age thirty, that "you can't teach an old dog new tricks," or that your memory in your golden years is half what it was in your youth. If that's what you think and believe, then you've been misled and misguided by too much myth-based advice. It's time to blow up those myths, and get the inside scoop on what really goes on inside your "aging" brain. Read on.

Myth 1: *Beginning around age thirty, your brain loses about 10,000 neurons a day.*

     Fact: For decades, a long-held belief was that we lose thousands of brain cells as we get older. However, new imaging technologies have now proclaimed this "fact" a downright myth. Yes, we do lose some brain cells, but not in the huge numbers previously believed.

Myth 2: *You're born with all the brain cells you'll ever have.*

     Fact: Another long-held dogma—now discredited— is that your brain stops producing new cells after infancy. The truth is that the aging brain is capable of generating new cells, particularly in the hippocampus, the center of learning and memory. In fact, research shows that the human brain can replenish cells in the hippocampus at the rate of hundreds of new cells every day.

     Your brain is also capable of forming new connections (dendrites and synapses) between neurons at any age as you learn new information and keep your brain active. In other words, brain connections get stronger with use.

Myth 3: *All memory declines with age.*

> **Fact:** Long-term memory, which houses your life stories and work knowledge, stays relatively intact. This means that older adults can process information more effectively and make better judgments because of their remembered experiences.
>
> On the other hand, short-term memory—remembering names, phone numbers, and so forth—tends to slide as a part of normal brain aging. Even so, short-term memory can be strengthened with practice and good habits.

Myth 4: *People use only a fraction of their brainpower.*

> **Fact:** Advertisers and the popular media have long perpetuated the myth that we use only a tiny portion of our brainpower—something like 10 percent. Actually, the origin of this myth dates back to the early 1800s when many scientists believed that brain functions were localized to particular regions of the brain and used independently for specific mental tasks. This belief subsequently turned out to be unfounded.
>
> Modern, state-of-the-art imaging techniques such as positron emission tomography (PET), which provides a picture of brain activity, have largely debunked the myth that humans use a small percentage of their brainpower. Scientists now know that much of the brain is active, although at varying degrees, during mental activities. Some parts may be working the hardest during particular tasks; others are less active but involved nonetheless.
>
> Suppose you're engaged in a conversation with another person and could observe your own brain activity. You'd see that the region responsible for speaking is highly active, while the part responsible for generating verbs—required for speech—is active, too. Still another part is active in hearing your own words and those of the

other person. At no time is just one brain region active all by itself. During any given mental task, many different brain regions are working in concert.

Myth 5: *You can't teach an old person new tricks.*

Fact: Age-related memory changes are primarily associated with attention problems, usually due to losses in hearing and vision, rather than with cognitive declines. The capacity to learn new information does not fall off with age. In fact, some memory functions such as vocabulary and the ability to reason improve with age. The brain never stops learning.

An elderly person, however, must be motivated to learn before new learning can take place. And, to retain information, additional practice is usually required.

Part Five

SPECIAL STRATEGIES TO
HELP YOU OUT

Addiction. Alzheimer's disease. Parkinson's disease. Stroke. Anxiety. Attention disorders. Menopause-related mood changes. They're all exceedingly scary conditions. What makes them so scary is the damage they can inflict on our brains and behaviors.

Even so, experts seem to concur that, depending on the illness, these diseases and conditions can be prevented, controlled, or even reversed—with a wide array of natural supplements, lifestyle changes, prescription medications, and more. This is the focus of Part 5: how to use complementary and conventional therapies to start living life to the fullest, starting right now.

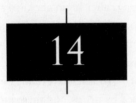

Different Therapies for Scary Conditions

Although they are potentially devastating conditions, addictions, Alzheimer's disease, Parkinson's disease, stroke, anxiety, attention disorders, and menopause-related mood changes can all be managed with a greater number of effective treatments than ever before, and many of these treatments are natural and gentle on your body. This chapter describes these scary conditions in greater detail and the most effective ways to combat them.

ADDICTION: THE MOST ADDICTIVE DRUGS AND 5 WAYS TO GET UNHOOKED

Not surprisingly, the most addictive drugs in our society are nicotine, alcohol, and illicit drugs such as cocaine and heroin. In the United States alone, there are approximately 47 million smokers, according to the

American Cancer Society; 8.2 million alcoholics; and 3.5 million illicit drug users, according to the National Institute on Drug Abuse (NIDA).

All three types of drugs alter brain chemistry in much the same way. Essentially, they produce their high by stimulating the production of dopamine—a joy-producing neurotransmitter—in the pleasure centers of the brain. When dopamine levels are jacked up, you feel euphoric for as long as the high lasts. (To a lesser extent, the levels of other neurotransmitters are increased by drugs, and these include serotonin, GABA, and norepinephrine.)

But as you move from voluntary to compulsory use (addiction), the continued use of these drugs tends to dull dopamine receptors on neurons and reduce their number. (Dopamine receptors are tiny structures mounted on cell walls that allow the neurotransmitter to enter cells.) Consequently, cells don't recognize or use dopamine properly, leaving too much of it in the pleasure centers of the brain.

Eventually, the pleasure centers adapt to the drug, and the addict will no longer feel satisfied—a condition known as tolerance—so increasingly larger doses of the drug are needed to produce the high. The addict develops not only a physical dependence on the drug but also a psychological one.

When an addict undergoes withdrawal from the drug, the brain is deprived of its only source of dopamine. As the body resets its dopamine system, all sorts of bodily reactions kick in: hypersensitivity to pain, tremors or jitters, nausea, cravings, extreme depression, to name just a few.

While it can be a long-term process, recovery from addiction is possible but usually requires multiple approaches. Bear in mind this advice from the NIDA: "No single treatment is appropriate for all individuals. Matching treatment settings, interventions, and services to each patient's problems and needs is critical."

If you're suffering from an addiction, here is a look at the steps you can take to beat it.

GET HELP

Decades of research demonstrate that many people can't overcome an addiction alone. It takes supportive psychotherapy, along with medical care and family support, to return to productive living. Happily, there are several forms of therapy that have proven effective in helping people recover from addictions. These are summarized in Table 14.1.

TABLE 14.1

Addiction-Busting Therapies

Therapy	Goals	How It Works
Aversion Therapy	Produce dislike (aversion) for the addictive substance.	A therapist repeatedly introduces the worst consequences of the behavior immediately after the pleasurable sensation occurs. That way, the negative and painful experience cancels out the pleasure. A therapist, for example, might show a smoker visuals of damaged lungs several seconds after he or she smokes—and do this repeatedly.
Behavioral Shaping	Encourage abstinence through the use of incentives, rewards, or positive reinforcement.	A therapist offers inducements that appeal to the patient if he or she refrains from drug use. *(Continued)*

THERAPY	GOALS	HOW IT WORKS
Brief-Intervention Therapy	Empower people with addictions to take responsibility for their problem and provide ways to do so.	Therapy involves one to three counseling sessions that focus on strategies designed to reinforce an addict's own commitment to change.
Coping Skills Treatment	Increase a person's ability to cope with situations that might lead to relapse.	Therapists provide skills training to reduce exposure to addictive substances; bolster motivation for abstinence by exploring the negative consequences of continued use; encourage self-monitoring to identify situations that encourage temptation; develop strategies to cope with cravings; work through thought processes that increase the risk of relapse; and prepare for emergencies.
Cue Exposure	Lessen the desire for the addictive substance, particularly in the presence of situations (cues) that trigger the craving.	Therapy systematically exposes the drinker to cues—such as social events, advertisements, or restaurants—that might trigger the desire to drink. During therapy, cues are not reinforced with the pleasure of having a drink.

DISCUSS MEDICATION THERAPY
WITH YOUR DOCTOR

According to the NIDA, medications can be an important component of treatment for many patients, especially when combined with counseling and other behavioral therapies. Numerous prescription medications are available to help recovering addicts overcome their addictions. These are listed in Table 14.2.

TABLE 14.2
Pharmacological Treatments for Substance Abuse

Drug	Uses	Therapeutic Benefits
Antabuse (disulfiram)	Alcoholism	When taken with alcohol, the drug produces unpleasant side effects, including headache, nausea, and vomiting.
Buprenorphine	Heroin addiction	Reduces craving for the narcotic by bonding to certain receptors in the brain and tricking the brain into thinking the cravings have been satisfied.
Catapres (clonidine hydrochloride)	Alcohol, nicotine, or tranquilizer withdrawal; narcotic detoxification	A high blood pressure medication that blocks norepinephrine to reduce feelings of stress and anxiety during withdrawal. *(Continued)*

Drug	Uses	Therapeutic Benefits
Depakene (valproic acid)	Alcohol withdrawal	An anticonvulsant that decreases alcohol withdrawal symptoms.
Levo-alpha-acetylmethadol	Heroin addiction	Reduces desire for heroin and is less potent than methadone.
Librium (chlordiazepoxide)	Alcohol withdrawal	Decreases symptoms of alcohol withdrawal, including anxiety and tremors.
Methadone	Heroin addiction	Reduces desire for heroin.
Narcan (naloxone)	Addiction to heroin and other drugs	Acts on receptors in the brain to reduce cravings.
Neurotonin (gabapentin)	Alcohol withdrawal	An anticonvulsant related to the neurotransmitter GABA and helps reduce withdrawal-related anxiety.
Nicorette (nicotine gum)	Smoking cessation	Reduces nicotine cravings and withdrawal symptoms. Helps you wean yourself from nicotine by gradually decreasing the dosage.

Drug	Uses	Therapeutic Benefits
Nicotine Patches (Habitrol, Nicoderm, Nicotrol, ProStep)	Smoking cessation	Reduces cravings and withdrawal symptoms by supplying a steady, specific amount of nicotine through the skin and into the bloodstream. Helps you wean yourself from nicotine by gradually decreasing the dosage.
Nicotrol Inhaler (nicotine inhalation system)	Smoking cessation	Provides a substitute source of nicotine to gradually help reduce dependence on the drug. Helps you wean yourself from nicotine by gradually decreasing the dosage. Includes a mouthpiece and cartridges.
ReVia (naltrexone)	Alcoholism and narcotic addiction	Acts on receptors in the brain to reduce alcohol and drug cravings.
Sabril (vigabatrin)	Alcohol withdrawal	A new anticonvulsant that increases levels of the neurotransmitter GABA in the brain by inhibiting an enzyme responsible for GABA's breakdown.
Tegretol (carbamazepine)	Alcohol withdrawal and cocaine addiction	An anticonvulsant that decreases withdrawal symptoms and helps treat addiction-related mood disorders. *(Continued)*

Drug	Uses	Therapeutic Benefits
Tenormin (atenolol)	Alcohol withdrawal	A beta-blocker that treats withdrawal-related anxiety.
Valium (diazepam)	Alcohol withdrawal	Decreases symptoms of alcohol withdrawal, including anxiety and tremors.
Zyban (bupropion hydrochloride)	Smoking cessation	Boosts levels of several brain neurotransmitters to produce a reduction of nicotine withdrawal symptoms and a weakening of the urge to smoke.

UNDERGO DETOXIFICATION

If you are chronically intoxicated with alcohol or any other drug, it may be necessary to undergo "detoxification," in which decreasing amounts of the drug are given as you are gradually and systematically taken off the drug altogether. Detoxification is best conducted in a hospital under medical supervision, because drug withdrawal can produce serious, sometimes fatal, side effects such as seizures.

Detoxification is designed to manage the acute symptoms of withdrawal, but by itself it does little to change long-term drug use. After detoxification, you must undergo others forms of therapy.

ENROLL IN A SELF-HELP GROUP

These include organizations such as Alcoholics Anonymous (AA) and Narcotics Anonymous (NA), which are fellowships of individuals with common addictive problems. The basic tenets of these groups are:

- Addiction is a physical, mental, and spiritual disease.
- The disease is believed to be incurable and progressive but can be arrested with abstinence.
- The symptoms of the disease are craving and loss of control.
- Drinking or substance abuse leads to physical and psychological illness but is not caused by these.
- Alcoholism and substance abuse are primarily spiritual illnesses characterized by a perception that the individual rather than a higher power is at the center of the universe.
- Addicts are seen as having defects of character brought on by their own selfishness and spiritual emptiness.

Change is brought about through motivation to kick the addiction, regular attendance at meetings, adherence to the Twelve Steps that are at the heart of the program, behavioral change (avoiding people, places, and things associated with the addiction), and reliance on a higher power.

Other types of self-help recovery groups are also beneficial because they provide social support, whether from friends, family, therapists, or other self-help group members. Social support is crucial to recovery.

TRY "WARM TURKEY"

This method is the opposite of "cold turkey" in which the addict abruptly quits. Cold turkey works well in smoking cessation.

By contrast, warm turkey emphasizes tapering down, rather than abstinence, along with counseling to teach addicts how to handle setbacks and to cope with various situations that may lead to relapses. A familiar example of warm turkey is use of a nicotine patch, applied in decreasing concentrations of the drug, to quit smoking.

KICK YOUR HABIT NATURALLY WITH 6 ADDICTION-BUSTING THERAPIES

Any effective intervention for addiction recovery should include a combination of the therapies previously discussed as well as certain alternative treatments. Used in conjunction with the earlier methods discussed, the following six natural, or holistic, therapies can be effective in the treatment of addictions and in reducing the symptoms of withdrawal. They also help to alleviate one of the worst instigators in addiction relapse—stress.

AURICULAR ACUPUNCTURE

Auricular acupuncture involves positioning several small needles in specific points in each ear. The needles are left in place for thirty to forty-five minutes. There is little or no pain at the time of insertion.

Remarkably, research shows that auricular acupuncture can be useful for promoting general relaxation, reducing the craving for drugs, and assisting addicts in staying abstinent. It has been successfully used to treat cocaine dependence, heroin addiction, smoking withdrawal, and addiction relapse. Advocates of auricular acupuncture emphasize that it should be used as part of a comprehensive program of care that employs counseling, education, and self-help groups.

There are more than 2,000 clinics worldwide now using auricular acupuncture to treat addictions. In the United States, one of the pioneering clinics is Lincoln Clinic in the South Bronx of New York, where the treatment has been used since the 1970s.

For information on auricular acupuncture, contact the Natural Acupuncture Detoxification Association at www.acudetox.com or 503-222-1362.

BIOFEEDBACK

Biofeedback employs a special machine that, through electrodes attached to your skin, monitors minute changes in your body's physiological reactions (temperature changes, heart rate, blood pressure, muscle tension, and so forth). While hooked up to the machine, you're simultaneously using visualization and relaxation to help consciously regulate these functions. As you relax, the machine provides instant feedback on how well you're controlling the various functions. The ultimate goal is to achieve the desired relaxation response but without the use of the machine.

According to a number of scientific investigations, addicts who are trying to abstain from drugs or alcohol often relapse because of the anxiety brought on by stressful events of everyday life. This observation has led some therapists to try biofeedback as a way to reduce anxiety in drug-abusing patients. In a study conducted at the Drug Dependence Treatment Service in Philadelphia, biofeedback was successful in reducing anxiety, depression, and drug cravings in a group of addicts. Other research has produced similar findings, leading some addiction experts to favor anxiety-reducing interventions like biofeedback to help reduce addictive behavior and the potential for relapse.

DIETARY THERAPY

Prolonged drug abuse or dependency wreaks havoc on health by destroying nutrients, preventing their absorption, and accelerating their excretion. Cocaine and heroin addiction, in particular, reduces the intake of nutritious foods and causes serious malnutrition, whereas marijuana increases the intake of food, particularly sweets, and may cause weight gain. In large amounts, alcohol flushes many nutrients from the body, including thiamine, vitamin B_6, and calcium. Smoking robs the body of vital, disease-fighting antioxidants.

Fortunately, such nutritional problems can be corrected with dietary therapy, which involves dietary changes and the use of high-potency nutritional supplements.

Dietary Guidelines for Alcohol Recovery

If you're recovering from alcoholism, do the following:

- Follow a diet higher in protein. Protein intake should comprise 20 to 25 percent of your total daily calories. Protein is required for tissue repair and regeneration, particularly if cirrhosis of the liver is present.
- Eat foods rich in vitamin A. These include carrots and sweet potatoes. Also, supplement with a multivitamin that contains vitamin A. This nutrient helps prevent respiratory infections, which are common in alcoholics.
- Take a supplemental B-complex vitamin. B-complex vitamins help prevent a host of alcohol-related diseases, including pellagra and tremors. They also reduce cravings for alcohol.
- Talk to your physician about whether you need an iron supplement. Iron helps reverse anemia, another consequence of alcoholism.
- Supplement with other vitamins and minerals. Most important are vitamins D, E, and K, and magnesium. Alcohol robs the body of these nutrients.

Dietary Guidelines for Drug-Addiction Recovery

A nutrient program designed to help those recovering from drug addiction should include supplementation with the following:

- B-complex vitamins to restore liver health.
- Calcium and magnesium to help control tremors.
- Vitamin C to help detoxify the body.
- Adequate protein (20 to 25 percent of your total daily calories) to help regenerate tissues.

Another nutritional agent that may be helpful during alcohol withdrawal is the amino acid tyrosine. Through a series of biochemical reactions, the body can convert the amino acids—tyrosine, in particular—

into dopamine and other brain chemicals. Experiments have shown that supplementing with amino acids reduced cravings for drugs and improved withdrawal symptoms considerably. Supplemental tyrosine thus appears to supply the brain with the amino acid building blocks it needs to manufacture and release dopamine naturally.

The usual supplemental dosage of tyrosine ranges from 500 to 1,000 milligrams daily. But check with your physician before using tyrosine to treat alcohol withdrawal.

Dietary Guidelines for Smoking Cessation

Smokers should increase their intake of the following nutrients:

- Vitamin C (as high as 5,000 milligrams daily or more), which is drastically depleted in smokers.
- B-complex vitamins to help support liver functioning.
- Vitamin E (400 IU daily) for protection against the severe oxidative damage caused by smoking.

HOMEOPATHY

Homeopathy is a medical system that uses minute doses of substances that in their original concentrations might induce symptoms of the disease being treated. Giving the small, usually diluted doses is designed to rally the immune system to fight off the disease.

Homeopathy does not cure drug or alcohol addictions but instead helps alleviate pain, anxiety, depression, and restlessness often associated with chemical dependency. Among the remedies used to treat these symptoms are tuberculinum, argentum, nitricum, and arsenicum.

Research into homeopathy and addiction is scant, but a few studies do show that it may be helpful in treating alcoholism and drug addiction.

For more information on homeopathy, contact the National Center for Homeopathy at www.homeopath.org, 877-624-0613, or 703-548-7790.

HYPNOSIS

Hypnosis—or hypnotherapy as it is known medically—has been used to help people break drug, alcohol, and smoking addictions. It appears to work by dispelling depression and anxiety and by helping people change their addictive behaviors.

One form of hypnosis that's effective is self-hypnosis, in which the therapist teaches the patient how to induce a hypnotic state. Audio- and videotapes are also used as tools in self-hypnosis.

In a case study published in a 1993 issue of the *American Journal of Clinical Hypnosis*, researchers from Ohio State University reported on a twenty-year-old woman who successfully used a tape to overcome a $500-a-day addiction to cocaine. The tape was actually a commercial weight-control tape.

For four months, she listened to it three times a day, mentally substituting the word "coke" in appropriate places. At the end of this period, she broke her addiction and has remained drug-free. The researchers noted: "Her withdrawal and recovery were extraordinary because hypnosis was the only intervention, and no support network of any kind was available."

Not everyone can be hypnotized, however, so results are often mixed.

YOGA

Practiced for more than 5,000 years, yoga incorporates an assortment of postures, or "asanas," coupled with deep breathing. It is often used as complementary therapy to free patients from drug addictions because it stimulates relaxation, eases muscular tension, and fosters positive mental health.

Clinical research with yoga as a complementary treatment for addiction has been impressive. Harvard researchers, for example, found that yoga was as effective in treating heroin addicts as traditional group therapy. Addicts who practiced yoga for seventy-five minutes once a week, while undergoing individual therapy, reduced their drug use and experienced fewer cravings than those who attended group and individual therapy only.

6 Herbal Detoxifiers for Alcohol and Drug Addiction

Alcohol and other drugs are toxins that damage organs, including the brain. One way to repair this damage is through detoxification, which involves mostly the drug-withdrawal process but can also include methods to restore organ health. An effective way to "detox" is to employ the following six herbs as a part of a total recovery program. Standard dosages are provided in Table 14.3 on page 303.

BURDOCK ROOT

Used since ancient times as a healing remedy, burdock root (*Arctium lappa*) is believed to be a blood purifier that cleanses the blood of toxins, including alcohol and drug residues. Burdock appears to be safe, although it may interfere with the absorption of iron and other minerals.

DANDELION ROOT

Dandelion—the stubborn weed that pops up in your lawn every spring—is actually a healthful herb, packed with vitamin A, vitamin C, and various minerals. It is believed to help repair liver damage, which can be induced by alcohol and drug abuse. Dandelion (*Taraxacum officinale*) is considered very safe.

GINSENG

If you're trying to cut back on your imbibing, consider supplementing afterward with ginseng, a medicinal herb that has been used for thousands of years as a restorative tonic. One type of ginseng—the *Panax* variety—has proven to be somewhat of a sobering-up agent. Researchers in Korea found that ginseng (3 grams per 140 pounds of body weight) enhanced blood alcohol clearance in male drinkers. In other words, the herb cleansed the body of alcohol in short order.

KUDZU

The roots and flowers of this plentiful and prolific plant (*Pueraria lobata*) have been used in China for more than 1,000 years as a treatment for alcoholism. In one Chinese study, the herb tamed alcohol cravings in 80 percent of the 300 people who took it, with no side effects. Harvard scientists tested the herb on lab hamsters bred to enjoy alcohol and discovered that it curtailed alcohol consumption by about 50 percent.

Kudzu blunts the urge to imbibe by accelerating your body's buildup of acetaldehyde, a factor in hangovers. You thus get your hangover practically right away—while you're drinking rather than the next day.

MILK THISTLE

Derived from a weedlike plant grown in the Mediterranean area, milk thistle (*Silybum marianum*) has been used to protect the liver since ancient times—a therapeutic use that has been validated by modern-day science. Milk thistle contains an active ingredient called silymarin, which works by binding to the surface of liver cells so that toxins can't get in.

Supplements containing standardized extracts of silymarin are used to treat liver disorders caused by alcohol and drug abuse, as well as cirrhosis, hepatitis, and other liver diseases, particularly in Europe. In fact, milk thistle is a German Commission E–approved herb for treating liver ailments.

RED CLOVER

Red clover (*Trifolium pratense*) is an age-old folk remedy for protection against numerous diseases. As an herbal detoxifier, it reportedly helps enhance blood circulation, cleansing the bloodstream of toxins. The herb works in this manner by improving "arterial compliance," the ability of an artery to expand and contract with the amount of blood flow so that circulation can proceed normally.

TABLE 14.3 Herbal Detoxifiers	
HERB	STANDARD DOSAGE*
Burdock Root	460 mg, 2 times daily
Dandelion Root	510 mg, 1 to 3 times daily
Ginseng	100 to 300 mg (standardized to 7% ginsenosides, 3 times daily)
Kudzu	30 to 120 mg, 2 to 3 times daily; or drink some kudzu tea the morning after to clear up a hangover.
Milk Thistle	280 to 420 mg daily
Red Clover	430 mg, 1 to 3 times daily

*Read label instructions for manufacturer's recommended dosage.

ALZHEIMER'S DISEASE:
PROMISING BREAKTHROUGHS

Among the most feared of all diseases is Alzheimer's disease. If it strikes, you gradually lose your mind, your memory, and the ability to recognize your loved ones. In the advanced stages of the disease, you become totally dependent on others for your care. Alzheimer's disease is unusual in that it can be definitively diagnosed only after death through an autopsy of the brain.

Happily, though, huge strides have been made in learning how to cope with this disease. For example, there are numerous, relatively simple lifestyle changes you can make now to hedge your bets against Alzheimer's disease. New medications have been developed to ease the symptoms and help sufferers lead more productive lives. And, finally, there are several herbal remedies available that appear to work as well as prescription drugs.

7 Top Lifestyle Strategies for Outwitting Alzheimer's Disease

One of the best ways to escape Alzheimer's appears to be through healthy living, pure and simple. That's one of the major findings of an ongoing, groundbreaking study being conducted by University of Kentucky scientist David Snowdon.

Called the Nun's Study, Snowdon's research has tracked 678 nuns of the School Sisters of Notre Dame—and analyzed the brains of those who are deceased—to learn why some got Alzheimer's and some did not. Snowdon's discoveries, combined with studies conducted by other investigators, provide some useful—and quite amazing—information on what you can do to outwit Alzheimer's disease. The first steps to take are ones we've mentioned before: Cut your risk of stroke by following lifestyle strategies such as exercising, avoiding tobacco, and eating a healthy diet; and reducing your risk of head injury by wearing protective headgear when you're riding a bike, and so on; continue active learning throughout your life; maintain a positive attitude; and stay socially connected. But those are not the only steps you can take. Here are three effective strategies you may never have seen before.

EAT A DIET HIGH IN FOLIC ACID

Nuns with high levels of folic acid showed little evidence of Alzheimer's in their brains after they died. Found in green leafy vegetables, folic acid battles the effects of homocysteine in the body, a protein that has been implicated in heart disease. Lots of folic acid in the diet is believed to reduce your risk of stroke and to guard brain cells from damage by homocysteine. For nutritional insurance, take in at least 400 micrograms of folic acid a day, the amount found in most multivitamins.

REDUCE THE FAT IN YOUR DIET

A large-scale meta-analysis (statistical study) found that the prevalence of Alzheimer's disease was lower in countries where fat and caloric content of diets was lower. Investigators theorize that the reason has to do with fat, which contributes to oxidative stress and inflammation—two processes that inflict free-radical damage to brain cells. Specific fats to limit include those found in margarine and other processed foods. In addition, eating fish, which contains brain-healthy fats, is associated with a lower risk of developing dementia.

TAKE ACETYL-L-CARNITINE

This vitaminlike substance plays several important roles in combating Alzheimer's disease. For example, acetyl-L-carnitine: promotes the uptake of the B-vitamin choline by cells and its subsequent formation into acetylcholine. Because patients with Alzheimer's disease are deficient in acetylcholine, scientists believe that supplementation with acetyl-L-carnitine may prove beneficial.

Acetyl-L-carnitine also restores memory and cognitive ability in Alzheimer's patients as well as in healthy adults. A team of researchers in Italy studied 130 Alzheimer's patients, randomly assigning them to receive either 2 grams of the supplement daily for a year or a placebo. By the end of the study, all the patients had deteriorated in mental function. But the supplement takers had less deterioration, particularly in memory, attention span, and verbal abilities.

The recommended dosage of acetyl-L-carnitine is up to 1,000 milligrams daily.

2 Surprise OTC Medicines That Reduce Your Risk

Two unlikely insurance policies against Alzheimer's disease may be sitting inside your medicine cabinet: aspirin and ibuprofen. Naturally, you know them best as the pills you pop to kill the pain of a headache or arthritis or reduce your fever when you're under the weather. But did you also know that these drugs, collectively known as nonsteroidal anti-inflammatory drugs (NSAIDs), may dramatically cut your odds of Alzheimer's disease by a whopping 60 percent or more?

This amazing risk reduction was first noticed in people who regularly took NSAIDs to ease the pain of arthritis. Arthritis sufferers have lower rates of Alzheimer's disease—an observation that led scientists to study how NSAIDs might help prevent this devastating brain disease. Since then, they've learned that people who take NSAIDs for two years or more have a greatly reduced risk of getting Alzheimer's disease. The most commonly used and effective NSAID is ibuprofen. Aspirin has a modest benefit.

HOW NSAIDS WORK

Among the characteristics of Alzheimer's disease is inflammation in the brain. Inflammatory reactions in the body can cause cells—including brain cells—to die. Aspirin and ibuprofen, because they're anti-inflammatory agents, reduce inflammation in tissues and thus preserve brain cells and synapses. They may also step up circulation to the brain and lower the production of free radicals, suspected of playing a role in Alzheimer's disease brain damage.

Ibuprofen may do a little more. An animal study conducted by researchers at the University of California at Los Angeles found that ibuprofen not only reduced inflammation, but it also lowered the number of amyloid plaques, harmful protein particles that build up inside and outside brain cells, destroying synapses.

THE SUPERASPIRINS AND ALZHEIMER'S DISEASE

Other anti-inflammatories, most notably the antiarthritic "super-aspirins" such Celebrex and Vioxx, are being studied to determine whether they have any benefits on memory, attention, reasoning, and other mental processes. These medications are known as cox-2 inhibitors because they block the action of an enzyme (cox-2) that builds up in arthritic joints, causing pain and inflammation. (Over-the-counter NSAIDs inhibit cox-2 as well, but they also block cox-1, which protects the lining of the stomach and intestines against stomach acids. When cox-1 is inhibited, ulcers are likely to form in the lining. Ulcers and stomach problems are a major side effect of NSAIDs, particularly in older adults.) Scientists are optimistic that cox-2 inhibitors, available by prescription, may delay the onset of Alzheimer's disease or prevent it from getting worse.

WHO SHOULD TAKE NSAIDS?

Considering the evidence in favor of NSAIDs, should you start taking them to drive down your risk of acquiring Alzheimer's disease? There's no clear-cut answer to that question yet. Nor do medical scientists know what dosage or how long to use NSAIDs to delay the development of Alzheimer's disease. However, clinical trials are under way to pinpoint the dosages and how to use NSAIDs safely.

SIDE EFFECTS OF NSAIDS

Keep in mind that NSAIDs are not without side effects, either. In addition to the aforementioned heartburn, nausea, and the development of stomach ulcers, side effects include stomach cramps or pain, bloating and gas, constipation, diarrhea, and dizziness. Ibuprofen, Celebrex, and Vioxx have been known to cause serious liver and kidney problems. The best advice is to talk to your family doctor about whether you're a good candidate for NSAID therapy to prevent Alzheimer's disease.

Smart Drugs

Technically known as "nootropics" (after a Greek word meaning "acting on the mind"), smart drugs are a collection of medicines designed to fight and treat dementia; cognitive decline associated with aging and Alzheimer's disease; and Alzheimer's disease itself. They work in various ways to help relieve the symptoms of declining mental capacity. Some are FDA-approved and available in the United States; others are available from overseas countries only, but can be obtained through pharmaceutical mail-order firms as long as you have a prescription from your physician.

Table 14.4 provides a current rundown of smart drugs, how they work, their side effects, and their availability.

TABLE 14.4
Smart Drugs

Drugs That Treat Non-Alzheimer's Dementia and Cognitive Decline

Drug	Actions	Side Effects	Availability
Eldepryl (selegiline hydrochloride)	Inhibits an enzyme that breaks down dopamine, elevating dopamine levels in the brain.	Abdominal pain, abnormal movements, anxiety, apathy, blurred vision	FDA-approved in U.S. for the treatment of Parkinson's disease.
Hydergine (ergoloid mesylates)	Protects brain cells against free radicals; improves blood and oxygen supply to the brain; enhances the use of glucose by brain cells.	Stomach upset, temporary nausea	FDA-approved in U.S. to treat people over age sixty with symptoms of mental decline.

Drug	Actions	Side Effects	Availability
Lucidril (centro-phenoxine)	Enhances the use of glucose by brain cells; reduces levels of brain-damaging toxins; improves memory and boosts mental energy.	Excitability, muscle stiffness, headache	Available in Europe.
Nimotop (nimodipine)	Prevents movement of calcium into cells of blood vessels, increasing supply of blood and oxygen to the brain.	Decreased blood pressure, headache, nausea	FDA-approved in U.S. to treat problems caused by ruptured blood vessels in the brain.
Nootropil (piracetam)	Increases the sensitivity of receptors in the brain responsible for learning and memory.	Insomnia, headache, nausea, stomach upset	Available in Europe.
Picamilon	Improves blood flow to the brain; enhances cognition.	Very few side effects, but should not be taken if you have kidney disease or a family history of stroke	Available in Russia.
Pyritinol	Enhances brain cell activity; restores cognitive function.	Skin rash, stomach upset	Available in Europe.
Trental (pentoxifylline)	Improves blood flow to the brain to help relieve symptoms of dementia.	Allergic reaction, anxiety, bad taste in mouth, vision problems, chest pain, constipation, depression, general body discomfort	FDA-approved in U.S.

(Continued)

	Drugs That Treat Alzheimer's Disease		
DRUG	ACTIONS	SIDE EFFECTS	AVAILABILITY
Aricept (donepezil hydrochloride)	Inhibits the action of an enzyme that degrades acetyl-choline in the brain and boosts levels of acetylcholine in the brain, thus improving a patient's ability to think and recollect information.	Diarrhea, fatigue, insomnia, loss of appetite, muscle cramps, nausea, vomiting	FDA-approved in U.S. for treating Alzheimer's disease.
Cognex (tacrine hydrochloride)	Same as above.	Abdominal pain, abnormal thinking, agitation, anxiety, chest pain, clumsiness, confusion, constipation, coughing, depression, diarrhea, dizziness, fatigue, flushing, frequent urination, gas	FDA-approved in U.S. for treating Alzheimer's disease.
Exelon (rivastigmine tartrate)	Same as above.	Stomach-related side effects, including nausea, vomiting, loss of appetite, weight loss	FDA-approved in U.S. for treating Alzheimer's disease.
Reminyl (galantamine hydrobromide)	Same as above.	Nausea, vomiting, diarrhea, anorexia, weight loss	FDA-approved in U.S. for treating Alzheimer's disease.

FUTURE ANTI-ALZHEIMER'S DRUGS YOU'LL BE HEARING MORE ABOUT

Taking what may be vital steps toward preventing and curing Alzheimer's disease, scientists are testing experimental drugs that could represent major breakthroughs in treatment. These are discussed below.

AN ALZHEIMER'S VACCINE

An experimental vaccine that can prevent memory loss in mice stricken with an Alzheimer's-like disease is being tested in people. The vaccine is a synthetic version of a protein called beta amyloid, which is responsible for the buildup of plaques in the brain. Scientists theorize that these plaques cause the loss of memory and personality that is characteristic of Alzheimer's disease.

When mice were inoculated with the synthetic beta amyloid vaccine, it blocked the formation of plaques in their brains. The vaccine triggered an immune reaction in the mice that cleared away these plaques. The vaccinated mice had fewer and smaller plaques in their brains.

So far, the vaccine appears safe in people, according to pharmaceutical company scientists who are conducting the human trials. These trials are being conducted under the sponsorship of American Home Products of Madison, New Jersey, and Eban Corporation of Dublin, Ireland.

ACAT INHIBITORS

Soaring cholesterol has been linked to an increased susceptibility to Alzheimer's disease, according to a Harvard study published in *Nature Cell Biology* in 2001. Harvard scientists have shown that cholesterol levels are directly linked to the amount of beta amyloid peptide produced in the body. Beta amyloid peptide is a key component of the plaque in the brain that is a hallmark of Alzheimer's disease.

The Harvard study also points out that an enzyme called ACAT, which is involved in cholesterol production, also governs the production of beta amyloid peptide. In their experiments, the scientists used cells specially designed to overproduce cholesterol and treated them with drugs called ACAT inhibitors, which block the action of the ACAT enzyme. The drugs dramatically reduced the production of beta amyloid peptide in the cells, hinting that these drugs may be effective weapons against Alzheimer's disease.

This research is similar to studies showing that people taking cholesterol-reducing drugs, which work by a different mechanism than ACAT inhibitors, reduce patients' chances of developing Alzheimer's disease and other dementias.

Because the Harvard experiment used only individual cells, the next step in the study of ACAT inhibitors is to test them in mice specially bred to have Alzheimer's disease. No human trials have yet been planned.

AN ALZHEIMER'S ANTIBIOTIC

Used to treat traveler's diarrhea, an antibiotic called clioquinol has the power to dissolve plaque in the brains of mice, according to researchers affiliated with Massachusetts General Hospital in Boston.

Basically, the drug traps the copper and zinc that are found in brain plaque. Both metals enable certain enzymes to snip beta amyloid peptide from a larger protein, causing more clumps of the peptide to form. Clioquinol not only dissolves plaques but also reduces the ability of the peptides to clump together. Mice given the antibiotic for nine weeks had 50 percent less amyloid deposits in their brains than untreated mice had. The drug's ability to prevent the accumulation of beta amyloid peptide in the brain is an important advance in treating Alzheimer's disease.

Years ago, clioquinol was yanked from the market by the FDA because a few people taking it developed a severe vitamin B_{12} deficiency. This deficiency, however, can be treated with supplementation.

Human trials testing the effectiveness of clioquinol in people with mild to moderate Alzheimer's disease are under way.

NEOTROFIN

Developed by NeoTherapeutics, Inc., of Irvine, California, Neotrofin is an experimental drug that stimulates the production and release of growth factors in the brain's memory centers. These growth factors encourage neurons to make connections with other neurons. In a large-scale investigation, the drug is being tested at fifty-one clinical sites around the United States. In previous human studies, Neotrofin has been shown to improve memory and behavior in patients with mild-to-moderate Alzheimer's disease.

DIMEBON

Approved in Russia as an antihistamine, a drug called Dimebon has recently been studied in Russia as an anti-Alzheimer's drug. In a preliminary study with rats, the drug targeted beta amyloid peptide and kept it from damaging brain cells. Further, in a small pilot study, fourteen Alzheimer's patients were treated with Dimebon for eight weeks and showed improvement in cognitive function, anxiety, and depression. It's too early to tell whether this Russian drug has potential in treating the disease, but you may be hearing more about it in the future.

ESTROGEN

In recent years, estrogen, the female hormone, has been in the spotlight as a potential treatment for Alzheimer's disease. Medical science turned its attention to the hormone when it became clear that postmenopausal women, whose bodies cease estrogen production, have 30-percent higher rates of the disease than men of similar age.

Estrogen may increase short-term memory and the ability to learn tasks and may decrease the risk of Alzheimer's disease, according to a study conducted by Columbia University's School of Public Health. Investigators studied more than 1,000 women aged seventy and older and found that those who had taken estrogen for just a year had lower odds of developing Alzheimer's disease than women who had never taken the hormone.

Further, the research team speculated that women who take estrogen for ten years may be able to cut their risk of the disease by 40 percent.

Another study found that, if you have Alzheimer's disease, taking estrogen may lessen its severity. Of 143 Alzheimer's patients, those who had been on estrogen were mentally sharper than their peers with the disease.

There's more: Estrogen may protect against age-related dementia. That's the finding of a meta-analysis (a statistical study) of ten studies that looked into the relationship between taking estrogen and the risk of dementia and Alzheimer's disease. The results of the meta-analysis suggest that taking estrogen may reduce a woman's risk of developing dementia by nearly 30 percent.

How exactly does estrogen exert its protective action? Researchers believe that estrogen may trigger neurons to sprout more branches, a benefit that translates into more brainpower. Other scientists think that estrogen reduces the formation of beta amyloid peptide, the brain-damaging protein linked to Alzheimer's.

The effect of estrogen requires more investigation, but it looks promising as a bonafide treatment for dementia and Alzheimer's disease.

HUPERZINE A: THE MIRACLE MEMORY BOOSTER AND ANTI-ALZHEIMER'S AGENT

If you find yourself blanking out more than usual, meet a dietary supplement known as huperzine A, a compound isolated from the herb club moss (*Huperzia serrata*). Originally from China, huperzine A has long been used as a folk medicine in that country to treat fever, inflammation, and short-term memory loss. More recently, it has been under investigation in the United States as a treatment for Alzheimer's disease.

Remarkably, huperzine A works in much the same way as do drugs currently prescribed to treat failing memory: It inhibits cholinesterase, the enzyme that breaks down acetylcholine, a neurotransmitter in the brain that is critical for memory and learning. By this action, huperzine A protects the brain's supply of acetylcholine from breakdown. In addition, huperzine A has been described in the medical literature as a "neuroprotective agent" because it appears to protect brain cells from damage induced by environmental toxins.

The supplement is marketed as Cerebra or Huperzine A. In clinical studies conducted thus far, huperzine has shown the following characteristics.

IMPROVES MENTAL STATUS IN ALZHEIMER'S PATIENTS

In a study conducted at Zhejiang Medical University in Shanghai, 103 patients with Alzheimer's took either 200 micrograms of huperzine A daily or a placebo. After two months, nearly 60 percent of the huperzine A–takers showed significant improvement in mental status compared to 36 percent who were given the placebo.

Further, researchers at the Chinese Academy of Sciences in Shanghai who have studied huperzine A feel that the supplement may have a longer duration of action in the body, compared to its drug counterparts Cognex and Aricept, and far fewer side effects.

PROTECTS AGAINST FREE RADICALS

One of the probable reasons behind the development and progression of Alzheimer's disease is brain damage caused by free radicals, unstable molecules that destroy cell membranes and lead to disease. A Chinese study of huperzine A found that the supplement reduced the cellular damage inflicted by free radicals in patients with Alzheimer's disease. Huperzine A's ability to fight free radicals may be the reason why it acts as a neuroprotective agent.

RESTORES MEMORY

Chinese scientists at the State Key Laboratory of Drug Research in Shanghai tested the memory-improving properties of huperzine A in rats whose memories had been impaired naturally by age or induced by scopolamine, a memory-damaging chemical. In the aged rats, huperzine A restored the animals' ability to remember how to navigate through a maze; in the scopolamine-treated rats, huperzine A restored their spatial memory, which governs the ability to remember directions.

ENHANCES LEARNING

Chinese researchers have also investigated the effect of huperzine A on learning and memory performance in teenage students. Thirty-four pairs of teenagers were given either 100 micrograms (in divided doses) daily or a placebo for four weeks. The students were then tested on a language lesson. The scores of those taking huperzine A were higher than the scores of those taking the placebo. The researchers concluded that the huperzine A capsules "enhance the memory and learning performance of adolescent students."

SUPPLEMENTING WITH HUPERZINE A

As with drugs prescribed for Alzheimer's disease, huperzine A will not reverse the disease but may slow its progression. People suffering early signs of Alzheimer's, or age-related memory disorders, should talk to their doctors about taking this supplement. Based on clinical trials, the normal daily dosage is 100 to 200 micrograms, taken in divided doses.

SAFETY OF HUPERZINE A

Short-term (twenty-eight days) research with huperzine A indicates that the compound has low toxicity. It is not yet known, however, whether it has any long-term side effects.

Even so, healthy people should not supplement with huperzine A on an ongoing basis. As noted above, it blocks the enzyme that breaks down acetylcholine, and some of this enzyme is required to prevent excessive amounts of acetylcholine from building up in the body. An excess of acetylcholine can cause untoward side effects.

Be sure to consult with your physician or health-care provider if you are considering supplementation with hyperzine A. Do not supplement with huperzine A if you are taking Aricept or Tacrine.

7 OTHER AMAZING
ANTI-ALZHEIMER'S HERBS

The following seven botanical medicines are also effective in treating the symptoms of Alzheimer's disease.

BLACK COHOSH

Black cohosh is among the herbs that can raise levels of estrogen in the body. Boosting estrogen, according to several studies, can help improve memory and mood in female Alzheimer's patients.

There is no established dosage for treating Alzheimer's disease, but for other conditions—namely, menopausal symptoms—the usual dosage is 20 to 40 milligrams of a standardized extract twice a day, for up to six months.

GINKGO BILOBA

Presently, ginkgo biloba is the herbal remedy most widely used to treat Alzheimer's disease. It improves blood flow to the brain, protects brain cells against free-radical damage, minimizes nerve-cell injury in oxygen-starved tissues, and protects cellular receptors used by neurotransmitters to gain entry into cells. In studies, ginkgo biloba has been shown to improve memory, attention span, mood, and cognitive performance.

The recommended dosage based on clinical trials is 120 to 160 milligrams of a standardized extract daily in two to three divided doses.

GINSENG

This herbal remedy is emerging as a possible treatment for Alzheimer's disease, even though it has not been well studied in humans. An animal study found that ginseng can facilitate the release of acetylcholine in the brain plus reduce inflammation.

In a study of Siberian ginseng, Russian investigators gave the herb to people with dementia and other mental problems stemming from ather-osclerosis and found that it improved their memories and enhanced their physical and mental vigor.

The recommended dosage is 100 to 300 milligrams (standardized to 7 percent ginsenosides) three times daily.

HORSEBALM

This herbal medicine is well endowed with two beneficial chemicals—carvacrol and thymol—that help prevent the breakdown of acetyl-choline.

The recommended dosage is 1 to 4 grams of the dried root taken three times daily, or 20 to 40 drops of the liquid extract taken three times daily.

STINGING NETTLE

Another estrogen-boosting herb is stinging nettle, a good source of natural boron. Boron naturally elevates estrogen in the body. Estrogen has been found to be protective against Alzheimer's disease.

Stinging nettle is normally used in connection with the treatment of prostate problems, rheumatoid arthritis, hay fever, and urinary tract in-fections.

There is no established dosage for treating Alzheimer's disease, but for other conditions the usual dosage is 120 milligrams of a root extract taken twice a day.

VINPOCETINE

Extracted from the periwinkle plant Vinca minor, vinpocetine has been shown to improve memory, learning, and overall cognitive perfor-mance in patients suffering from mild-to-moderate dementia. It is con-sidered a neuroprotective herb.

The herb works in several impressive ways. It dilates blood vessels, ensuring unobstructed blood flow to the brain; guards against abnormal blood clotting; prevents hypoxia (lack of oxygen) in the brain; and snuffs out free radicals in the brain. Because of these actions, vinpocetine is considered to have potential in treating Alzheimer's disease.

The recommended dosage based on clinical trials is 15 to 45 milligrams a day.

WILLOW BARK

Willow bark is an aspirinlike herb that acts as an anti-inflammatory agent. It contains salicin, a natural compound that is responsible for the herb's anti-inflammatory and pain-relieving actions.

Research suggests that people who have taken a good deal of anti-inflammatory drugs throughout their lives have a lower incidence of Alzheimer's disease. Accordingly, many herbalists feel that taking willow bark, the herbal version of aspirin, could be protective as well.

The recommended dosage varies; check the product label for dosage information.

PARKINSON'S DISEASE: THE BEST NEW THERAPEUTIC CHOICES

More than 1 million people in the United States suffer from a progressive disorder of the central nervous system known as Parkinson's disease. Most are over age fifty, although a version of the disease called "young-onset" Parkinson's can strike people under age forty.

In Parkinson's disease, there is a degeneration of nerve cells in the substantia nigra, a region of the brain that produces dopamine, the neurotransmitter that sends signals within the brain to allow smooth movement of the muscles. Dopamine is lost, causing nerve cells to become overactive. As a result, patients are unable to control their movements, and walking, arm movement, and facial expression become impaired.

Symptoms show up in the following ways:

- shaking at rest.
- stiffness of limbs and trunk.
- slowness of movement.
- reduction of facial expressions.
- impaired balance and coordination.
- shuffling gait.
- difficulties in speech, swallowing, and chewing.

Since the 1970s, the standard treatment for Parkinson's disease has been the administration of the drug levodopa, a precursor of dopamine. Dopamine cannot be directly replaced because of the brain's protective blood-brain barrier, which bars most substances from entering it. Levodopa, however, can pass through this barrier and is converted to dopamine in the brain. Treatment with levodopa does not cure the disease nor does it prevent its progressive changes. Further, there are untoward side effects associated with levodopa.

Your physician may prescribe levodopa in combination with another drug, carbidopa, in a medication marketed as Sinemet. This combination helps alleviate the side effects of levodopa and makes the drug more potent. About 80 percent of Parkinson's patients take this drug.

A problem with both drugs, however, is that they may become less effective within two to five years. Side effects include low blood pressure upon standing, hallucinations, and delirium. Your physician will work with you to find the right dosage to minimize these side effects.

Fortunately, therapies for treating Parkinson's disease have made great advances and now include a wider choice of medications than ever before. What follows is a look at some of the best therapeutic choices for treating this disease.

DOPAMINE AGONISTS

Approved for use alone or in conjunction with levodopa, these drugs mimic dopamine's action in the brain. While on these medications, you require less levodopa. The most familiar dopamine agonists are Parlodel (bromocriptine) and Celance (pergolide). Newer versions are Requip (ropinirole hydrochloride) and Mirapex (pramipexole dihydrochloride).

ELDEPRYL

Also called Deprenyl, this drug works by delaying the breakdown of naturally occurring and levodopa-produced dopamine. This allows the buildup of dopamine in surviving nerve cells. This drug is often prescribed for patients with early Parkinson's disease.

There is a long list of side effects associated with this medication, according to *The PDR Family Guide to Prescription Drugs*. Among the side effects are abdominal pain, abnormal movements, anxiety, apathy, and blurred vision.

TASMAR AND COMTAN

Tasmar and Comtan represent a new class of drugs for treating Parkinson's disease. They work by inhibiting the action of an enzyme that breaks down the levodopa in Sinemet. They must be taken with Sinemet or levodopa because they have no effect on Parkinson's disease when taken alone.

According to *The PDR Family Guide to Prescription Drugs*, common side effects include abdominal pain, acid indigestion, breathing difficulty, chest pain, confusion, constipation, and drowsiness.

ARTANE AND COGENTIN

In Parkinson's disease, the short supply of dopamine creates a surplus of acetylcholine in the brain. Both of these drugs reduce the amount of acetylcholine in the brain and help correct the imbalance between the two neurotransmitters. They are usually taken with levodopa. A problem with these drugs, however, is their serious side effects, particularly in the elderly. The drugs cause urinary retention and mental confusion and are thus not prescribed for people over age sixty-five or seventy.

According to *The PDR Family Guide to Prescription Drugs*, common side effects are blurred vision, dry mouth, nausea, and nervousness.

SYMMETREL

Generally prescribed for mild cases of Parkinson's, this drug is an antiviral medication that appears to work by reducing acetylcholine and by stimulating the release of dopamine from storage sites in the brain. It is used alone or in combination with Sinemet.

According to medical studies, common side effects include difficulty concentrating, dizziness or lightheadedness, headache, irritability, loss of appetite, and nausea.

ESTROGEN

In postmenopausal women, estrogen is one of the drug therapies for preventing osteoporosis and the risk of bone fractures. It may also reduce the risk or slow the progression of Parkinson's disease, according to Mayo Clinic research. These studies show that women on estrogen are 40 percent less likely to develop the disease, and women with Parkinson's disease who took estrogen showed improvements in memory, motor skills, and thinking.

Another piece of proof that estrogen may be helpful in Parkinson's is that women are only half as likely to get the disease as men.

Estrogen is not yet approved as a treatment for Parkinson's disease, but, based on the latest evidence, it may become one in the future.

DEEP-BRAIN STIMULATION

This relatively new procedure involves the surgical implantation of a multi-electrode lead in the brain. The lead is then connected to a pulse generator, which is similar to a cardiac pacemaker, implanted near the collarbone. When a tremor begins, you activate the device by operating a special magnet that adjusts the electrical current.

The device stimulates the thalami, two walnut-sized areas deep within the brain that help control sensory information and movement. A recently released study by French neurosurgeons found that deep-brain stimulation can relieve the symptoms of Parkinson's disease (particularly tremor) for up to eight years. Normally, you still must take medication if you undergo deep-brain stimulation, although sometimes the dosage can be cut back.

SURGERY

Two types of surgery are available for Parkinson's disease: pallidotomy, which destroys a small portion of the globus pallidus (believed to be overactive in Parkinson's patients), and thalamotomy, which destroys a specific set of cells in the thalamus.

Both surgeries provide welcome relief from symptoms. The positive effects of pallidotomy may wear off after two years, however, necessitating future surgeries. Designed for the 5 to 10 percent of Parkinson's patients with disabling arm or hand tremor, thalamotomy reduces or eliminates the problem in as many as 90 percent of patients.

Overlooked Nutrient for Parkinson's Disease

In the Netherlands, researchers looked into the relationship between vitamin E and Parkinson's disease and found that high levels of the vitamin were linked to a low rate of the disease in more than 5,300 people. Their findings hint that vitamin E may be protective against Parkinson's disease.

Vitamin E is an antioxidant, meaning that it protects cells from damage. It occurs naturally in vegetable oils, whole-grain cereals, dried beans, and green leafy vegetables—yet its content is not high. Consequently, many nutritionists feel that vitamin E supplements are more effective than foods as a means of getting adequate vitamin E.

Supplementing with 400 IU daily is an excellent way to receive the extra amount you may need.

15

Stroke: It Doesn't Have to Happen

Despite its amazing powers, the brain is vulnerable to various illnesses and accidents. One of these is stroke (also called a "brain attack"), a disturbance to the brain's blood supply. Stroke occurs when the blood supply to the brain is cut off, either by bleeding from an artery, blockage by plaque (fatty deposits that build up in blood vessels), or because of a blood clot. A disturbance like this lasting more than a few seconds can damage or kill brain cells. Physicians call this area of dead cells an "infarct." Without prompt medical treatment, cells in the surrounding tissue will also die. If a stroke victim receives treatment within a six-hour window, there is less chance of further damage.

After a stroke, the victim may lose control of certain abilities, depending on which area of the brain has been affected. The consequences of stroke are listed in Table 15.1.

TABLE 15.1 Effects of Stroke	
BRAIN REGION AFFECTED	**CONSEQUENCES**
Cerebellum	Abnormal reflexes of the head and torso; coordination and balance problems; dizziness
Left Hemisphere	Language and speech problems; right-side paralysis
Right Hemisphere	Problems with spatial reasoning and perception
Brain Stem	Loss of control of involuntary functions, including breathing, blood pressure, and heartbeat; impairments in eye movements, hearing, speech, and swallowing

TYPES OF STROKE

Each year, approximately 400,000 to 600,000 Americans suffer a stroke, and nearly 150,000 people die as a result. Stroke is the third leading cause of death, the leading cause of disability among adults, and a major factor in late-life dementia.

The three major types of stroke are discussed below.

THROMBOTIC STROKE

The most common type of stroke is a thrombotic stroke, in which a fatty deposit forms in the inner wall of an artery and results in the formation of plaque. The plaque builds up, narrowing the artery and blocking blood flow to the brain. A blood clot (thrombus) may then form on the plaque, further restricting the flow of blood, oxygen, and nutrients to the brain.

EMBOLIC STROKE

An embolic stroke occurs when a blood clot formed elsewhere in the body is carried by the blood and lodges in an artery leading to the brain, choking off blood flow. When traveling through the bloodstream, the clot is called an embolus.

HEMORRHAGIC STROKE

A less common type of stroke is the hemorrhagic stroke. It is caused when an artery supplying blood leaks into the brain. The leaking artery prevents needed oxygen and nutrients from reaching the brain, and nerve tissue dies off as a result.

One type of hemorrhagic stroke can occur when an artery that has weakened over time bulges (called an aneurysm) and suddenly ruptures.

8 RECOMMENDATIONS TO PREVENT STROKE

The good news about stroke is that it is largely preventable by taking the following eight relatively simple measures to protect your heart and blood vessels.

CONTROL YOUR BLOOD PRESSURE

Elevated blood pressure (hypertension) can damage the blood vessels feeding your brain, choking off brain-nourishing blood and oxygen and increasing your risk of full-blown stroke. High blood pressure also increases your chances of having "mini-strokes"—unnoticed strokes that ultimately can contribute to a decline in faculties.

Studies indicate that people with hypertension perform poorly on tests that measure learning, memory, and other cognitive skills. You can help control blood pressure by eating a low-fat diet high in fruits, vegetables, whole grains, and beans; exercising; managing stress; and having your blood pressure checked on a regular basis.

QUIT SMOKING

Cigarette smoking is linked to an increased risk of stroke. But if you quit now, you'll do your heart and blood vessels a world of good. Studies show that the risk of stroke for people who have quit smoking for two to five years is lower than for people who still smoke.

CURTAIL ALCOHOL INTAKE

Excessive alcohol intake has been linked to stroke risk as well. To be on the safe side, consume alcohol in moderate portions (no more than one to two small drinks daily, if at all). Moderate consumption may protect against stroke by elevating levels of beneficial phytochemicals that break up clots in the blood.

EXERCISE REGULARLY

Exercise strengthens the heart and blood vessels and improves circulation to the brain. Research shows that people who engage in even light or moderate physical activity have a 40-percent less chance of stroke than couch potatoes do.

EAT WELL

Choose foods low in saturated fat and cholesterol and eat lots of stroke-reducing fruits and vegetables. A Harvard study revealed that drinking citrus juices and eating cruciferous vegetables such as broccoli, cauliflower, and Brussels sprouts can reduce stroke risk by as much as 32 percent. High-fiber foods also help prevent stroke.

SUPPLEMENT WITH MAGNESIUM

The arteries in your brain require twice as much magnesium as arteries elsewhere in your body. If an insufficient amount of magnesium makes it to the cells of the arterial walls, arteries may contract suddenly, leading to stroke. For stroke prevention, some medical experts recommend taking a daily supplement of about 250 milligrams, in addition to what you obtain from food.

CONSIDER LOW-DOSE ASPIRIN THERAPY

Aspirin has been approved by the FDA to help reduce the risk of stroke if you've had a previous clot-induced stroke or have had a warning sign called a transient ischemic attack (TIA). (TIA is discussed further below.)

Aspirin prevents platelets—tiny clotting substances in blood—from abnormally clumping together in a process called platelet aggregation. Platelet aggregation triggers the formation of dangerous blood clots that can lead to heart attack or stroke.

The recommended dosage of aspirin for stroke prevention is 50 to 325 milligrams daily.

If you have had a hemorrhagic stroke, however, the aspirin-a-day regimen may be dangerous. That's because aspirin diminishes the clotting ability of the blood. Therefore, the bleeding that is characteristic of a hemorrhagic stroke is less likely to be stopped by the clotting of your blood.

TREAT SLEEP APNEA

Very loud snoring may signal a disorder called obstructive sleep apnea, in which the sleeper stops breathing for a couple of seconds. Research shows that people with sleep apnea have dangerously low levels of oxygen in their blood, with rising levels of carbon dioxide—a condition that can cause blood clots or stroke. Because sleep apnea is a serious disorder, sufferers should seek proper medical care. Solutions range from the use of a masklike compressor that maintains air flow at night to surgical corrections that open up the size of the airways.

5 Warning Signs of Stroke

Think of stroke as a brain attack and seek emergency treatment at the first appearance of symptoms. These include:

1. Rapid onset of blurred vision or decreased vision, particularly in one eye.
2. Difficulty in speaking or understanding simple statements.
3. Sudden numbness, weakness, or paralysis of the face, arm, or leg, especially on one side of the body.
4. Sudden dizziness, trouble walking, loss of balance, or an unexplained fall.
5. Severe headache with no known cause (can be a sign of an impending hemorrhagic stroke).

MINI-STROKES: MORE DANGEROUS THAN YOU KNOW

Sometimes, the warning signs of stroke last for only a few moments, then disappear. This may indicate a mini-stroke, known medically as a transient ischemic attack (TIA). It is caused by a temporary deficiency in the blood supply to the brain. Most frequently, TIAs are due to atherosclerosis, characterized by the formation of plaques in arteries. TIAs are diagnosed through medical examinations and tests, including CT scans or MRIs to provide images of the arteries under evaluation.

TIAs are dangerous because they are strong omens of stroke. In fact, a third of people who experience TIAs have a stroke within five years; another third will experience additional TIAs. You should not ignore a TIA, but see a doctor right away.

Factors that increase your risk of TIA include high blood pressure, some forms of heart disease, smoking, diabetes, and advanced age.

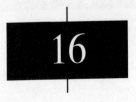

The Many Faces of Anxiety

If you're like most people, you've felt uptight from time to time... the butterflies before a big business presentation... the stress of an impending deadline... worry over mounting bills. While almost everyone feels anxious at one time or another, roughly 18 million Americans suffer from anxiety so severe and seemingly permanent that it interferes with their daily lives.

4 ANXIETY DISORDERS

If you're experiencing a level of anxiety that interferes with your daily life, you could be suffering from one of the following four anxiety disorders.

GENERALIZED ANXIETY DISORDER

About 8 percent of the population suffers from general anxiety disorder, and it affects as many men as women. Generally, it is characterized by ongoing, but irrational, fears that something bad is going to happen. Other symptoms include feeling upset, apprehensive, depressed, irritable, or uneasy. You also may have trouble concentrating on the normal tasks at hand. Your body may react to the anxiety on a physical level with symptoms such as a galloping pulse, clammy skin, shortness of breath, muscular tension, tremors, nausea, lightheadedness, insomnia, and fatigue.

Research has revealed that people suffering from general anxiety disorder may have an imbalance of an important brain chemical called GABA. When treated with drugs that increase GABA activity, anxiety tends to simmer down.

Besides physiological imbalances, deep-seated emotional problems or long-term stress may be at the root of a generalized anxiety disorder. For example, you may have chronic low self-esteem or tend to look at the world in a negative way. Unresolved stress such as an abusive marriage, loss of a loved one, or constant money woes can also trigger this condition. Table 16.1 lists recommended treatments for generalized anxiety disorder.

TABLE 16.1 Recommended Treatments for Generalized Anxiety Disorder	
Natural Therapies*	• Kava (100 mg, 3 times daily) • GABA (200 mg, 4 times daily) • 5-HTP (100 to 300 mg, 3 times daily) • Theanine (100 to 400 mg daily) • Nutritional supplements: niacinamide (500 to 800 mg daily) and calcium (1,000 to 2,000 mg daily). Some research indicates that both nutrients may be helpful in reducing symptoms of anxiety. *(Continued)*

Natural Therapies*	• Homeopathy • Aromatherapy • Relaxation and meditation • Exercise
Prescription Medications*	• Antianxiety drugs, including BuSpar (buspirone), beta-blockers, Effexor (venlafaxine), and Atarax (hydroxyzine) • Benzodiazepine drugs, including Valium (diazepam) and Serax (oxazepam) • Antidepressants, particularly selective serotonin reuptake inhibitors (SSRIs) such as Prozac (fluoxetine), Zoloft (sertraline), or Paxil (paroxetine)
Counseling	• Cognitive therapy • Group therapy

*Several of these recommended treatments—kava, homeopathy, aromatherapy, antianxiety drugs—are discussed elsewhere throughout this book.

PANIC DISORDER

Suddenly, without warning and for no apparent reason, you are gripped with intense terror. You literally freeze, unable to move. Within minutes, your heart starts racing, you're gasping for breath, your chest squeezes in pain, you're shaking and sweating. You feel like you're going to die or go crazy. Then, as quickly as these horrible feelings came on, they leave—until the next episode catches you unaware.

Though symptoms vary from individual to individual, this scenario is typical of a "panic attack," a very real and frightening psychological event that characterizes panic disorder. It may last anywhere from ten minutes to a half-hour. Nearly 3 million Americans suffer from this debilitating problem.

No one is yet sure exactly what causes panic disorder, but there are some fairly strong scientific hunches. People suffering from panic disorders, for example, may have a chemical imbalance in the brain or an overactive amygdala, the portion of the brain that controls such emotions as fear and anxiety. Or panic disorder may have a genetic link, since it tends to run in families. Also, a panic attack may be a symptom of an underlying disease. In fact, more than forty diseases can trigger paniclike reactions. Table 16.2 lists recommended treatments for panic disorder.

TABLE 16.2 Recommended Treatments for Panic Disorder	
Natural Therapies*	• GABA (200 mg, 4 times daily) • 5-HTP (100 to 300 mg, 3 times daily) • Inositol (12 grams daily) • Relaxation therapy
Prescription Medications*	• Antianxiety drugs, including BuSpar (buspirone), beta-blockers, Effexor (venlafaxine), and Atarax (hydroxyzine) • Antidepressants, particularly selective serotonin reuptake inhibitors (SSRIs) such as Prozac (fluoxetine), Zoloft (sertraline), or Paxil (paroxetine)
Counseling	• Cognitive therapy • Group therapy

*Several of these recommended treatments—kava, homeopathy, aromatherapy, antianxiety drugs—are discussed elsewhere throughout this book.

PHOBIAS

Few of us like to see a snake slither across our path. And who doesn't clench the armrest when an airplane flight gets turbulent? Fears like these are common, but if they become so intense that you won't walk in your garden or board an airplane you may be suffering from a phobia.

Basically, a phobia is the fear of a place, situation, or object. Phobias run the gamut from the simple, such as fear of snakes or spiders, to the emotionally paralyzing—fear of being in public places (a phobia known as agoraphobia), for example. There are literally hundreds of different kinds of phobias, and every person has one or two.

A phobia is a concern only if it regularly interferes with and compromises daily living. A phobic person will go to great lengths to avoid the situation he or she fears. Table 16.3 lists the recommended treatments for phobias.

TABLE 16.3	
Recommended Treatments for Phobias	
Natural Therapies*	• Kava (100 mg, 3 times daily) • Nutritional supplements: niacinamide (500 to 800 mg daily) and calcium (1,000 to 2,000 mg daily). Some research indicates that both nutrients may be helpful in reducing symptoms of phobia. • Meditation • Exercise
Prescription Medications*	• Benzodiazepine drugs, including Valium (diazepam) and Serax (oxazepam) • Antidepressants, particularly selective serotonin reuptake inhibitors (SSRIs) such as Prozac (fluoxetine), Zoloft (sertraline), or Paxil (paroxetine)
Counseling*	• Cognitive therapy • Group therapy • Exposure therapy

*Several of these recommended treatments—kava, homeopathy, aromatherapy, antianxiety drugs—are discussed elsewhere throughout this book.

OBSESSIVE-COMPULSIVE DISORDER (OCD)

People who suffer from this disorder exhibit compulsions—rituals they must perform before they can begin another activity. Examples of ritualistic behavior include repetitive hand washing, excessive neatness, checking and rechecking to make sure something isn't forgotten, or performing an activity in a series of senseless steps. If the rituals can't be completed as desired, the sufferer may feel an overwhelming sense of anxiety or despair.

Obsessions may involve the mind as well. The obsessive–compulsive may be plagued with persistent thoughts of violence or sex or fears of becoming infected with germs. Table 16.4 lists the recommended treatments for obsessive-compulsive disorder.

TABLE 16.4 Recommended Treatments for Obsessive-Compulsive Disorder	
Natural Therapies*	• Kava (100 mg, 3 times daily) • St. John's wort (300 mg, 3 times daily) • Inositol (12 grams daily) • Exercise
Prescription Medications*	• Antidepressants, particularly selective serotonin reuptake inhibitors (SSRIs) such as Prozac (fluoxetine), Zoloft (sertraline), or Paxil (paroxetine)
Counseling	• Cognitive therapy • Exposure therapy • Combination of therapy and antidepressants

*Several of these recommended treatments—kava, homeopathy, aromatherapy, antianxiety drugs—are discussed elsewhere throughout this book.

7 Natural Paths to Calm

Whether you're suffering from an anxiety disorder or just a bad case of the nerves, there are numerous holistic options that will help keep you calmer and more at peace. Described below, these include herbal, vitamin, amino acid, homeopathic, and aromatherapy solutions.

GAMMA-AMINOBUTYRIC ACID (GABA)

GABA, the brain's natural tranquilizer, is available as a supplement, used to induce relaxation. Taken prior to bedtime, it produces a deep, more restful sleep. GABA works as an "inhibitory" neurotransmitter, meaning that it blocks anxiety messages from being transmitted from nerve cell to nerve cell.

The standard dosage for easing anxiety is 200 milligrams taken four times a day on an empty stomach. In dosages that exceed the recommended amount, GABA can increase anxiety.

5-HYDROXY-TRYPTOPHAN (5-HTP)

Although best known as a natural antidepressant, 5-HTP is often recommended for reducing anxiety and improving sleep quality. It works by increasing levels of serotonin, a feel-good neurotransmitter. In an eight-week study, 5-HTP was compared with Anafranil (clomipramine) in forty-five people suffering from anxiety disorders. The results showed that 5-HTP was nearly as effective as Anafranil.

The standard dosage of 5-HTP is 100 to 300 milligrams taken three times daily. This supplement should not be taken if you are using prescription antidepressants that elevate serotonin because the combination may hike serotonin to dangerous levels. 5-HTP also interacts adversely with a medication used to treat Parkinson's disease, carbidopa (Sinemet), and the combination can cause serious skin problems. Nor should you take 5-HTP if you suffer from heart disease, stroke, or high blood pressure.

KAVA

The most popular herbal remedy for treating anxiety is kava, which works relatively fast and has few short-term side effects. Case in point: In a 1991 study, fifty-eight patients suffering from anxiety of non-mental origin were divided into two groups—a kava group that took a kava extract (100 milligrams, three times daily) and a placebo group. The experiment lasted four weeks, and after weeks one, two, and four of treatment, the subjects were assessed using a reputable test to evaluate anxiety. In just one week, the kava-supplementers showed a significant reduction in anxiety symptoms and were dramatically better by the end of the study. (Those in the placebo group didn't fare as well.) No one experienced any of the possible side effects, which include restlessness, tremor, headache, stomach complaints, and drowsiness.

INOSITOL

Inositol, a member of the B-complex family, is critical to brain-cell chemistry and is used by various types of receptors to help transmit messages. With the exception of niacin, there is more inositol in the body than any other vitamin.

Inositol has been investigated as a treatment for panic disorder. In one study, twenty-one patients with panic disorder were treated with 12 grams a day of inositol or a placebo for four weeks. The results were promising. The inositol-treated group had fewer panic attacks, but when they did have one it was less severe. Little change was observed in the placebo group. The researchers concluded that "the fact that inositol is a natural component of the human diet makes it a potentially attractive therapeutic for panic disorder."

There's more. Their research continued with a look into whether inositol could help people suffering from obsessive-compulsive disorder. In 1996, thirteen patients with this disorder were given 18 grams of inositol daily or a placebo for six weeks. Remarkably, inositol significantly helped obsessive-compulsive sufferers, too.

Why did inositol work so powerfully in treating panic disorder and obsessive-compulsive disorder? One possible explanation is that inositol appears to regulate normal levels of the brain chemical serotonin. And the other incredible news about inositol is that it produces no untoward side effects.

Inositol is certainly worth a look if you're plagued by either of these anxiety disorders. For anxiety, natural health practitioners recommend a dosage of 12 grams daily.

THEANINE

An amino acid extracted from green tea, theanine produces a tranquilizing effect on the brain without causing drowsiness. It works by increasing levels of GABA, an antianxiety neurotransmitter, in the brain to deliver a sense of calm and well-being. Theanine also boosts levels of dopamine, another neurotransmitter with mood-lifting effects.

This natural relaxant appears to have other benefits as well, verified by animal studies. Studies with rodents show that it enhances the ability to learn and remember and protects brain cells from damage that leads to dementia.

Theanine is sold in capsules as a dietary supplement. The standard dosage is 100 milligrams once daily for general relaxation; or 100 milligrams taken four times a day for an ongoing mood-elevating effect.

HOMEOPATHY

Homeopathy, a medical system that uses minute doses of natural substances to stimulate a patient's immune system, is increasingly being used to treat mental disorders. Researchers at Duke University studied the effects of homeopathic remedies on patients suffering from phobia, panic disorder, and depression, with impressive results. Symptoms improved by more than 50 percent. The researchers concluded that "homeopathy may be useful in the treatment of affective and anxiety disorders in patients with mildly to severely symptomatic conditions."

If you're not familiar with homeopathy, which remedies are best? Generally, there are three homeopathic medicines used to treat anxiety disorders. They are discussed below.

Aurum Metallicum

Similar to the therapeutic gold compounds used to treat arthritis, aurum metallicum is used to treat anxiety, depression, postpartum depression, alcohol withdrawal, and rheumatoid arthritis. It consists of a finely ground powder mixed with milk sugars. Follow the label for dosage instructions.

Calms Forte

This is a formulation of various calming herbs (passionflower, milky oats, and chamomile) and minerals (mainly calcium and magnesium). It comes in a package of thirty-two caplets. Follow the label for dosage instructions.

Sepia

Derived from the ink of the cuttlefish, sepia is considered a leading homeopathic remedy for mental disorders, including anxiety, irritability, and depression. Like most homeopathic remedies, sepia comes in several strengths. Follow the label for dosage instructions.

AROMATHERAPY

Aromatherapy employs essential oils to treat emotional problems, such as stress and anxiety, as well as a number of other ailments. When something, or someone, smells good, our bodies respond positively to the aroma by releasing feel-good substances similar to endorphins, used to combat anxiety. What's more, these scents waft into the limbic region, or emotional center, of the brain, to produce feelings of calm. Here are several oils that, when diffused into the air, can induce tranquility. For a quick look, see Table 16.5 on page 341.

Chamomile Oil

From a distance, the flowers of chamomile resemble little yellow apples tucked in the grass—which is why the ancient Greeks dubbed the plant "chamaimelon" from *khamai* ("on the ground") and *melon* (apple). Chamomile is also spelled "camomile."

As an aromatic oil, chamomile is prized for its ability to dispel nervous tension, reduce anxiety, and lessen stress. In a study conducted at the University Department of Experimental Psychology in Cambridge, researchers instructed subjects to inhale chamomile oil and discovered that the oil had a positive effect on mood and judgment.

Clary Sage Oil

In the Middle Ages, this herb was used to heal eye problems, hence the name "clary," which originates from a word meaning "clear eyes." Today, the herb is considered a treatment for menstrual problems because it contains an estrogenlike plant hormone that helps relieve cramps and prevent hot flashes. Clary sage also stimulates the adrenal glands and thus greatly relieves stress.

Aromatherapists use clary sage to calm nervous anxiety, settle panic states, and reduce stress. A study conducted at Oxford University found that clary sage, used in aromatherapy, reduced fear, anxiety, and pain in women during labor and reduced the need for painkillers during delivery. Chamomile oil was also effective.

Lavender Oil

The aroma of lavender oil, extracted from the lavender (*Lavandula*) herb, has long been known to have a calming effect on the body. In fact, chemical analyses of lavender, along with animal experiments, have discovered that the herb contains compounds that exert a light sedative effect.

One study has tested this effect in people, with some intriguing results. Researchers from the University of Leicester in central England found that insomniacs in a nursing home slept as well when lavender oil was diffused into the air as they did while taking sleeping pills, including tranquilizers. Further, the people were less restless during sleep than they were while taking drugs. Scientists speculate that sedative compounds in lavender stimulate olfactory nerves in the nose that connect to brain areas that bring on sleep.

Lavender is approved by German Commission E for insomnia. Alternative health-care practitioners also recommend lavender for treating people with dementia because of its calming effect.

Orange Oil

Extracted from fresh orange peel, orange oil gives off a pleasant, refreshing aroma that reportedly induces relaxation. Writing in the medical journal *The Lamp*, nurse Pam Tobin noted that, because orange oil is sedating, relaxing, and calming, it is an excellent oil to use in massage therapy to prevent agitation in people suffering from dementia.

In addition, aromatherapists believe that orange oil can be employed for treating stress, anxiety, and depression when used in massage, added to bathwater, or diffused into the air.

Vanilla Oil

If you've ever passed a bottle of vanilla extract under your nose, you're familiar with its delightful aroma. In aromatherapy, vanilla oil is known for its ability to calm and relax the body when diffused into the air or used as a massage oil. Clinically, vanilla oil does seem to help people cope with stressful situations. Case in point: At Memorial Sloan-Kettering Cancer Center in New York City, patients exposed to vanilla fragrance while undergoing magnetic resonance imaging (MRIs) scans reported less anxiety than those exposed to non-scented air. Vanilla oil can be combined with orange oil and diffused into the air for a doubly relaxing effect.

TABLE 16.5
Aromatherapy Prescriptions

Oil*	Uses
Chamomile Oil	Eases nervous tension, anxiety, and stress; improves mood and judgment
Clary Sage Oil	Treats anxiety, panic states, and stress
Lavender Oil	Exerts a calming effect; acts as a mild sedative
Orange Oil	Induces relaxation; treats anxiety, stress, and depression; prevents agitation in dementia patients
Vanilla Oil	Induces relaxation; treats anxiety and stress

*For information on how to use essential oils, refer to "Sniff Your Way to Better Brainpower" in Chapter 5.

4 Nonaddictive Antianxiety Medications

People with severe anxiety are routinely treated with prescription medications. And, in most cases, that's as it should be, since anxiety can be so debilitating and seemingly permanent that it interferes with normal living.

Some of the most widely prescribed antianxiety drugs are the benzodiazepines, which include diazepam (Valium), clorazepate (Tranxene), oxazepam (Serax), lorazepam (Ativan), and alprazolam (Xanax). Each is more alike than different. They are recommended as specific doses, for short-term use only, and can be effective for helping people get through stress-producing situations.

Benzodiazepines produce their calming effect by interacting with a group of brain cells located in the limbic system, the area of the brain that controls emotions. Once inside cells, benzodiazepines intensify the action of a brain neurotransmitter called GABA, which prevents anxiety messages from being transmitted from nerve cell to nerve cell and thus maintains a calming effect on the body.

Such drugs have worked well for millions of people, restoring their sanity and enabling them to return to productive living. But, while their use can be an effective part of treating and managing anxiety, these drugs are not without complications. Many are highly addictive, leading to dependency and abuse. Some increase the risk of accidental injury, produce worrisome sedation, and have other intolerable side effects.

Fortunately, other antianxiety drugs are available, and they're just as effective as benzodiazepines but with fewer side effects and less potential for addiction. If you're being treated for anxiety, you may want to ask your physician about the following four alternatives.

BUSPAR

Approved in 1986, BuSpar (buspirone) affects the action of the calming neurotransmitter serotonin. Specifically, the drug lowers serotonin levels in people who have too much and elevates levels in those who have too little. Studies show that BuSpar works as well as the benzodiazepines for managing anxiety but has not been found useful for panic attacks. Additionally, BuSpar is nonsedating and nonaddictive.

According to *The PDR Family Guide to Prescription Drugs*, some common side effects may include chest pain, dizziness, dream disturbances, headache, lightheadedness, and nausea. A drawback of this drug is that it may take one to two weeks to start working.

BETA-BLOCKERS

Beta-blockers are actually a family of cardiovascular drugs. The best known is propanolol (Inderal), which was approved in 1967 to treat irregular heartbeats. Since then, its use has expanded to include the prevention of second heart attacks, plus the treatment of angina, high blood pressure, migraine headaches—and anxiety.

Beta-blockers interfere with the action of certain nerve systems in the body that stimulate the activity of the heart, thereby alleviating malfunctions like irregular heartbeats. What's more, they subdue the force and rate of heart contractions. The drug's action on nerve systems somehow relieves anxiety.

Medical experts note that taking a beta-blocker one hour before an anticipated stressful event can reduce anxiety significantly. These drugs do not normally produce sedation and are not habit-forming.

According to *The PDR Family Guide to Prescription Drugs*, side effects may include stomach cramps, congestive heart failure, constipation, diarrhea, breathing problems, dry eyes, hair loss, nausea, hallucinations, and several others.

EFFEXOR

Effexor (venlafaxine) is a "serotonin-norepinephrine reuptake inhibitor," meaning that it increases levels of both serotonin and norepinephrine in the brain. It is prescribed not only for anxiety but also for depression. There is an extended release (Effexor XR) version of the drug, designed to be taken just once a day.

Clinical studies with Effexor show that the drug not only relieves anxiety but also helps patients regain a normal life both at work and at home. Effexor does not cause drowsiness or addiction.

According to *The PDR Family Guide to Prescription Drugs*, side effects may include abdominal pain, abnormal dreams, abnormal ejaculation or orgasm, blurred vision, chills, constipation, cough, diarrhea, and dizziness. Effexor may also raise blood pressure.

ATARAX

Atarax (hydroxyzine) is an antihistamine sometimes prescribed to treat anxiety and tension. It is also useful in alleviating anxiety that results from physical illness. The drug works by suppressing activity in areas of the central nervous system to produce a calming effect.

Atarax does cause drowsiness. Fortunately, though, this common side effect is temporary, disappearing within a few days or after reducing the dosage.

Other common side effects listed in the *The PDR Family Guide to Prescription Drugs* include dry mouth, twitches, tremors, and convulsions.

THE HIGH ANXIETY OF POSTTRAUMATIC STRESS DISORDER: THE CAUSES, THE CURES

Over the course of a lifetime, one in every two people will experience a life-threatening trauma, according to the Madison Institute of Medicine, Inc., an organization involved in treating various mental disorders. The traumatic experience could involve rape, sexual abuse, war, a natural disaster, fire, major car accident, plane crash, robbery, captivity, or an act of terrorism such as that which occurred in the United States on September 11, 2001.

In the aftermath of such an event, it is normal to feel anxiety, be emotionally numb, have nightmares, suffer amnesia, or experience other unusual symptoms. For most people, these symptoms diminish within a few weeks. But for others, they linger for months or years, interfering with normal life. In such cases, the victim is said to have "posttraumatic stress disorder" (PTSD).

This disorder was once called "shell shock" or "battle fatigue," but it is not limited to soldiers harmed by war. Any trauma beyond the range of normal human experience can induce PTSD in survivors of the trauma. Even so, veterans are its main victims, with as many as 800,000 Vietnam vets suffering from PTSD.

Its specific symptoms, which can be identified by an experienced clinician, are listed in Table 16.6. These may surface immediately after the

TABLE 16.6
Common Symptoms of PTSD

INTRUSIVE SYMPTOMS	AVOIDANCE SYMPTOMS	AROUSAL SYMPTOMS
• Persistent recollections of the traumatic event in thoughts, images, daydreams, and nightmares • Acting and feeling as if the event were recurring (through flashbacks, hallucinations, or delusions) • Mental distress in reaction to reminders of the event • Physiological reactions (rapid heartbeat, elevated blood pressure, etc.) in response to these reminders	• Avoiding feelings, thoughts, conversation associated with the event • Avoiding activities, people, or places that recall the event • Problems in recalling the event • Sense that life will be brief, or lack of fulfillment or meaning in life	• Insomnia • Angry outbursts or irritability • Lack of concentration • An extreme sense of being on guard • Increased "startle response" (easily startled)

Adapted from: Morrison, J. *DSM-IV Made Easy: The Clinician's Guide to Diagnosis* (New York: The Guilford Press, 1995); Flannery, R. B. 1999. Psychological trauma and posttraumatic stress disorder. *International Journal of Emergency Mental Health* 1: 135–140.

trauma or be delayed by six months or longer. In people diagnosed with this disorder, seemingly benign incidents or associations—a loud noise, a certain odor, even a locale—can spark a PTSD attack, and the horror of the trauma comes back, unbidden, in torrents of panic.

THE BRAIN AND PTSD SYMPTOMS

It has been scientifically theorized that the amygdala, an almond-shaped structure in the brain, may be involved in generating certain PTSD responses. Normally, the amygdala helps us react appropriately to threatening situations. But in PTSD sufferers, those reactions can go haywire. That's because the amygdala somehow pairs innocuous environmental cues (like a noise or smell) with a traumatic memory, triggering a pathological reliving of the terror.

Other research suggests that trauma may harm the hippocampus. Two studies have found that people with traumatic histories have smaller hippocampi than normal, and this may set off symptoms.

TREATING PTSD

Fortunately, PTSD is a treatable condition. Studies show that many patients recover within a relatively short time after the trauma, with up to two-thirds of patients recovering within five months. In a minority of trauma victims, however, PTSD may last for many years and, indeed, for life.

Four therapies that have been shown to be effective in treating PTSD are summarized below.

Exposure Therapy

This form of therapy helps you confront feared objects, situations, people, memories, and images in a safe way. Your therapist may ask you to recount the traumatic memories until they lose their grip over you. This can be done by recounting them aloud, writing about them, reading about them, or recording them on tape to be listened to repeatedly.

Another form of exposure therapy encourages you to confront your fear in real-life situations, such as visiting the place where the trauma occurred, and doing so over and over again until the discomfort fades.

Anxiety Management

Anxiety management combines a set of techniques designed to help you cope better with PTSD symptoms. These techniques include *breathing training* to reduce hyperventilation (which produces sensations that make you more anxious); *relaxation* to reduce muscular tension; assertiveness training to teach you how to directly express your feelings, needs, or opinions; *positive thinking* and *self-talk* so that you learn to replace destructive thoughts with positive ones; and *thought stopping* in which you learn how to turn off discomforting thoughts.

Cognitive Therapy

Cognitive therapy helps you understand how your thoughts lead to anxiety, depression, anger, or irrational behavior. You learn how to slip out of self-defeating thought patterns and think more positively and realistically about the world around you.

Medication Therapy

Medications are often used in conjunction with the previously mentioned treatments used to treat PTSD. As of May 2000, the only FDA-approved medication for treating the disorder is sertraline (Zoloft), a selective serotonin reuptake inhibitor (SSRI), but other medications are used as well. The major medications used to treat PTSD are as follows:

- Elavil (amitriptyline)
- Xanax (alprazolam)
- Valium (diazepam)
- BuSpar (buspirone)
- Zoloft (sertraline)
- Paxil (paroxetine)
- Tofranil (impramine)
- Norpramin (desipramine)

GETTING HELP

If you have been diagnosed with PTSD or think you may have it, talk to a doctor. Although it can take time for your symptoms to improve, with the proper treatment you can recover and move forward with your life.

Novel Treatment for PTSD: Eye Movement Desensitization and Reprocessing (EMDR)

An innovative approach to treating PTSD is Eye Movement Desensitization and Reprocessing (EMDR), developed by Francine Shapiro, Ph.D., a licensed psychotherapist and senior research fellow at the Mental Research Institute in Palo Alto, California. She is also the author of *EMDR: The Breakthrough Therapy for Overcoming Anxiety, Stress, and Trauma* (Basic Books, 1997). EMDR is based on the theory that traumatic memories are somehow sealed away in the nervous system and unable to be processed or recalled in a normal, nontroubling way.

Dr. Shapiro discovered EMDR quite by accident. She noticed that when troubling thoughts and emotions came into her mind, her eyes would begin moving laterally as well as diagonally. After purposely making the same eye movements while focusing on distressful memories, Dr. Shapiro found that these memories became less disturbing and began eventually fading away. She began using the technique on trauma victims and discovered that it could alleviate PTSD in many of the cases. To date, EMDR has been used successfully to help millions of trauma survivors.

WHAT HAPPENS DURING AN EMDR SESSION?

Basically, EMDR works like this: During a session, you're instructed to visualize a traumatic memory while mentally reliving the negative emotions attached to it. At the same time, the therapist waves his or her hand, or a plastic rod, rapidly back and forth in front of your eyes as you try to follow it with your eyes. This portion of the session—referred to as desensitization—is followed by a period in which you conjure up positive thoughts and feelings, while the therapist waves a hand or rod and takes you through another series of repetitive eye movements.

In many cases, EMDR relieves traumatic distress and removes the anxiety associated with traumatic memories—benefits that have been substantiated by scientific experiments. Recent clinical research has found that in studies of people suffering from rape, combat stress, loss of a loved one, accidents, and natural disasters, 84 to 90 percent of victims no longer experienced PTSD after only three sessions of EMDR.

HOW IT WORKS

How, then, does EMDR work its wonders? No one really knows for sure, not even the 22,000 therapists in the United States who currently use EMDR. The general consensus is that traumatic events are processed by the brain in a fashion different from the way normal events are processed. By stimulating the brain's memory-processing system, EMDR defuses the traumatic memory and converts it into a normal, less distressful remembrance. The net effect is that patients can respond more positively to painful memories.

EMDR does have its detractors, and many psychologists feel that it is just one of numerous therapies that can be used to treat PTSD. Those therapies include antianxiety drugs and counseling. As yet, though, few healing tools have been found that truly conquer the intense fear and anxiety of a PTSD episode as well as EMDR does. Unfortunately, EMDR does not work for everyone.

LOCATING AN EMDR PRACTITIONER

EMDR is worth a try, particularly since it is not harmful and does not involve medication with prescription drugs. If you want to try EMDR, find a therapist trained and licensed in its use. One key source of information is the EMDR Institute, P.O. Box 51010, Pacific Grove, California 93950; (408) 372-3900; www.emdr.com.

17

Attention Deficit Hyperactivity Disorder (ADHD): Do You Have It?

Inability to pay attention, constant fidgeting, impulsive behavior—these are a few of the signs of attention deficit hyperactivity disorder (ADHD), a condition in which attention-regulating centers in the brain go haywire. There is also an imbalance in dopamine and possibly other neurotransmitters in the brain. The net effect is inattention, hyperactivity, impulsivity, or a combination of all three.

First described in 1902, ADHD has historically been considered a childhood condition and is one of the most common behavioral disorders in children. However, recent data suggest that ADHD persists into adult life in approximately 30 to 50 percent of adults who had the disorder as children.

Could you be one of them? To find out, read "18 Signs You Should Ignore" on page 351. This list of symptoms is based primarily on guidelines from the *Diagnostic and Statistical Manual of Mental Disorders*, Fourth Edition (DSM-IV), considered the most valid standard for diagnosing the disorder. (A diagnosis, however, should be made by a psychologist or psychiatrist who is knowledgeable in ADHD, in concert with a physician. A physician can rule out medical conditions that mimic ADHD, such as thyroid disease, certain types of seizures, hearing problems, head injury, and liver disease.)

18 Signs You Shouldn't Ignore

If you have ADHD, you will exhibit either inattention symptoms or hyperactivity-impulsivity symptoms (or both) that have lasted for at least six months to a degree that interferes with your job and your quality of life.

INATTENTION SYMPTOMS

Suspect ADHD, if at least six of the following symptoms of inattention often apply to you:

- Fails to pay close attention to details or makes careless errors in tasks, on the job, or in other activities.
- Has trouble maintaining concentration.
- Doesn't seem to listen well.
- Neither follows through nor completes jobs (but not because you oppose the job or don't understand the instructions).
- Can't get organized or set priorities.
- Dislikes activities that require sustained mental effort.
- Loses materials needed for tasks, jobs, or other activities.
- Is easily distracted.
- Is forgetful, missing appointments, social commitments, deadlines, and other activities.

HYPERACTIVITY-IMPULSIVITY SYMPTOMS

Suspect ADHD if at least six of the following symptoms often apply to you:

HYPERACTIVITY SYMPTOMS

- Has difficulty relaxing.
- Feels chronically restless.

- Has trouble engaging in leisure-time activities.
- Feels chronically on the edge or on the go.
- Talks excessively.

IMPULSIVITY
- Answers questions before they have been completely asked.
- Blurts out comments that are rude or insulting.
- Displays a hot, explosive temper, with angry outbursts.
- Displays mood changes ranging from euphoria to despair (the mood changes cannot be explained by a mood or personality disorder).

WHAT CAUSES ADHD?

Most researchers believe that ADHD is a genetic disorder, particularly since it tends to run in families. In other words, you can inherit ADHD.

But nongenetic factors are involved as well. Premature birth, maternal alcohol and tobacco use, exposure to high levels of lead in early childhood, and brain injury account for between 20 and 30 percent of ADHD cases among children.

TREATMENT OPTIONS

ADHD can be treated successfully, using a combination of natural remedies, prescription medications, counseling, and lifestyle changes. These are discussed below.

NATURAL HELP FOR ADHD:
10 CONCENTRATION-BOOSTING SUPPLEMENTS
If you're someone who believes in taking your health into your own hands, you may want to try one of the following dietary supplements. They could help boost your concentration and help you main-

tain your focus. However, the amount of research dedicated to natural remedies for attention problems has been minimal. The little that exists has been conducted mostly in children. Even so, supplementation may work just as well for adults. Prior to taking supplements or giving them to your child, always get your physician's or pediatrician's approval.

American Ginseng/Ginkgo Biloba

Recently, researchers at the University of Alberta in British Columbia tested the combined extracts of American ginseng (200 milligrams daily) and ginkgo biloba (50 milligrams daily) in thirty-six children (aged three to seventeen) who either had been diagnosed with ADHD or were suspected of having the disorder. American ginseng was chosen for the study because it has a higher concentration of a particular ginsenoside suspected of having a more positive effect on cognitive performance. Ginsenosides, which are plant steroids, are the main active constituents of the ginseng root.

By the end of the month-long trial, the supplement had improved symptoms of ADHD, including social problems, hyperactivity, and impulsivity, in a majority of the children. The results of this study are preliminary, but stay tuned: Current knowledge about these herbs suggests that they represent an avenue of research clearly worth pursuing.

The recommended dosage of ginseng for adults is 100 to 300 milligrams (standardized to 7-percent ginsenosides), three times daily; ginkgo, 120 to 160 milligrams of a standardized extract daily in two to three divided doses. Possible side effects of ginseng include headache, increased blood pressure, insomnia, and asthma attack. Possible side effects of ginkgo include headache, irritability, restlessness, and gastrointestinal disorders.

Amino Acid Combinations

Often recommended to treat ADHD are combinations of amino acids, usually formulated in a single supplement product. Generally, these supplements contain the following nutrients:

- GABA, which has a calming effect on the brain.
- Glycine, required for the healthy functioning of the central nervous system.
- Taurine, which balances and regulates neurotransmitters in the brain to enhance attention, cognitive performance, and feelings of well-being.
- Glutamine, which elevates levels of GABA in the brain.
- Phenylalanine, which boosts alertness and mood.
- Tyrosine, a building block of several neurotransmitters that helps reduce anxiety.

Combined amino acid supplements contain varying amounts of amino acids. You should follow the label instructions for the recommended dosage.

DHA

Less-than-adequate levels of DHA, a fat found mostly in fish and flaxseed, are correlated with attention problems in children, according to a Purdue University study. Researchers found significantly lower levels of DHA in children with ADHD compared to controls. This finding suggests that increasing DHA in a child's diet, whether through supplementation or increased servings of fish, may be beneficial in treating ADHD.

The recommended dosage of DHA is 100 milligrams a day for healthy adults who obtain some DHA from fish and other sources. If you eat little or no fish, 200 milligrams a day is recommended.

Glyconutrient Supplements

Glyconutrients are a blend of specific complex carbohydrates. Supplements marketed as glyconutrients are designed to support cellular communication so that organs, glands, and the immune system can function optimally.

One such supplement—Ambrotose complex manufactured by Mannatech, Inc.—was clinically tested in seventeen children diagnosed with

ADHD. Twelve of the children were on prescribed doses of Ritalin (methylphenidate); the rest were not taking any medication.

For six weeks (the duration of the study), all the children took Ambrotose supplements (one capsule per 10 pounds of body weight the first day and one capsule per 20 pounds of body weight thereafter). After three weeks, another Mannatech supplement was given to the children: phyto-Bears, which contains flash-dried fruits and vegetables and is free of artificial preservatives, colorants, or chemical stabilizers. The dosage was five capsules a day before school.

By the end of the six-week experiment, the glyconutrient supplement had decreased the number and severity of symptoms associated with ADHD, whether or not the children were taking Ritalin. (The addition of Phyto-Bears did not reduce symptoms any further.) It is not yet clear exactly how glyconutrients work to reduce symptoms. The authors point out that there is a need for further studies that examine how naturally occurring food substances such as saccharides combat ADHD.

Mineral Supplements

Natural health-care practitioners often recommend calcium and magnesium supplementation for quelling hyperactivity because both minerals have a calming effect on the body. In support of this practice, a Polish study found that calcium, magnesium, zinc, copper, and iron levels were abnormally low in hyperactive children aged four to thirteen, compared to a healthy control group. Other studies have corroborated these findings. Although researchers noted that "it is necessary to supplement trace minerals in children with hyperactivity," check with your pediatrician or physician first.

Probiotics

By age five, the average child in the United States has taken multiple rounds of antibiotics to treat various types of bacterial infections. Although antibiotics can wipe out bacterial illnesses, their overuse leads to a condition called dysbiosis, a risk factor for ADHD. Dysbiosis is a condition in which there is an imbalance of healthy bacteria in the intestinal tract. Antibiotics tend to kill off this healthy bacteria, along with harmful bacteria, and the result is dysbiosis. Its symptoms include diarrhea, gas, bloating, and poor absorption of nutrients.

A growing number of health-care practitioners thus believe that the health of the intestinal tract plays a significant role in ADHD and that children prescribed antibiotics should also take supplemental nutrients called "probiotics." Probiotic supplements help restore and maintain healthy intestinal bacteria in the aftermath of antibiotic usage. Examples of probiotic supplements are those containing either *L. acidophilus* or *B. bifidum* or both, as well as fructo-oligosaccharides, a special type of complex carbohydrate. All three of these substances promote the growth of healthy bacteria in the intestinal tract. Probiotics are safe and not associated with any side effects. Even so, talk to your pediatrician about supplementation and appropriate dosage.

Another supplement often recommended to combat dysbiosis is olive leaf extract, possibly because one of its active ingredients, oleuropein, may keep body-invading bacteria at bay. It appears to curb the growth of various bacterial strains, specifically those that attack the intestines and urinary tract.

Pycnogenol

Extracted from the bark of French maritime pine trees, pycnogenol is a natural complex of about forty antioxidants. Among its various health benefits, this agent may help normalize levels of neurotransmitters and rebalance brain chemistry.

Writing in the *Journal of the American Academy of Child and Adolescent Psychiatry*, Steven Heimann, M.D., of Evansville, Indiana, reported on how pycnogenol decreased hyperactivity, impulsiveness, and school behavioral problems in a ten-year-old boy with ADHD. According to Dr. Heimann, "a growing number of parents with ADHD-afflicted children are requesting that practitioners provide information about pycnogenol, if not an outright prescription."

Although there is not much information on the correct dosage levels for treating ADHD in adults or children, therapeutic dosages for other conditions range from 25 to 100 milligrams daily.

Pyruvate

Pyruvate or, more specifically, pyruvic acid is marketed as a natural weight-loss supplement, but several recent studies, evaluating weight loss, have found favorable side effects: increased alertness, decreased fatigue, and improved mood.

No one knows why these occurred, however. But it may have something to do with pyruvate's ability to increase the metabolic rate and allow more energy to be produced in the body at rest.

The recommended dosage of pyruvate ranges from 2 to 6 grams a day.

SAM-e

S-adenosyl-L-methionine (SAM-e) is a natural antidepressant available without a prescription in pharmacies and health-food stores. The body synthesizes this compound from methionine, an amino acid, and adenosine triphosphate, a molecular fuel. Bodily levels of SAM-e, however, fall when mood dips.

SAM-e is a "methyl donor." When helped by vitamin B_{12} and folic acid, it gives a piece of itself (a methyl group) to tissues and organs. This dispersal supports various vital processes, one of which is an increase in levels of serotonin and dopamine. The net benefit is to elevate mood and lift depression.

SAM-e has been tested as a treatment for adult ADHD, with impressive results. In one small study of eight men with ADHD, six subjects experienced less anxiety and felt more confident and less confused while taking the supplement.

The recommended dosage is up to 800 milligrams daily.

Vitamin B_6 (Pyridoxine)

This B-complex vitamin is involved in the metabolism of neurotransmitters, including serotonin (which is often low in hyperactive children), dopamine, and adrenaline. This may explain why vitamin B_6 has been shown to help improve hyperactivity.

In one study, researchers investigated vitamin B_6 supplementation in hyperactive children, aged eight to thirteen, who were also taking prescribed doses of Ritalin. High and low dosages of vitamin B_6 were used in the study, averaging 12.5 milligrams per kilogram of body weight a day and 22 milligrams per kilogram of body weight a day for twenty-one weeks. The vitamin dramatically boosted blood levels of serotonin and was slightly more effective than Ritalin in reducing symptoms. It is important to add here that this study was conducted quite a while ago— 1979—and the findings have not been replicated in recent years, so it's unclear whether vitamin B_6 can be considered a bonafide treatment for ADHD.

MEDICATION THERAPY

Your doctor can prescribe medication for treating adult ADHD. There are two classes of drugs commonly prescribed: antidepressants and stimulants.

Antidepressants

Antidepressants increase the concentration of neurotransmitters in the central nervous system. The net effect is to control the emotional aspects of the disorder and improve the mood problems that often accompany it.

Among the classes of antidepressants available, tricyclic antidepressants (TCAs) appear to be most effective in treating ADHD in adults. Like most prescription mood drugs, TCAs work on brain chemicals. TCAs, in particular, slow the rate at which certain neurotransmitters— namely, serotonin, norepinephrine, and dopamine—reenter the brain. This action increases the concentration of the neurotransmitters throughout the rest of the central nervous system, alleviating feelings of depression and controlling emotional outbursts.

Drugs in this family include Tofranil (imipramine), Norpramin (desipramine), Pamelor (nortriptyline), and Elavil (amitriptyline). Another antidepressant that may be effective is Wellbutrin (bupropion), which has more stimulant properties than the TCAs. Each type of TCA has its own potential side effects; you should check with your physician or pharmacist for a complete list.

Stimulants

In ADHD, there is an imbalance in the synthesis of dopamine and norepinephrine in the cerebral cortex, and stimulants stabilize these neurotransmitters. Stimulants commonly used to treat ADHD include Dexedrine (dextroamphetamine) and Ritalin (methylphenidate). Considered first-line treatment for the disorder, these drugs improve attention and concentration, plus reduce impulsivity in adults with the disorder. Nearly 100 percent of adult patients respond to treatment with these stimulants. Dexedrine, however, is highly addictive, and Ritalin has a high potential for abuse.

Another stimulant used to treat ADHD is Cylert (pemoline). It increases the risk of hepatitis, however, and should be considered only when other stimulants have failed to work. Many physicians shy away from prescribing Cylert.

In some cases, your physician may wish to prescribe a combination of an antidepressant and a stimulant.

The most common side effects of these drugs are listed in Table 17.1.

TABLE 17.1

Side Effects of Drugs Used to Treat ADHD

Stimulants	Side Effects
Cylert (pemoline)	Insomnia, liver damage
Dexedrine (dextroamphetamine sulfate)	Excessive restlessness, overstimulation, high abuse potential; should not be taken if you suffer from agitation, cardiovascular disease, glaucoma, overactive thyroid gland, or substance abuse
Ritalin (methylphenidate)	Inability to fall asleep, nervousness, high potential for abuse
	(Continued)

TCA Antidepressants	Side Effects *
Elavil (amitriptyline)	Abnormal movements, anxiety, black tongue, blurred vision, breast development in men, breast enlargement in women, coma, confusion, constipation, delusions
Norpramin (desipramine)	Abdominal cramps, agitation, anxiety, black tongue, red or blue spots on skin, blurred vision, breast development in men, breast enlargement in women, confusion, constipation; should not be taken if you have suffered a heart attack
Pamelor (nortriptyline)	Abdominal cramps, agitation, anxiety, black tongue, blurred vision, breast development in men, breast enlargement in women, confusion, constipation, delusions
Tofranil (impramine)	Abdominal cramps, agitation, anxiety, black tongue, bleeding sores, blood disorders, blurred vision, breast development in men, breast enlargement in women, confusion
Non-TCA Antidepressant	Side Effects
Wellbutrin (bupropion)	Abdominal pain, agitation, anxiety, constipation, dizziness, dry mouth, excessive sweating, headache, loss of appetite, nausea

*For a complete list of drug side effects, see *The PDR Family Guide to Prescription Drugs*™, available online at www.pdr.net.

Monitor How Well Your Medication Is Working

Observe your behavior to see if your medication is significantly helping with inattention, impulsivity, irritability, mood changes, emotional outbursts, restlessness, forgetfulness, and other symptoms. Write down any positive or adverse effects of your medication. If the medication is not helping, talk to your doctor about adjusting the dosage or changing the medication.

COUNSELING

Adults with ADHD often suffer from low self-esteem, feelings of failure, poor social skills, and relationship problems. Individual counseling can help you work through and solve such issues. If married, you may have significant problems in your relationship due to forgotten commitments, impulsive actions, and emotional outbursts. Marital therapy can help you and your spouse enhance communication, resolve conflict, and solve problems.

The good news is that adults with ADHD rarely require more than six months to a year of psychotherapy to resolve various issues associated with the disorder.

In addition to counseling, consider joining a support group of other adults with ADHD. In a support group, you can get the encouragement, positive feedback, and understanding you need to deal with the disorder. Ask your psychotherapist or physician about support groups in your area. If there isn't one, consider starting a group.

LIFESTYLE STRATEGIES

If you suffer from adult ADHD, some simple lifestyle changes can make a world of difference in your behavior, attitude, and mood. Here are several suggestions.

Employ Self-Management Strategies

If you suffer from ADHD, the following organizational strategies and memory aids will minimize symptoms:

- Make lists and computerized schedules to help you better organize your life and set priorities.
- Avoid procrastination.
- Place a large calendar with important dates and deadlines in a visible location.
- Reduce distractions by removing clutter from your desk, moving to a windowless office, or going to a quiet, isolated place.
- Arrive at work early to complete tasks before coworkers arrive and the phones start ringing.
- Break down projects into small manageable steps, each with its own deadline.
- Take breaks when needed. If you get upset or feel overstimulated, give yourself a time-out. Leave the situation or go to a quiet place to calm down.

Try the Feingold Diet

Developed by noted pediatrician Benjamin Feingold, M.D., this diet is used primarily to help children with ADHD, but it may be beneficial for adults, too. Basically, the diet eliminates foods containing artificial dyes and flavors (mainly petroleum-based additives); BHA, BHT, and TBHQ (petroleum-based preservatives); and salicylate-containing foods and nonfood products. These substances are believed to aggravate symptoms of ADHD.

Salicylates, in particular, may suppress the production of an enzyme called phenol sulfotransferase (PST), which is involved in processing neurotransmitters. Foods that contain salicylates include almonds, apples, apricots, cherries, all berries, peaches, plums, prunes, tomatoes, cucumbers, and oranges.

For information on this diet, contact the Feingold Association at (800) 321-3287 or www.feingold.org.

Exercise

Many clinicians advocate regular exercise for adults with ADHD. Exercise helps increase concentration, relieve stress, work off aggression, and energize the body. Further, it eases depression by elevating bodily levels of feel-good endorphins.

Maintain a Sense of Humor

Try to joke with yourself, your family, and your friends about some of your symptoms. Having a sense of humor helps ease tension and makes others more understanding and forgiving about your behavior.

Remember, ADHD Is a Neurological Disorder

ADHD stems from your genes and has to do with how your brain is wired. It is neither a moral failing nor a character flaw.

Educate Yourself About Adult ADHD

Self-help organizations such as Children and Adults with Attention Deficit Disorder (CHADD; (800) 233-4050 or www.chadd.org) can provide information about the disorder. CHADD publishes a magazine called *Attention!*, which contains informative, up-to-date articles on ADHD. You can subscribe to the magazine by contacting the organization or by logging on to its Web site.

Another great organization is National Attention Deficit Disorder Association, which you can contact at (847) 432-ADDA or www.add.org. This organization has numerous articles available online that cover nearly all aspects of adult ADHD.

An organization offering a wealth of information on adult ADHD is Attention Deficit Disorder Resources. You can contact the organization at (253) 759-5085 or www.ADDult.org.

Creativity: A Never-Ending Gift

Whether it's coming up with a powerful advertising slogan for your biggest client or deciding what to serve for dinner tonight, creative thinking is an integral part of our thought life, day in and day out. It's the secret of business success, the power behind solving those little problems that nag us every day, and the source of greater happiness. (After all, who hasn't felt the personal joy of dreaming up a great idea?) The list of creativity's gifts goes on and on.

A 9-POINT PLAN TO NURTURE AND STIMULATE YOUR CREATIVE THINKING

To be creative, you don't have to be a writer, an artist, a musician, or an inventor; every person on Earth has creative potential. The key is to unlock your creative potential so that you can be more successful and live life more fully. Here's how.

TAKE YOUR BODY AND BRAIN FOR A WALK

One of the greatest creative thinkers of all time—Albert Einstein— took frequent walks to solve problems. And no wonder. Walking gets creative juices flowing in at least three ways. First, it increases and improves oxygen flow to the brain, energizing brain cells for sharper mental performance. Second, some scientists believe that exercise, in general, triggers the release of various brain chemicals that enhance creativity. Third, others speculate that exercise may subdue activity in the left half of the brain, the part that deals with logic, and stimulate the right half, which is responsible for creative thought.

TAKE FREQUENT BREAKS TO REENERGIZE YOUR BRAIN

If you're a "desk potato"—that is, sitting at your desk all day—your powers of concentration and creativity will dissipate and your productivity will dip. Rather than sit still, get up and move around, at least once an hour, to get blood flowing to your brain. You'll be more alert and productive as a result.

CAPTURE IDEAS THAT POP INTO YOUR MIND

If you don't, they will vanish from your mind. Artists should carry sketchpads; writers and inventors should carry notepads; everyone, in fact, should have pen and paper in order to capture ideas.

TAKE ADVANTAGE OF THE
FOUR-STAGE CREATIVE PROCESS

In 1962, an investigator named Graham Wallas studied well-known scientists and innovators and discovered that they went through four stages of creative problem solving: (1) the preparation stage, which consists of formulating the process, studying previous work on it, and thinking intensely about it; (2) the incubation stage, in which there is no visible work on the problem but rather a "mulling over" to let the subconscious work on it; (3) the illumination stage, in which important insights are gained about the problem (put another way, the "light bulb goes on in your head"); and (4) the verification stage, in which the idea is tested and evaluated.

Practically speaking, here's how this might work if you're wrestling with how to design a new addition on your house. First, you'd research other similar designs, study them, and think hard and long about how they may or may not fit your needs. Second, you'd put the project aside and let your subconscious conjure up ideas. Third, workable ideas would start bubbling up from the subconscious, and, four, you'd go to work, putting them on paper.

DAYDREAM

Henry Ford once hired an efficiency expert to evaluate the running of his company. The expert's report was favorable, although he expressed reservations about one employee. "It's that man down the corridor," he said. "Every time I go by his office, he's just sitting there with his feet on his desk. He's wasting your money."

"That man," replied Ford, "once had an idea that saved us millions of dollars. At the time, I believe his feet were planted right where they are now."

Whether you're grappling with a way to solve a business problem or thinking up an idea for a novel, just relax, close your eyes, and let your mind wander freely. Don't edit your thoughts. You'll be surprised at the creative ideas that come into your mind.

LOOK AT A CHALLENGE OR A PROBLEM FROM A DIFFERENT PERSPECTIVE

When Jonas Salk was asked about how he invented the polio vaccine, he responded, "I pictured myself as a virus or a cancer cell and tried to sense what it would be like."

This is an example of "divergent thinking," an essential component of creativity. It involves the ability to quickly come up with different solutions and alternatives to a problem, plus the ability to be "original." Essentially, originality describes the difference between your ideas and those of most other people.

GET ADEQUATE SLEEP

Research shows that even one night of sleep loss negatively affects divergent thinking. British investigators assessed twelve subjects who went thirty-two hours without sleeping, along with twelve controls who slept normally. Sleep loss significantly impaired performance on a test that measured originality and other measures of divergent thinking. Convergent thinking, on the other hand, was found to be more resilient to short-term sleep loss.

EXPAND YOUR HORIZONS

Hallmark Cards has the world's largest creative staff, with 700 artists and writers who generate more than 15,000 original designs for cards and related products annually. To inspire them, the company brings in visiting writers and artists every year from around the world. Guests have included actress Betty White, author Betty Friedan, *New Yorker* cartoonist Gahan Wilson, and the animal-free circus Cirque de Soleil. Hallmark also sends its writers and artists to faraway places such as Paris, London, and Bologna as well as to locales such as the Southwest and Pacific Northwest for research. The whole idea is to spark innovation by exposure to new people and places.

You can do the same. Go to creativity conferences and workshops, meet people in various creative fields, travel, visit museums, read magazines and books for inspiration, and so forth. By getting out of your box, you start "thinking outside the box."

BELIEVE THAT YOU'RE CREATIVE

In a three-month study of creativity, psychologists examined the characteristics of creative people. Education, family background, and a variety of personal preferences were all considered possible contributors to individual creativity. However, the single common denominator that determined their creativity was attitude. The creative people simply believed that they were creative. Have faith in your abilities.

Creativity on the Job

When 500 American CEOs were asked what businesses must do to survive in the twenty-first century, the top answer was "practice creativity and innovation." If you want to foster creativity in your workplace, here are some suggestions from Stephen Schwambach, Ph.D., a psychologist, pastor, and author.

CULTIVATE AND ENCOURAGE AN OUTRAGEOUS SENSE OF HUMOR

Humor may not be the same thing as creativity, but, without a doubt, it is one of creativity's best friends. Enter a room full of uptight, humorless killjoys, and nine times out of ten you'll find that creativity has long ago crept quietly out the door.

BUILD AN ENCOURAGING ENVIRONMENT

Creativity thrives in an atmosphere of lively, effusive encouragement. It dies under the harsh spotlight of fault-finding criticism. Breakthrough solutions often arise from the yeasty mixture of a dozen or more cockamamy ideas. If even one person at the table is sitting there with a frown of disapproval on his or her face every time something off the wall is suggested, there will be no volatile brew to spark the new. In most cases, the wise planner schedules brainstorming sessions at different times than evaluation meetings—and often with entirely different people in attendance.

With that in mind, don't be afraid to invite outsiders, people not trained in your field. They may help you see things from a different angle.

TAP IN TO THE POWER OF PLAY

Rather than restricting your creative meetings to the company board-room, try gathering on blankets you've spread out on a nearby park lawn; going for a pre-meeting walk through a museum; taking a bus ride to grab a curbside hot dog, followed by an impromptu picnic; and gathering at a group member's home for darts, billiards, and coffee—all while the ideas flow.

In addition, give group members something to do with their hands. Studies have shown that when adults have something to play with while they meet, their minds can come up with some highly creative ideas. Experiment with soft, squeezable balls, a Slinky or two, and finger puzzles of various sorts.

Part Six

SMART CHOICES AND
BEST SOURCES

All across this country and on scores of Internet sites are places and resources you need for medical care and up-to-date information on mind,
mood, and memory. Listed here are hospitals, clinics, psychiatric facilities,
Web sites, books, manufacturers of smart supplements, brain-building
products, and more. It's not meant as a comprehensive guide, but it will
give you a good start on where to get the help you need. Keep in mind,
too, that phone numbers and Web sites are subject to change.

Top Alzheimer's Clinics and Research Centers

If searching for an Alzheimer's clinic for you or a loved one, check out a nearby university medical center or large hospital. These institutions are most likely to offer cutting-edge treatment in addition to opportunities to participate in clinical trials.

Most of the clinics listed below are funded by the National Institute on Aging (NIA). Researchers at these centers are working to translate research advances into improved care and diagnosis for Alzheimer's patients while, at the same time, focusing on the long-term goal of finding a way to cure and possibly prevent Alzheimer's disease.

For more information, you may contact any of the centers on the following state-by-state list. Where available, Web sites are provided.

ALABAMA

The Alzheimer's Disease Center, University of Alabama, Birmingham

Director's Telephone: (205) 934-3847

Information: (205) 934-2178

www.main.uab.edu/show.asp?durki=11627

Established in 1991, this center is dedicated to research into Alzheimer's disease, and provides comprehensive diagnostic and medical services to patients. NIA funded.

ARIZONA

Behavioral Neuroscience and Alzheimer's Clinic, Tucson

(520) 626-6524

www.azumc.com/specialtycare/types/alzheimers.htm

This clinic focuses on patients with Alzheimer's disease and other dementias (particularly the loss of cognitive ability as well as memory problems). Anyone older than sixteen years of age can be evaluated.

CALIFORNIA

ALZHEIMER'S DISEASE CENTER, UNIVERSITY OF CALIFORNIA, DAVIS
Director's Telephone: (916) 734-6280
www.alzheimer.ucdavis.edu/adc

ALZHEIMER'S DISEASE CENTER, UNIVERSITY OF CALIFORNIA, IRVINE
Director's Telephone: (949) 824-5847
www.alz.uci.edu

The three centers listed above provide diagnostic services that include
memory testing, laboratory evaluation, neurological exams, brain
scans, and medical history. Patients with symptoms of memory loss,
disorientation, and confusion may be enrolled in the program and are
eligible to participate in research studies. Additional services include
patient and family education, referrals to community and health services, and support groups. NIA funded.

ALZHEIMER'S DISEASE CENTER, UNIVERSITY OF CALIFORNIA,
LOS ANGELES
Director's Telephone: (310) 206-5238
www.adc.ucla.edu

Established in 1990, this center provides a formal program in research and
clinical care. It has been involved in numerous studies of experimental
drugs for the treatment of Alzheimer's disease. NIA funded.

ALZHEIMER'S DISEASE CENTER, UNIVERSITY OF CALIFORNIA,
SAN DIEGO
Director's Telephone: (858) 534-4606
Information: (858) 622-5800
www.adrc.ucsd.edu

Researchers at this center have been instrumental in making a number of
discoveries related to the basic biology and treatment of Alzheimer's disease. Established in 1984, the center enrolls volunteers with the disease
and related dementias as well as normal control subjects. NIA funded.

ALZHEIMER'S DISEASE RESEARCH CENTER, STANFORD UNIVERSITY
Information: (650) 852-3287
www.stanford.edu/yesavage/ACRC.html

ANDRUS GERONTOLOGY CENTER, UNIVERSITY OF
    SOUTHERN CALIFORNIA
Director's Telephone: (213) 740-1758
Information: (213) 740-7777
www.usc.edu/dept/gero/ADRC

This program conducts research into the disease and offers diagnostic and
    medical care to patients. One of its goals is to increase participation of
    Hispanics, African-Americans, and other minorities in drug trials.
    NIA funded.

SAN FRANCISCO ALZHEIMER'S AND DEMENTIA CLINIC,
    SAN FRANCISCO
(415) 673-4600
www.sfcrc.com

This clinic is devoted to the investigation, diagnosis, treatment, and manage-
    ment of Alzheimer's disease and is directed by Jerome Goldstein, M.D., a
    board-certified medical neurologist with a special interest in the treat-
    ment of this disease. Ongoing research programs into the disease are con-
    ducted at the clinic.

GEORGIA

EMORY ALZHEIMER'S DISEASE CENTER, EMORY UNIVERSITY, ATLANTA
Information: (404) 728-6950
www.emory.edu/WHSC/MED/ADC

In addition to extensive research into Alzheimer's disease, this center of-
    fers diagnostic services, classes and small-group discussions, and other
    services designed to improve patients' quality of life. NIA funded.

ILLINOIS

COGNITIVE NEUROLOGY AND ALZHEIMER'S DISEASE CENTER, NORTH-
    WESTERN UNIVERSITY, CHICAGO
Director's Telephone: (312) 908-9339
www.brain.nwu.edu

The emphasis at this center is on research and on training professionals to
    work with patients and their caregivers. NIA funded.

RUSH ALZHEIMER'S DISEASE CENTER, RUSH-PRESBYTERIAN-
   ST. LUKE'S MEDICAL CENTER, CHICAGO
Director's Telephone: (312) 942-3350
Information: (312) 942-4463
www.rush.edu/patient/radc
This center is devoted to the care and evaluation of patients with Alzheimer's disease; the education of professional and family caregivers; and
   research into the causes, treatment, and prevention of the disease and related dementias. NIA funded.

INDIANA

INDIANA ALZHEIMER'S DISEASE CENTER, INDIANA UNIVERSITY,
   INDIANAPOLIS
Director's Telephone: (317) 274-7818
Information: (317) 278-2030
www.pathology.iupui.edu/ad
This program identifies people with Alzheimer's disease and evaluates
   them with a number of laboratory, medical, psychological, and memory tests on an annual basis. Participants have access to information;
   voluntary participation in drug trials; and follow-up medical, social,
   and educational support services. NIA funded.

KENTUCKY

SANDERS-BROWN RESEARCH CENTER ON AGING, UNIVERSITY OF
   KENTUCKY, LEXINGTON
Director's Telephone: (606) 323-6040
www.coa.uky.edu
This center supervises research projects, evaluates patients, provides med-
   ical care, and offers educational programs. NIA funded.

MARYLAND

ALZHEIMER'S DISEASE CENTER, THE JOHNS HOPKINS
  MEDICAL INSTITUTIONS
Director's Telephone: (410) 955-5632
www.alzresearch.org
This center is focused on discovering the causes of Alzheimer's disease,
  finding effective treatments, and helping those afflicted with the disease and their families. NIA funded.

MASSACHUSETTS

ALZHEIMER'S DISEASE CENTER, BOSTON UNIVERSITY, BEDFORD
Director's Telephone: (781) 687-2632
Information: (781) 687-2916
www.xfaux.com/alzheimer
This program is a research, education, and resource center serving the
  needs of people with Alzheimer's disease and the professionals who
  treat them. NIA funded.

ALZHEIMER'S DISEASE CENTER, HARVARD MEDICAL SCHOOL/
  MASSACHUSETTS GENERAL HOSPITAL, BOSTON
Director's Telephone: (617) 726-1728
www.hms.harvard.edu/aging/adrc.html
This center is focused on improving the diagnosis of Alzheimer's disease
  and developing more effective treatments for it. Each year, researchers
  enroll approximately 200 patients with dementia to participate in clinical trials. NIA funded.

MICHIGAN

MICHIGAN ALZHEIMER'S DISEASE RESEARCH CENTER, UNIVERSITY OF
MICHIGAN, ANN ARBOR

Information: (734) 764-2190

www.med.umich.edu.madrc

Established in 1989, this center is devoted to research, clinical care, and educational activities in Alzheimer's disease and related disorders. Through its programs, individuals and families in Michigan have access to the most advanced diagnostic techniques and treatments as well as to current research findings. NIA funded.

MINNESOTA

MAYO ALZHEIMER'S DISEASE RESEARCH CENTER, MAYO CLINIC,
ROCHESTER

Information: (507) 284-1324

www.mayo.edu/research/alzheimers_center

The purpose of this center is to provide care to patients and promote research and education on Alzheimer's disease. NIA funded.

MISSOURI

ALZHEIMER'S DISEASE RESEARCH CENTER, WASHINGTON UNIVERSITY,
ST. LOUIS

Director's Telephone: (314) 286-2881

Information: (314) 286-2881

www.biostat.wustl.edu/adrc

The purpose of this center is to conduct research into Alzheimer's disease, provide training to health-care professionals, and offer educational support to patients and their caregivers. NIA funded.

NEW YORK

ALZHEIMER'S DISEASE RESEARCH CENTER, MOUNT SINAI SCHOOL OF
   MEDICINE/BRONX VA MEDICAL CENTER, NEW YORK CITY
Director's Telephone: (212) 824-7008
Information: (212) 241-8329
www.mssm.edu/psychiatry/adrchome.html
This center provides evaluation of memory problems, counseling for patients with memory disorders and their families, and research into the
   cause and treatments of Alzheimer's disease. The program also offers
   support groups. NIA funded.

ROCHESTER ALZHEIMER'S DISEASE CENTER, UNIVERSITY OF ROCHESTER
Information: (716) 275-2581
www.urmc.rochester.edu/adc/index.html
This center is devoted to finding more effective ways of treating Alzheimer's disease through research. NIA funded.

TAUB INSTITUTE FOR RESEARCH ON ALZHEIMER'S DISEASE AND THE
   AGING BRAIN, COLUMBIA UNIVERSITY, NEW YORK CITY
Director's Telephone: (212) 305-3300
Information: (212) 305-6553
pathology.cpmc.columbia.edu/adhome.html
The mission of this program is to develop ways to identify people at risk
   for Alzheimer's disease and devise new therapies to prevent or delay
   disorders of the aging brain. It offers advanced diagnostic and clinical
   care and opportunities to participate in clinical trials. NIA funded.

WILLIAM AND SYLVIA SILBERSTEIN AGING AND DEMENTIA RESEARCH
CENTER, NEW YORK UNIVERSITY SCHOOL OF MEDICINE, NEW
YORK CITY

Director's Telephone: (212) 263-5703

Information: (212) 263-5700

aging.med.nyu.edu

Services of the center include comprehensive diagnostic evaluations, clinical trials of new treatments, management of behavioral symptoms, and counseling. To be eligible, participants must be at least fifty years of age. NIA funded.

NORTH CAROLINA

JOSEPH AND KATHLEEN BRYAN ALZHEIMER'S DISEASE RESEARCH
CENTER, DUKE UNIVERSITY, DURHAM

Director's Telephone: (919) 286-3228

www.medicine.mc.duke.edu/adrc

Established in 1985, this center provides state-of-the-art care and research for Alzheimer's disease patients and their families. In addition, the center offers community outreach programs; support services for families and caregivers; and research on the diagnosis, management, and treatment of the disease. NIA funded.

OHIO

UNIVERSITY ALZHEIMER CENTER, CASE WESTERN RESERVE UNIVERSITY, UNIVERSITY HOSPITALS OF CLEVELAND

Director's Telephone: (216) 844-6400

Main Telephone: (800) 252-5048

www.ohioalzcenter.org

This center carries out memory and aging studies and collaborates with researchers across the country and throughout the world to find a cure for Alzheimer's disease. NIA funded.

OREGON

OREGON ALZHEIMER'S DISEASE CENTER, OREGON HEALTH SCIENCES
    UNIVERSITY, PORTLAND
Director's Telephone: (503) 494-6976
Information: (503) 494-6976
www.ohsu.edu/som-alzheimers
This center has a clinic that provides comprehensive care to people with
    Alzheimer's disease and is staffed by neurologists, psychologists,
    nurses, and psychiatrist, all experienced in the disease and its treat-
    ment. Opportunities are available for patients to participate in clinical
    trials. NIA funded.

PENNSYLVANIA

ALZHEIMER'S DISEASE RESEARCH CENTER, UNIVERSITY OF
    PITTSBURGH
Director's Telephone: (412) 624-6889
Information: (412) 692-2700
www.adrc.pitt.edu
This center coordinates and supports research into Alzheimer's disease,
    provides a memory disorders clinic that evaluates and treats individ-
    uals over the age of forty who are experiencing memory impairment,
    conducts community outreach programs, and provides education
    programs for health-care professionals and families of patients. NIA
    funded.

PENN ALZHEIMER'S DISEASE CENTER, UNIVERSITY OF PENNSYLVANIA,
    PHILADELPHIA
Director's Telephone: (215) 662-6399
Information: (215) 662-4708
www.uphs.upenn.edu/ADC
This center is dedicated to identifying the causes of Alzheimer's, discover-
    ing effective treatments, and finding a cure for the disease and other
    dementias.

TEXAS

ALZHEIMER'S DISEASE RESEARCH CENTER, BAYLOR COLLEGE OF
MEDICINE, HOUSTON

Information: (713) 798-6660

www.bcm.tmc.edu/neurol/struct/adrc/adrc1.html

This center conducts research into Alzheimer's disease and diagnoses and
treats patients with the disease and related disorders. Patients are seen
for the diagnosis of memory problems, confirmation of diagnosis, and
participation in research studies. Counseling and support groups are
available as well. NIA funded.

ALZHEIMER'S DISEASE RESEARCH CENTER, UNIVERSITY OF TEXAS,
SOUTHWESTERN MEDICAL CENTER, DALLAS

Director's Telephone: (214) 648-3239

Information: (214) 648-3198

www.swmed.edu/alzheimer

This center provides a thorough diagnostic evaluation of adult memory
problems and conducts ongoing research to improve the diagnosis,
treatment, and care-giving techniques involved in Alzheimer's disease.
NIA funded.

WASHINGTON

ALZHEIMER'S DISEASE CENTER, UNIVERSITY OF WASHINGTON, SEATTLE

Main Telephone: (206) 762-1010, ext. 3491

www.depts.washington.edu/adrcweb

This center focuses on research into the disease but is also committed to
implementing treatment techniques that improve patient care and
function. NIA funded.

Top Memory Clinics

If you're having frequent memory problems and want to know what's up, you can be assessed and treated at a memory clinic. Although memory clinics do assess people for Alzheimer's disease, they focus on diagnosing a broader range of memory impairments, including those connected with head injury, epilepsy, stroke, substance abuse, and other medical and psychological disorders that can produce memory loss.

The services of memory clinics vary, but generally they specialize in testing, diagnosing, assessing, and treating dementia and other related memory disorders. Some memory clinics are involved in testing new drugs and may offer the chance to participate in clinical drug trials.

More and more memory clinics are cropping up in the United States. If there is no clinic near you, don't worry. A major hospital or medical center can provide many of the same services.

The listings below include phone numbers and, where available, Web sites.

ARIZONA

Memory Disorders Clinic, University Medical Center, Tucson
(502) 626-2357
www.azuma.com/specialtycare/types/alzheimers.htm

CALIFORNIA

Memory and Aging Center, San Francisco Medical Center
(415) 476-6880
www.ucsf.edu/research/centers.html

Memory Assessment Clinic, University of California, Irvine
(949) 824-2382
www.alz.uci.edu/clinic.html

Memory Disorders Clinic, University of California, Los Angeles
(310) 206-5238
www.adc.ucla.edu/about_adrc.html

FLORIDA

INTERNET INFORMATION ON MEMORY CLINICS IN FLORIDA
IS AVAILABLE AT:
www.myflorida.com/doea/healthfamily/contacts/elderissues/
doeamemorydisordersclinics.html

BRAIN BANK, MOUNT SINAI MEDICAL CENTER, MIAMI BEACH
(305) 674-2543

EAST CENTRAL FLORIDA MEMORY DISORDER CLINIC, MELBOURNE
(407) 768-9575

LEE MEMORIAL HEALTH SYSTEM MEMORY DISORDER CLINIC, FORT
MYERS
(941) 772-6538

MAYO CLINIC JACKSONVILLE, JACKSONVILLE
(904) 223-2000

NORTH BROWARD MEMORY DISORDER CENTER, POMPANO BEACH
(954) 786-7392

ORLANDO REGIONAL MEDICAL CENTER MEMORY DISORDER CLINIC,
NEUROSCIENCE CENTER, ORLANDO
(407) 237-6336

ST. MARY'S MEDICAL CENTER MEMORY DISORDER CLINIC, INTRA-
COASTAL HEALTH SYSTEM, INC., WEST PALM BEACH
(506) 844-6300

SARASOTA MEMORIAL MEMORY DISORDER CLINIC, SARASOTA
(941) 917-7197

TALLAHASSEE MEMORIAL HEALTHCARE MEMORY DISORDER CLINIC,
TALLAHASSEE
(850) 681-5001

University of Florida Memory Disorder Clinic, J. Hillis
    Miller Medical Center, Gainesville
(352) 392-3491

University of Miami Memory Disorder Clinic (M-801), Miami
(305) 547-4082

University of South Florida Memory Disorder Clinic, Tampa
(813) 974-3100

West Florida Memory Disorder Clinic, West Florida Regional
    Medical Center, Senior Health Services, Pensacola
(850) 494-4885

Wien Center, Mount Sinai Medical Center, Miami Beach
(305) 674-2543

MARYLAND
The Johns Hopkins University School of Medicine, Baltimore
(410) 955-5000
www.hopkinsmedicine.org/medicalschool

MASSACHUSETTS
Memory Disorders Unit, Brigham and Women's Hospital,
    Boston
(617) 732-8060
**neuro.oas.mgh.harvard.edu/alzheimers/patient_resources/patient_
resources.html**

Memory 101, Beth Israel Deaconess Medical Center, Harvard
    Medical School, Cambridge
(617) 426-5500
www.bidmc.harvard.edu

MINNESOTA

THE MEMORY CENTER
The Minneapolis Clinic of Neurology, Ltd.
(763) 588-0661
www.minneapolisclinic.com

MEMORY DISORDERS CLINIC, RAMSEY
(800) 323-2949

NEW YORK

MEMORY ENHANCEMENT PROGRAM, MOUNT SINAI SCHOOL OF MEDI-
   CINE, NEW YORK CITY
(212) 241-2665
www.mssm.edu

OHIO

MEMORY DISORDERS CLINIC AT OHIO STATE UNIVERSITY MEDICAL
   CENTER, COLUMBUS
(614) 293-8531
neurology.med.ohio-state.edu/cognitive/memory-disorders-clinic.html

OREGON

THE MEMORY ASSESSMENT CLINIC, OREGON HEALTH SCIENCES
   UNIVERSITY, PORTLAND
(503) 494-6976
www.ohsu/som-alzheimers/memory_cl.html

PENNSYLVANIA

MEMORY DISORDERS CLINIC, UNIVERSITY OF PENNSYLVANIA HEALTH
   SYSTEM
www.uphs.upenn.edu/ADC/clinicalcare/mdc/clinical_services.htm

Memory Disorders Clinic, University of Pittsburgh
(412) 692-2700
www.adrc.pitt.edu

VERMONT

The Memory Clinic, Southwestern Vermont Health Care,
 Bennington
(802) 442-6361
www.svhealthcare.org

WISCONSIN

Dean Memory Disorders Clinic, Madison
(608) 255-8800

Family Medicine Clinic, Eau Claire
(715) 839-5175
www.uwdoctors.org/clinic/documents/eauclaire.shtm

Froedtert Memory Disorders Clinic, Milwaukee
(414) 454-5220

Gunderson Memory Disorders Clinic, LaCrosse
(608) 782-7300

Marshfield Clinic Neurosciences, Marshfield
(800) 699-3377
www.marshfieldclinic.org

Memory Assessment Clinic—Lakeview Center, Wausau
(715) 261-6092; (715) 261-6070; (888) 486-9545
www.medsch.wisc.edu.wai/clinics.wausau.html

Memory Center—Affinity Health System, Oshkosh
(920) 303-3560
www.medsch.wisc.edu.wai/clinics.oshkosh.html

MEMORY DIAGNOSTIC CENTER OF NORTH WEST WISCONSIN,
   CUMBERLAND
(715) 822-6107
www.medsch.wisc.edu.wai/clinics.cumberland.html

MEMORY DIAGNOSTIC CENTER OF SOUTH CENTRAL
   WISCONSIN, MADISON
(800) 421-4420
www.medsch.wisc.edu.wai/clinics.madison.html

MEMORY DISORDERS CLINIC, MARSHFIELD
(800) 782-8581
www.medsch.wisc.edu.wai/clinics.marshfield.html

NORTHERN WISCONSIN MEMORY DIAGNOSTIC CENTER, RHINELANDER
(715) 369-6534
www.medsch.wisc.edu.wai/clinics.rhinelander.html

BEST PSYCHIATRIC HOSPITALS

On a regular basis, *U.S. News & World Report* ranks hospitals in the United States according to their specialties. The rankings serve "as a resource for consumers who are seeking maximum care in the diagnosis, treatment, and management of a difficult medical problem," the editors said in a prepared statement.

Those hospitals excelling in psychiatric care are listed below and were ranked solely on their reputation. (Psychiatric hospitals treat a range of mental problems, including mood and anxiety disorders.) To make the list, a hospital had to be named by at least 3 percent of the number of board-certified specialists who responded to the magazine's surveys over the past three years. The survey was conducted by the National Opinion Research Center (NORC) at the University of Chicago.

For other hospitals that made the list but are not in the top ten below, see the magazine's Web site: **www.usnews.com/usnews/nycu/health/hosptl/specpsyc.htm.**

MASSACHUSETTS GENERAL HOSPITAL, BOSTON

Among the psychiatric programs at Massachusetts General Hospital is the Mood and Anxiety Disorders Institute. Clinical services range from onetime evaluations or consultations to long-term treatment. To schedule an appointment or consultation, call (617) 724-6748. Web site: **www.mghmadi.org.**

NEW YORK–PRESBYTERIAN HOSPITAL, THE UNIVERSITY HOSPITALS OF COLUMBIA AND CORNELL, NEW YORK CITY

Psychiatric services are offered through the Columbia Department of Psychiatry and include consultations, evaluations, outpatient care, day treatment, crisis intervention, and inpatient treatment for numerous emotional problems and psychiatric disorders.

Worth mentioning is that Columbia's psychiatrists are among the best in America. Leading surveys such as *New York Magazine*'s List of Best Doctors rank Columbia doctors as among the top in the country.

For information about psychiatric programs, call (212) 305-6001. Web site: **www.nyp.org.**

MCLEAN HOSPITAL, BELMONT, MASSACHUSETTS

McLean Hospital is internationally recognized for its research on schizophrenia and bipolar disorders through its Bipolar Psychotic Disorders Program. The program provides partial hospitalization, in which patients spend most of their days on the McLean campus and participate in intensive, personalized treatment; outpatient clinics that provide individual and group therapy; inpatient acute care, for those who need an individualized program of care; and continuing care, in which patients can live in special residential apartments to work on living skills and build a support peer system. For information on this program, call (800) 333-0338.

McLean Hospital also houses the Massachusetts General Hospital Obsessive–Compulsive Disorders Institute. The program provides individual and group therapy, medication therapy, and behavioral therapy. For information on the institute, call (617) 855-3279. Web site: **www.mcleanhospital.org.**

C. F. MENNINGER MEMORIAL
HOSPITAL, TOPEKA, KANSAS

Menninger has been among the top psychiatric hospitals in the United States since *U.S. News & World Report* began its poll in 1991. The institution offers an individualized residential program for adults with difficult-to-treat mental illnesses, including schizophrenia, and longstanding mood disorders.

There are three levels of care: intensive residential care for patients with the most serious symptoms; intermediate residential care for patients who require less nursing supervision and are able to participate in therapeutic group activities; and basic residential care for patients who can live in a fairly independent atmosphere.

Menninger encourages family involvement and provides educational presentations and materials to family members. Family therapy is available for an additional fee.

For information about the residential program, call (800) 351-9058. Web site: **www.menniger.edu.**

JOHNS HOPKINS HOSPITAL, BALTIMORE

Johns Hopkins Hospital has a number of programs that set it apart. Among them: the Anxiety Disorders Clinic and the Affective Disorders Clinic.

The Anxiety Disorders Clinic offers psychiatric evaluations, second opinions, consultations, and psychological as well as pharmacological treatments for individuals suffering from anxiety. The clinic treats patients with generalized anxiety, panic, social anxiety, obsessive-compulsive symptoms, posttraumatic stress, and premenstrual syndrome (PMS). For information regarding treatment, call (410) 955-6111 or (410) 955-2324. To make an appointment, call (410) 583-2610.

The Affective Disorders Clinic treats patients with depression and bipolar disorder. It provides a twelve-bed inpatient unit, two outpatient treatment programs, a consultation clinic, and an adolescent consultation clinic for depressed and bipolar patients ages twelve to eighteen. For information, call (410) 955-5212. Web site: **www.hopkinsmedicine.org/medicalschool.**

UCLA NEUROPSYCHIATRIC INSTITUTE AND HOSPITAL, LOS ANGELES

Located on the UCLA campus in Westwood, this institution is one of the world's leading centers for comprehensive patient care, research, and education in mental health. It offers a full range of treatment options for patients who need inpatient care, outpatient treatment, or partial-day services. For information, call (310) 825-0511. Web site: **www.npi.ucla.edu.**

YALE–NEW HAVEN PSYCHIATRIC HOSPITAL, NEW HAVEN, CONNECTICUT

This hospital is a seventy-six-bed facility providing specialized psychiatric care to adults and children. Its services include a special geriatric psychiatry unit, a partial-day program providing group therapy, intensive outpatient care, a crisis intervention unit, and a children's psychiatric inpatient unit. For information, call (203) 688-3182. Web site: **www.ynhh.org.**

MAYO CLINIC, ROCHESTER, MINNESOTA

This world-famed medical center provides comprehensive treatment programs in psychiatry and psychology. For information, call (507) 284-2511. Web site: **www.mayoclinic.org.**

DUKE UNIVERSITY MEDICAL CENTER,
DURHAM, NORTH CAROLINA

Among the notable programs offered in psychiatry at Duke University Medical Center are the Anxiety Disorders Clinic and the Mood Disorders Clinic. The Anxiety Disorders Clinic evaluates and treats adult patients with anxiety disorders, including obsessive-compulsive disorder, panic disorder, generalized anxiety disorder, post-traumatic stress disorder, social phobia, major depression, and more. Treatment includes clinical testing, pharmacological therapy, individual and group therapy, and inpatient psychiatric treatment. For information on this program, call (919) 684-0100.

The Mood Disorders Clinic treats patients with bipolar disorder, major depression, panic and generalized anxiety disorder, and other mood disorders. Treatment involves clinical testing, pharmacological therapy, state-of-the-art electroconvulsive therapy, individual and group therapy, inpatient psychiatric treatment, and specialized treatment programs for elderly patients. For information on this program, call (919) 684-0100. Web site: **www.mc.duke.edu.**

UNIVERSITY OF PITTSBURGH MEDICAL CENTER,
PITTSBURGH, PENNSYLVANIA

The Western Psychiatric Institute and Clinic located in Pittsburgh is the psychiatric specialty hospital of the University of Pittsburgh Medical Center and is considered one of the nation's foremost university-based psychiatric facilities. The facility offers inpatient hospitalization, detoxification, psychiatric clinical trials, outpatient psychiatric and psychological treatment programs, electroconvulsive therapy, and more. For more information, call (800) 533-UPMC. Web site: **www.upmc.edu.**

Best Hospitals for Brain and Nervous System Disorders

The following hospitals have frequently made the top ten in *U.S. News & World Report*'s ranking for best hospitals for the treatment of brain and nervous system disorders, technically known as "neurology." These hospitals have specialists who excel in treating stroke and diagnosing memory loss.

For other hospitals that have made the list but are not in the top ten, see the magazine's Web site: **www.usnews.com/usnews/nycu/health/hosptl/specneur.htm.**

MAYO CLINIC, ROCHESTER, MINNESOTA

Under its Division of Cerebrovascular Diseases, the Mayo Clinic provides its highly successful Mayo Stroke Center and its Cerebrovascular Clinic, in addition to many other programs. With its numerous inpatient and outpatient activities, this division constitutes the largest practice of cerbrovascular disease in the United States.

Established in 1966, the Mayo Stroke Center is dedicated to identifying and treating patients at high risk for stroke and reducing those risks. At the Cerebrovascular Clinic, the staff works with patients with stroke and stroke-related illnesses such as high blood pressure, heart disease, and diabetes.

For information on the Division of Cerebrovascular Diseases, call (507) 284-2511. Web site: **www.mayoclinic.org.**

MASSACHUSETTS GENERAL HOSPITAL, BOSTON

In neurology, Massachusetts General Hospital offers an array of top-notch programs for the treatment of stroke, Alzheimer's disease, brain tumors, epilepsy, Huntington's disease, multiple sclerosis, and neuromuscular disorders, to name just a few. For information, call (617) 726-2000. Web sites: **www.mghmadi.org** and **www.mgh.harvard.edu.**

JOHNS HOPKINS HOSPITAL, BALTIMORE

The Neuropsychiatry Service of Johns Hopkins Hospital is an internationally known team of neuropsychiatrists, geriatricians, nurses, occupational therapists, and psychologists providing care to more than 800 people a year. They treat patients with chronic brain conditions such as Alzheimer's disease, Parkinson's disease, stroke, multiple sclerosis, epilepsy, head trauma, mental retardation, and other conditions. The team also treats people who suffer from symptoms such as memory loss, depression, lack of motivation, agitation, explosive spells, and other complaints.

Specific treatments include medications, behavior management, education, and counseling. In addition, patients have the opportunity to participate in clinical trials of new treatments.

For information, call (410) 955-6158. Web sites: **www.hopkinsmedicine.org/ medicalschool** and **www.med.jhu.edu/jhhpsychiatry/master1.htm.**

NEW YORK–PRESBYTERIAN HOSPITAL, NEW YORK CITY

The hospital offers a comprehensive program of inpatient and outpatient care. Patient neurology care is provided at a seventy-six-bed facility, along with twelve intensive-care-unit beds on a separate floor.

Outpatient care clinics are designed for patients with Parkinson's disease and other movement disorders, neuromuscular diseases, multiple sclerosis, epilepsy, and memory disorders. There is also a Pediatric Neurology Clinic.

For information, call (888) 694-5700 or (212) 305-6001. Web site: **www.nyp.org.**

UNIVERSITY OF CALIFORNIA, SAN FRANCISCO MEDICAL CENTER

The Neurology Department at this institution is widely recognized as one of the leading neuroscience centers in the United States. Among the neurology services at this facility is the Memory and Aging Center. It provides evaluation, advice, medical treatment, follow-up, and the possibility of participating in research studies. Generally, patients are referred by health-care providers, social service agencies, or family members. You may also refer yourself. For further information or to make an appointment, call (415) 476-6880.

The medical center also houses the Parkinson's Disease Clinic and Research Center. It exists to provide comprehensive and compassionate care for patients and families affected by this disease, to discover the causes and effective treatments for Parkinson's disease, and to educate health-care providers, patients, caregivers, and the general public about the disease. Patients have access to a variety of services, including physical therapy, occupational therapy, swallowing and speech evaluations, and surgical treatments. For information about the Parkinson's Disease Clinic and Research Center or to schedule an appointment, call (415) 353-2273. For information about participating in current research studies, call (415) 476-9276, ext. 3.

Other neurology services include treatment for multiple sclerosis, pain management, and various neurological diseases. The phone number for the Department of Neurology is (415) 476-1487. The Medical Center Web site: **www.ucsf.edu.**

CLEVELAND CLINIC, CLEVELAND, OHIO

Among the many notable programs at the Cleveland Clinic is the Cerebrovascular Center. It has one of the largest groups of experts solely dedicated to the care and management of stroke. This includes a team of board-certified neurologists, neurosurgeons, vascular surgeons, radiologists, stroke rehabilitation specialists, and more. They treat more than 2,000 stroke patients each year—one of the highest stroke-related patient volumes in North America.

For information, call (800) 223-2273. Web site: **www.clevelandclinic.org.**

HOSPITAL OF THE UNIVERSITY OF PENNSYLVANIA, PHILADELPHIA

Established in 1874, the Department of Neurology at this hospital was the first such department in the United States and provides care for patients with diseases of the brain, spinal cord, nerve, or muscle, as well as neurological cancers and eye-related neurological disorders.

The department offers some fourteen programs in neurological care. Among them are the Stroke and Critical Care Neurology program, the Memory Disorders program, and the Parkinson's Disease and Movement Disorders Center.

In the Stroke and Critical Care Neurology program, patients receive state-of-the-art care from a team of neurologists, neurosurgeons, radiologists, neuronurses, and others. Family education is a priority as well.

The Memory Disorders program provides comprehensive assessment and treatment for patients with memory, language, and visual and thinking difficulties. Underlying causes of such problems commonly include Alzheimer's disease, stroke, brain injury, and Parkinson's disease.

The Parkinson's Disease and Movement Disorders Center not only treats patients with Parkinson's disease but also those with Tourette's syndrome, Huntington disease, and various movement disorders. This center is one of the largest of its kind in the United States.

To schedule an appointment in any of these programs, call (800) 789-PENN. Web site: **www.aphs.upenn.edu.**

UCLA MEDICAL CENTER, LOS ANGELES

The Department of Neurology at the UCLA Medical Center offers comprehensive consultation, diagnosis, and treatment for adult patients with disorders of the brain, spinal cord, nerves, and muscles, as well as behavioral problems related to the brain and nervous system. These programs include treatment for people with Alzheimer's disease, memory disorders, and stroke.

Other programs include headache management, a general neurology program, multiple sclerosis treatment, a neuro-oncology program, movement disorders program, seizure disorder center, post-polio program, and neurological rehabilitation, to name just a few.

To contact the UCLA Medical Center, call: (800) UCLA-MD1. Web sites: **www.healthcare.ucla.edu** and **www.adc.ucla.edu/about_adrc.html.**

BARNES-JEWISH HOSPITAL, ST. LOUIS, MISSOURI

The Neurology and Neurosurgery Services at Barnes-Jewish Hospital include diagnosis and treatment of many neurological disorders including dementia, stroke (through its Stroke Center), Parkinson's disease, movement disorders, epilepsy, and many other conditions.

The hospital has a twenty-bed neurological/neurosurgical intensive care unit, one of the largest and most sophisticated in the United States. There is also a thirty-one-bed neurology division and a twenty-five-bed neuroclinical division in addition to other beds for epilepsy, movement disorders, and sleep disorders.

For information on neurological services at Barnes-Jewish Hospital, call (314) 747-3000. Web site: **www.barnesandjewish.org.**

BRIGHAM AND WOMEN'S HOSPITAL, BOSTON

The Department of Neurology at Brigham and Women's Hospital provides care to patients with diseases of the brain, spinal cord, nerves, and muscles. Specialists offer evaluation, consultation, and management in the areas of memory disorders, neuromuscular diseases, stroke, movement disorders, seizure disorders, sleep disorders, brain tumors, and headache. For information, call (617) 732-5355. Web site: **www.brighamandwomens.org.**

Top 100 Hospitals for Stroke Care

The following hospitals have been recognized in a study released by the HCIA-Sachs Institute, a top provider of health-care information, as the nation's top 100 hospitals for stroke care. They are listed below by state. Check your local telephone book for listings.

ALABAMA
BMC — Montclair, Birmingham

ARIZONA
Tucson Medical Center, Tucson

CALIFORNIA
Dominican Santa Cruz Hospital, Santa Cruz
Salinas Valley Memorial Hospital, Salinas

CONNECTICUT
Hospital of St. Raphael, New Haven

FLORIDA
Bon Secours-Venice Hospital, Venice
Charlotte Regional Medical Center, Punta Gorda
Community Hospital of New Port Richey, New Port Richey
Englewood Community Hospital, Englewood
Indian River Memorial Hospital, Vero Beach
Largo Medical Center, Largo
Lee Memorial Hospital, Fort Myers
Leesburg Regional Medical Center, Leesburg
Marion Community Hospital DBA Ocala Regional Medical
    Center, Ocala
Martin Memorial Medical Center, Stuart
Mease Countryside Hospital, Safety Harbor
Morton Plant Hospital, Clearwater
Munroe Regional Medical Center, Ocala
North Florida Regional Medical Center, Gainesville

Oak Hill Hospital, Spring Hill
Palm Beach Gardens Medical Center, Palm Beach Gardens
Palms of Pasadena Hospital, St. Petersburg
St. Anthony's Hospital, St. Petersburg
Sarasota Memorial Hospital, Sarasota
Seven Rivers Community Hospital, Crystal River
West Florida Regional Medical Center, Pensacola

GEORGIA
Middle Georgia Hospital, Macon
West Georgia Health System, La Grange

IDAHO
St. Luke's Regional Medical Center, Boise

ILLINOIS
St. Francis Hospital, Blue Island
St. John's Hospital, Springfield

INDIANA
Community Hospital East, Indianapolis
Lutheran Hospital of Indiana, Fort Wayne
Parkview Memorial Hospital, Fort Wayne
St. Mary's Medical Center, Evansville
St. Vincent Hospital & Health Care Centers, Inc., Indianapolis

IOWA
St. Luke's Methodist Hospital, Cedar Rapids

KANSAS
Wesley Medical Center, Wichita

KENTUCKY
Hardin Memorial Hospital, Elizabethtown
Murray-Calloway County Hospital, Murray
Norton Hospital, Louisville
St. Joseph Hospital, Lexington

LOUISIANA
Willis–Knighton Health System, Shreveport

MARYLAND
Greater Baltimore Medical Center, Baltimore

MASSACHUSETTS
Massachusetts General Hospital, Boston

MICHIGAN
Harper University Hospital, Detroit
Henry Ford Health System, Detroit
Marquette General Hospital, Marquette
Northern Michigan Hospital, Petoskey
William Beaumont Hospital, Royal Oak
William Beaumont Hospital, Troy

MISSOURI
Boone Hospital Center, Columbia
St. Francis Medical Center, Cape Girardeau
St. Luke's Hospital, Kansas City

MONTANA
St. Vincent Hospital & Health Center, Billings

NEBRASKA
Bryan Memorial Hospital, Lincoln

NEW JERSEY
The Medical Center at Princeton, Princeton
Underwood Memorial Hospital, Woodbury

NEW YORK
Albany Medical Center Hospital, Albany
Mary Imogene Bassett Hospital, Cooperstown
North Shore University Hospital, Manhasset

NYU Health Center, New York City
St. Joseph's Hospital Health Center, Syracuse
St. Peter's Hospital, Albany

NORTH CAROLINA
First Health Moore Regional Hospital, Pinehurst
Pitt County Memorial Hospital, Greenville

OHIO
Bethesda Hospital, Cincinnati
Kettering Memorial Hospital, Kettering
The Toledo Hospital, Toledo

OREGON
Kaiser Sunnyside Hospital, Clackamas

PENNSYLVANIA
Allegheny General Hospital, Pittsburgh
The Bryn Mawr Hospital, Bryn Mawr
Geisinger Medical Center, Danville
Good Samaritan Hospital, Lebanon
Hamot Medical Center, Erie
Jefferson Hospital, Pittsburgh
Lehigh Valley Hospital, Allentown
Mercy Hospital, Scranton
Northwest Medical Center, Oil City
Pocono Medical Center, Stroudsburg
St. Clair Memorial Hospital, Pittsburgh
Thomas Jefferson University Hospital, Philadelphia

SOUTH CAROLINA
Hilton Head Medical Center & Clinics, Hilton Head Island
Medical University of South Carolina, Charleston

SOUTH DAKOTA
Sioux Valley Hospital, Sioux Falls

TENNESSEE
CENTENNIAL MEDICAL CENTER, NASHVILLE

TEXAS
BAYLOR UNIVERSITY MEDICAL CENTER, DALLAS
McALLEN MEDICAL CENTER, McALLEN
MEMORIAL HERMANN BAPTIST BEAUMONT, BEAUMONT
METHODIST HOSPITAL, HOUSTON
MOTHER FRANCES HOSPITAL, TYLER
ST. MARY HOSPITAL, PORT ARTHUR
SCOTT & WHITE MEMORIAL HOSPITAL, TEMPLE

VIRGINIA
CARILION MEDICAL CENTER, CARILION ROANOKE MEMORIAL
    HOSPITAL/COMMUNITY HOSPITALS, ROANOKE
INOVA FAIRFAX HOSPITAL, FALLS CHURCH
MEMORIAL REGIONAL MEDICAL CENTER, RICHMOND

WASHINGTON
PROVIDENCE ST. PETER HOSPITAL, OLYMPIA

WEST VIRGINIA
BECKLEY ARH, BECKLEY

WISCONSIN
UNIVERSITY OF WISCONSIN HOSPITAL & CLINICS, MADISON
WAUSAU HOSPITAL, WAUSAU

Where to Buy Supplements, Herbs, and Other Nutraceuticals

Below is a list of manufacturers and distributors that carry brain- and mood-support supplements. You can use this information to obtain additional product information directly from the companies. None of the companies listed had any input in the writing or production of this book but are listed because they are well-known manufacturers. Addresses, phone numbers, and Web sites are subject to change.

BIOTICS RESEARCH
www.bioticsresearch.com
L-Phenylalanine, L-Tyrosine, Taurine, Garlic Plus, Ginkgo Biloba, V.H.P. (valerian, hops, passionflower)

COUNTRY LIFE
101 Corporate Drive
Hauppauge, New York 11788
Fax: (631) 232-5051
www.country-life.com
Nature's Elements

ECLECTIC INSTITUTE
14385 S. E. Lusted Road
Sandy, Oregon 97055
(888) 799-4372
www.eclecticherb.com
Garlic, Ginkgo, Hops, Kava, Oats, Passionflower, Skullcap, St. John's Wort, Valerian, Valerian-Passionflower, Kava-California Poppy, Chewable Ginkgo, Chamomile

ENZYMATIC THERAPY
825 Challenger Drive
Green Bay, Wisconsin 54311
(800) 558-7372
www.enzy.com

Anti-Anxiety, HyperCalm, Kava-30, Kava-55, KavaTone, KidCalm, Melatonin Complex, Relaxcin, Rest'N, Sleep Ease, St. John's Wort Complex, St. John's Wort Extract, St. John's Wort Plus with Kava, St. John's Wort-100, Stress-End, Trimax, Valerian-400

GENERAL NUTRITION, INC.
Customer Resources Department
300 Sixth Avenue
Pittsburgh, Pennsylvania 15222
(888) 462-2548
www.gnc.com
Cognita, Sleep Formula, SAM-e, and various prebiotic and probiotic supplements; and many homeopathic remedies

GERO VITA INTERNATIONAL
4936 Yonge Street
Toronto, Ontario M2M 6S3 Canada
www.giv.com
Mind Extender, BrainPower, Focusil, Neocel, CerebreX

HerbShop.com
www.herbshop.com
5-HTP, Happy Camper, Kava, Nutri-Calm, St. John's Wort

J. R. CARLSON LABORATORIES, INC.
15 College Drive
Arlington Heights, Illinois 60004-1985
(847) 255-1600
(888) 234-5656
www.carlsonlabs.com
Nutra Support Memory, Garlic 600, Super Omega-3 Fish Oils, Super-DHA, Kava, St. John's Wort, Ginkgo Biloba Plus

LIFE EXTENSION FOUNDATION
1100 West Commercial Boulevard
Fort Lauderdale, Florida 33309
(800) 544-4440
www.lef.org

Acetyl-L-Carnitine, CDP Choline, Choline Bitartrate, Choline Cooler, Cognitex, Cognitex with Pregnenolone, DMAE Caps, DMAE-Ginkgo Capsules, DMAE Powder, Huperzine A with Vitamin E, Lecithin Granules, Lecithin with B5 and BHA, NADH, PC-Ginkgo Extract, Phosphatidylserine Caps, Super Ginkgo Extract, Vinpocetine

MADIS BOTANICALS
375 Huyler Street
South Hackensack, New Jersey 07606
(201) 440-5000
www.pureworld.com
American Ginseng PE, KavaPure PE, KavaPure PE 30%, KavaPure PE 40%, KavaPure SG 70 mg, Panax Ginseng PE 8%, Passionflower PE 4%, Siberian Ginseng PE 0.7 %, St. John's Wort PE 0.3%, St. John's Wort PE 0.3% UV, Valerian PE 0.8%

MARTEK BIOSCIENCES
6480 Dobbin Road
Columbia, Maryland 21045
(800) 662-6339
www.martekbio.com
Neuromins DHA, Neuromins 200, Neuromins for Kids, Neuromins PL

MEGAFOOD
P.O. Box 325
Derry, New Hampshire 03038
(603) 432-5022; (800) 848-2542
www.mega.food.com
Essentials for Stress, Un-Stress Daily Foods

NATROL, INC.
Chatsworth, California 91311
(800) 326-1520
www.natrol.com
Melatonin (1 mg), Melatonin (3 mg), Melatonin Liquid, Melatonin Timed Release, Sleep N Restore, 5-HTP, DHEA, GarliPure, Siberian Ginseng, Ginkgo Biloba, Kava, St. John's Wort

NATURAL ORGANICS (Nature's Plus supplements)
548 Broadhollow Road
Melville, New York 11747-3708
(631) 293-0030
www.naturesplus.com
Ginkgo Combo, Ultra Ginkgo, Ginkgo Biloba Extended Release, Ginkgo Biloba, Choline 600-mg Extended Release, NeuroGenic, Neuro-Boost Spray, Huperzine Rx-Brain, Phosphatidyserine/DMAE Complex, Fuel for Thought Neuro Nutrition, St. John's Wort (250 mg), St. John's Wort (300 mg), Herbal Kidz Smartkidz

NATURE'S ANSWER
75 Commerce Drive
Hauppauge, New York 11788
(800) 439-2324
www.naturesanswer.com
Brainstorm, Chamomile Flower, Garlic Bulb, Garlic Super Complex, Ginseng (11 varieties), Kava Extract, Kava Root, Mood Balance, Passionflower Herb, Skullcap Herb, Slumber, St. John's Wort Flowering Tips, St. John's Wort Herb Extract, St. John's Wort Herb Extract Super, Tense Ease, Valerian Root

NATURE'S LIFE
7180 Lampson Avenue
Garden Grove, California 92841
Fax: (714) 379-6501
www.natlife.com
Melatonin (3 mg), Menopause Formula, SAM-e Complex, Super Lecithins

NATURE'S WAY
10 Mountain Springs Parkway
Springville, Utah 84663
(801) 489-1500
www.naturesway.com
Choline, Ex-Stress Formula, Ex-Stress Liquid, 5-HTP, Ginkgo Extract, Ginkold, Hops, Insomnia, Lecithin, Lecithin Concentrate, Melatonin, MentAlert Formula, Organic St. John's Wort, Phosphatidylserine, Skullcap, Silent Night Formula, Silent Night

Nutramax Laboratories, Inc.
2208 Lakeside Boulevard
Edgewood, Maryland 21040
(410) 776-4000; (800) 925-5187
www.senior-moment.com
Senior Moment

Pharmaton
www.pharmaton.com
Ginsana, Ginkoba, Movana

Schiff Vitamins
(800) 526-6251
www.schiffvitamins.com
Melatonin, Garlic, DHEA, 5-HTP, St. John's Wort

Solgar
500 Willow Tree Road
Leonia, New Jersey 07605
(877)-SOLGAR-4
www.solgar.com
*Siberian Ginseng, Whole American Ginseng, Korean Ginseng, Ginkgo Leaf,
Super Ginkgo, Kava Root, Valerian Root*

Source Naturals
19 Janis Way
Scotts Valley, California 95066
(831) 438-1144; (800) 815-2333
www.sourcenaturals.com
*Melatonin, NightRest, St. John's Wort, Kava Extract, Attentive Child, Acetyl-L-
Carnitine, Calm Thoughts, DMAE, GABA, Ginkgo, Higher Mind, Mega Mind,
Mental Edge, Phosphatidyl, Positive Thoughts, ThiaMind, Vincamine*

SPRING VALLEY HERBS AND NATURAL FOODS
1738 South Glenstone
Springfield, Missouri 65804
(417) 882-1033; (800) 967-3982
www.springvalleyherbs.com
L-5-HTP, Super Stress Complex, Stress Formula with 500 C, Ginkgo Biloba Extract, Ginseng Extract (Korean Panax), Ginseng Extract (Siberian), Odorless Garlic, Brain Support, Mood Support, Kava Root Extract-Plus, KavaPure, St. John's Wort Extract, St. John's Wort Extract Plus, Valerian Root, Lecithin Capsules, Lecithin Granules, Phosphatidyl Choline, Phosphatidyl Serine Complex

SUNDOWN HERBALS
www.rexallsundown.com
Garlic, Ginkgo Biloba, Ginseng, Korean Ginseng, Siberian Ginseng, Valerian Root, St. John's Wort Extract, Kava

TWINLABS
2120 Smithtown Avenue
Ronkonkama, New York 11779
(631) 467-3140; for product information: (631) 630-3486
www.twinlab.com
MaxiLife Brain Protector, MaxiLife Choline Cocktail with Caffeine, MaxiLife Choline Cocktail without Caffeine, MaxiLife Citicholine, DMAE Caps, DMAE-H3, Executive Stress Caps, Neurovites

BEST BRAIN WEB SITES

ADDICTIONS

- *American Council for Drug Education.* A substance-abuse prevention and education agency that develops programs and materials based on the most current research into substance abuse. Web site: www.acde.org.
- *National Clearinghouse for Alcohol and Drug Information (NCADI).* Information service of the Center for Substance Abuse Prevention. World's largest resource for the latest information on substance abuse. Web site: www.health.org.
- *National Council on Alcoholism and Drug Dependence, Inc.* Provides education, information, help, and hope to those struggling with addictions. Web site: www.ncadd.org.
- *National Institute on Alcohol Abuse and Alcoholism.* Offers publications on alcoholism, information on research, and links to related sites. Web site: www.niaa.nih.gov.
- *National Institute on Drug Abuse (NIDA).* Offers information on common drugs of abuse, trends, and statistics; an online catalog; information on research; and links to other helpful sites. Web site: www.nida.nih.gov.

ALZHEIMER'S DISEASE

- *Alzheimer's Association.* Dedicated to research on the causes, cure, and prevention of the disease; provides educational and support services to patients, their families, and caregivers. Web site: www.alz.org.
- *Alzheimer's Disease Review.* An online journal that discusses the most current research and advances in treating the disease. Web site: www.mc.uky.edu/ad-review.
- *Alzheimer Page.* An educational service of Washington University's Alzheimer's Disease Research Center in St. Louis, Missouri. Web site: www.biostat.wush.edu/alzheimer.
- *Alzheimer Web.* A resource for researchers and for anyone interested in research developments partaining to the disease. Web site: www.home.mira.net/-dhs/ad.html.

- *National Institute on Aging, Alzheimer's Disease Education and Referral Service*. Provides information on Alzheimer's research, publications, and links to related physical and mental health resources. Also provides referral information. Web site: www.alzheimers.org.

ANXIETY

- *Anxiety Coach*. Information about anxiety disorders and how to treat them. Provides links to related sites and a reading list. Web site: www. anxietycoach.com.
- *Anxiety Disorder Association of America*. Promotes the prevention, treatment, and cure of anxiety disorders. Web site: www.adaa.org.
- *National Anxiety Foundation*. Provides information on anxiety disorders for patients and professionals. Web site: www.lexington-on-line.com/naf.html.
- *National Institute of Mental Health*. Offers information for consumers and professionals about panic disorder, obsessive-compulsive disorder, posttraumatic stress disorder, phobias, and general anxiety problems. Web site: www.nimh.nih.gov/anxiety.

BRAIN AND MEMORY INFORMATION

- *All the Tests*. Filled with fun, challenging mental tests of all kinds, including think and memory tests. Web site: www.AllTheTests.com.
- *Amazing Brain*. Advanced information on the brain. Web site: Tqjunior. advanced.org/4371/index.htm.
- *ArcAngel*. A basketball training system in which you learn to improve shooting via visualization and repetition. Web site: www.arcangel.org.
- *Atlas on the Brain*. Online atlas of the brain from Harvard University. Web site: www.med.harvard.edu/AANLIB.
- *Brain Backgrounders*. Online series of articles that answer basic brain questions. Web site: www.sfn.org/backgrounders/.
- *Brain Channels*. A Web site that provides brain-enhancement products, late-breaking brain-research news, education, entertainment, brain teasers, and more. Web site: www.brainchannels.com.
- *Brain.com*. Loaded with information on the brain, from nutrition to inTelephoneligence tests to brain-enhancement products. Web site: www.brain.com.

- *Brainconnection.com*. An online source of information about the brain and neuroscience research for teachers, parents, and students. Web site: www.brainconnection.com.
- *The Brain Store*. A virtual storefront for ordering learning resources and materials based on the latest brain research application. Web site: www.thebrainstore.com.
- *Dana*. A gateway to brain information and brain disorders, as well as current brain research. Also includes "Brainy Kids Online" for children, parents, and teachers. Web site: www.dana.org.
- *Digital Anatomist*. Features an interactive brain atlas, with 2D and 3D images. Web site: www.biostr.washington.edu/.
- *MemoryZine*. Offers memory training products designed for self-paced learning at home or at the office. Also includes educational information and the latest brain research. Web site: www. memoryzine.com.
- *Mensa*. Take the organization's Web site test to see how you rate inTelephonelectually. (A high score on the test does not qualify you for membership, however. Mensa membership tests are administered at colleges and universities around the country.) Web site: www. mensa.org.
- *NASA's Cognition Lab*. Provides a tutorial for a great mental workout. Web site: www.olias.arc.nasa.gov/cognition/tutorials/index.html.
- *New Horizons*. Provides links to an excellent series of articles by leading brain specialists and researchers. Web site: www.newhorizons.org/blab.html#intro.
- *Super Memory*. A Web site devoted to improving memory, self-growth, creativity, and time management. Web site: www.supermemo.com.
- *Total Memory*. Dr. Cynthia Green's Web site featuring memory exercises and other valuable information. Web site: www.totalmemory.com.

DEPRESSION

- *Depressed Anonymous*. A 12-step program of recovery for individuals with depression. Web site: www.depressedanon.com.
- *Depression After Delivery*. Provides information about postpartum mood and anxiety disorders and links to related resources. Web site: www.depressionafterdelivery.com.

- *Depression Clinic.* A comprehensive site providing information on the causes of depression, medication, treatment, and more. Web site: www. depressionclinic.com.
- *National Depressive and Manic-Depressive Association (NDMDA).* An educational resource for patients, families, professionals, and the public on the nature of depressive and manic-depressive illness. Web site: www.ndmda.org.
- *National Foundation for Depressive Illness, Inc. (NAFDI).* Provides information for the public and for professionals about depression and the availability of treatment. Web site: www.depression.org.
- *National Mental Health Association.* Offers resources to improve the mental health of individuals and help them achieve victory over mental illnesses. Web site: www.nmha.org.

PHOBIAS

- *Social Anxiety Support.* Provides information on social anxiety, offers forums and chat rooms, plus twenty-four-hour help. Web site: www. socialanxietysupport.com.

POSTTRAUMATIC STRESS DISORDER (PTSD)

- *International Society for Traumatic Stress Studies.* A valuable source for information on PTSD. Web site: www.istss.org.
- *Posttraumatic Stress Disorder (PTSD) Alliance.* Serves as an educational support tool for individuals with PTSD and their loved ones, those at risk of PTSD, and professionals who work with trauma survivors. Web site: www.ptsdalliance.org.

MISCELLANEOUS

- *Alternative Medicine.* The National Institutes of Health (NIH) has formed The Office of Alternative Medicine, which can be accessed online. It provides consumer information on various aspects of complementary and alternative medicine. Web site: www.oam.nih.gov.
- *Life Extension Foundation.* This is the world's largest organization dedicated to finding scientific methods of preventing and treating disease. You can find helpful information on the most effective ways to treat a wide range of diseases and medical conditions. Web site: www.lef.org.

TOP BRAIN BOOKS

Aging with Grace: What the Nun Study Teaches Us About Leading Longer, Healthier, and More Meaningful Lives by David Snowden, Ph.D. (Bantam Doubleday, 2001).

The Anxiety Cure: An Eight-Step Program for Getting Well by Robert L. DuPont, Elizabeth DuPont Spencer, and Caroline M. DuPont (John Wiley & Sons, 1998).

Anxiety, Phobias, and Panic: A Step-by-Step Program for Regaining Control of Your Life by Reneau Z. Peurifoy (Warner Books, 1995).

Brain Builders! A Lifelong Guide to Sharper Thinking, Better Memory, and an Age-proof Mind by Richard Leviton (Prentice Hall Press, 1995).

Brain Fitness: Anti-Aging Strategies for Achieving Super Mind Power by Bob Goldman, Ronald Klatz, and Lisa Berger (Main Street Books, 1999).

Brain Longevity: The Breakthrough Medical Program That Improves Your Mind and Memory by Cameron Stauth (Warner Books, 1999).

The Brain Wellness Plan: Breakthrough Medical, Nutritional, and Immune-Boosting Therapies by Jay Lombard and Carl Germano (Kensington Publishing Corporation, 1998).

Building Mental Muscle: Conditioning Exercises for the Six InTelephoneligence Zones by David Gamon, Ph.D. (Allen D. Bragdon Publisher, 1999).

Change Your Brain, Change Your Life: The Breakthrough Program for Conquering Anxiety, Depression, Obsessiveness, Anger, and Impulsiveness by Daniel G. Amen (Times Books, 2000).

The Diet Cure: The Eight-Step Program to Rebalance Your Body Chemistry and End Food Cravings, Weight Problems, and Mood Swings—Now by Julia Ross (Penguin, 2000).

Feeling Good: The New Mood Therapy by David D. Burns, M.D., and Aaron T. Beck (Wholecare, 1999).

Female and Forgetful: A Six-Step Program to Help Restore Your Memory and Sharpen Your Mind by Elisa Lottor, Ph.D., M.D., and Nancy P. Bruning (Warner Books, 2002).

Food & Mood: The Complete Guide to Eating Well and Feeling Your Best by Elizabeth Somer (Owl Books, 1999).

Getting Your Life Back: The Complete Guide to Recovery from Depression by Jesse H. Wright and Monica Ramirez (Basco, 2001).

Improve Your Memory by Ronald W. Fry (Career Press, 2000).

The Memory Book by Harry Lorayne and Jerry Lucas (Ballantine Books, 1996).

Menopause and the Mind: The Complete Guide to Coping with Cognitive Effects of Perimenopause and Menopause, Including Memory Loss, Foggy Thinking, and Verbal Slips by Claire L. Warga, Ph.D. (Touchstone Books, 2000).

Mind Boosters: A Guide to Natural Supplements That Enhance Your Mind, Memory, and Mood by Ray Sahelian, M.D. (St. Martin's Press, 2000).

Mood Food: Brighten, Heal, and Elevate Your State of Mind by Jane Eldershaw (Sourcebooks, Inc., 2001).

The Omega-3 Connection: The Groundbreaking Anti-Depression Diet and Brain Program by Andrew Stoll, M.D. (Free Press, 2001).

One-Minute Brain Teasers: Official American Mensa Puzzle Book by Alan Stillson (Sterling Publications, 2001).

Owner's Manual for the Brain: Everyday Applications from Mind-Brain Research by Pierce J. Howard (Bard Press, 2000).

Parkinson's Disease: A Complete Guide for Patients and Families by William J. Wiener, M.D., and Lisa M. Shulman, M.D. (Johns Hopkins University Press, 2001).

Smart Moves by Carla Hannford, Ph.D. (Great Ocean Publishers, 1995).

Stroke-Free for Life: A Complete Guide to Stroke Prevention and Treatment by David O. Wiebers, M.D. (Cliff Street Books, 2001).

Super Brain Power by Jane Marie Stine (Prentice Hall Press, 2000).

Super Brain Power: 28 Minutes to a Supercharged Brain by Dane Spotts (Lifequest Publications, 1999).

The 36-Hour Day: A Family Guide to Caring for Persons with Alzheimer's Disease, Related Dementing Illnesses, and Memory Loss Later in Life by Nancy L. Mace and Peter V. Rabins, M.D. (Warner Books, 2001).

Thoughts and Feelings: Taking Control of Your Moods and Your Life by Matthew McKay, Martha Davis, Ph.D., and Patrick Fanning (New Harbinger Publications, 1998).

Total Memory Workout by Cynthia R. Green, Ph.D. (Bantam Books, 1999).

The User's Manual for the Brain by Bob G. Bodenhamer and L. Michael Hall, Ph.D. (Crown House Publishing, 2001).

Your Memory: How It Works and How to Improve It by Kenneth L. Higbee, Ph.D. (Marlowe & Co., 2001).

Your Miracle Brain by Jean Carper (HarperCollins, 2000).

SMART PRODUCTS

SMART GAMES

- *Bright Brain*. Designed for kids, this brain-enrichment kit promises to boost your child's learning by 30 percent. The program consists of fifteen specific "neural activators" that increase the ability to read, learn, think, write, and pay attention in school. Geared for the early primary school learner, ages four to eight. Available from Brain.com.
- *Cranium™ Board Game*. This game challenges players mentally in order to advance around the board. Available from Brain.com.
- *Who Wants to Be a Millionaire*. Based on the hit TV show, this game features questions that range in difficulty from $100 up to $1 million. Like the real show, it includes "ask the audience" and "phone a friend." Available in stores and from Brain.com.

SMART SOFTWARE

- *Best Intentions*. This program is designed to help you improve your "prospective remembering"—remembering tasks you have that you have yet to do, such as meeting deadlines and appointments, taking medications, running errands, returning rental videos, buying birthday cards, and recalling phone numbers. Available from MemoryZine.com.
- *Facts & Figures*. This program incorporates various strategies that help you remember lists, find misplaced items, improve your spatial memory, and improve your recall of facts and figures. Available from MemoryZine.com.
- *Galaxy of Brain Games*. A collection of ten challenging games designed to test your mind as well as your reflexes. Designed for all age groups. Available from BrainChannels.com.
- *Mind Rover*. With this game, you design small robots to play against those designed by other players in challenging mental battles. Available from Brain.com.
- *MyLifeZone™*. A twelve-week program that teaches you how to tap into your subconscious mind to boost your brainpower, improve your memory, and speed up your reaction time. Available from Brain.com.

- *Names & Faces*. Incorporating the latest techniques in memory improvement, this program teaches you how to learn the names of others and recall them when necessary. Available from MemoryZine.com.
- *Nature of Memory*. This program helps you learn about memory, assess your memory readiness, and learn about new memory aids. Available from MemoryZine.com.
- *ThinkFast!™ for Peak Mental Performance*. Available on CD or electronic download, this program contains mental exercises designed to improve mental performance, boost memory, increase attention, and accelerate decision-making. Available from Brain.com.

SMART MUSIC

The following products are collections of musical arrangements produced by the Center for Psychoacoustical Research, where experts in the fields of audiology, psychology, education, and music develop music for enhancing health and learning. Available from Brain.com.

- *Concentration*. Designed to sharpen your focus and mental attention, these twelve baroque masterpieces stimulate the brain with high-frequency sounds.
- *Thinking*. Featuring rearranged works by Beethoven, Schubert, Debussy, and others, this collection is designed to enhance relaxation while stimulating the brain to maintain concentration.
- *Learning*. Designed to accelerate learning and enhance creativity, these arrangements of baroque masterpieces feature gentle sounds of nature.
- *Productivity*. These seventeen movements from classical musicians are designed to stimulate the nervous system to promote alertness.
- *Relax*. Selections from Schumann, Beethoven, Vivaldi, and others are designed to calm the mind and unwind the body.
- *De-Stress*. A movement from Mahler's Fourth Symphony is combined with sounds of foghorns and ocean waves to help release tension and induce sleep.

The following smart music products are available from Amazon.com: *Brainwave Suite; Brainwave Journey; Brainwave Music;* and *Meditation System.*

References

A majority of the information in this book comes from medical literature in both the popular magazines and scientific journals; professional textbooks; interviews with experts; Internet sources; and computer searches of medical databases of research abstracts.

Introduction: You're the Boss of Your Brain

Bisacre, M. (ed.) et al. *The Illustrated Encyclopedia of the Human Body*. New York: Exeter Books, 1984.

Colburn, D. 1999. The infinite brain. *The Washington Post*, September 28, p. Z12.

Editor. 1998. Inside the human brain. *Science World*, November 16. Online: www.findarticles.com.

Editor. 1997. The principles of nerve cell communication. *Alcohol & Research World*, March 22, pp. 107–108.

Editor. 1994. Smart glue: Brain research. *The Economist*, October 15, pp. 114–115.

Farndon, J. *The Big Book of the Brain*. New York: Peter Bedrick Books, 2000.

Geary, J. 1997. A trip down memory's lanes. *Time*, May 5. Online: www.time.com.

Greenfield, S. A. *The Human Brain*. New York: Basic Books, 1997.

Henig, R. M. *How a Woman Ages*. New York: Ballantine Books, 1997.

Pesman, C. *How a Man Ages*. New York: Ballantine Books, 1984.

Raver, A. 1995. The healing power of gardens. *Saturday Evening Post*, March 13, pp. 42–45.

Sahelian, R. 1999. 5 brain chemicals and why they're important. *Better Nutrition*, March. Online: www.findarticles.com.

Stickney, N. 1997. Your body's control center. *U.S. Kids*, January 1, pp. 36–37.

Treays, R. *Understanding Your Brain*. Tulsa, Oklahoma: EDC Publishing, 1996.

Part 1: The Foundations of Great Mental Fitness

CHAPTER 1: HOW TO BOOST YOUR BRAINPOWER

15 Lifestyle Secrets

Black, P. 1999. Keeping memory lane unclogged. *Business Week*, March 8, p. 116.

Editor. 2000. Age-proofing your brain. *Consumer Reports*, August, pp. 62–64.

Editor. 1998. Recharge your life. *Essence*, June, pp. 36–39.

Heavey, B. 1998. Be a head master. *Men's Health*, April, pp. 78–79.

Koontz, K. 2000. Use it or lose it. *Vegetarian Times*, August. Online: www.findarticles.com.

Kotulak, R. 1996. Keeping the brain sharp as we age. *Saturday Evening Post*, November 21, pp. 50–55.

Leinwald, D. 2001. Studies show Ecstasy can damage brain. *USA Today*, July 20, p. 3A.

Myslinski, N. R. 1998. Now where did I put those keys? Tips for better memories. *The World & I*, November, p. 160.

Norton, A. 2001. High-fat diets linked to poorer brain function. Reuters News Service, February 22. Online: www.pdr.net.

Popova, N. K. 2000. Serotonin metabolism in the rat brain during water deprivation and hydration. *Rossiiskaia Fiziologicheskii Zhurnal Imeni I. M. Sechenova* 86:140–147.

Zintl, A. 2000. Mothers: Instant energy. *Parenting*, August, p. 104.

6 Nutrients to Eat Every Week

Editor. 1998. Guide to the smart nutrients. *Natural Health*, March/April. Online: www.findarticles.com.

Pierre, C. 2001. The new science of eating to get smart. *Prevention*, July, pp. 122–129.

Sizer, F., and E. Whitney. *Nutrition Concepts and Controversies*, 7th ed. Belmont, California: West/Wadsworth, 1997.

Stains, L. R. 1998. Super immunity. *Prevention*, March, pp. 100–110.

2 Proteins That Improve Your Thinking

Kanarek, R. B. et al. 1990. Effects of food snacks on cognitive performance in male college students. *Appetite* 14:15–27.

Zeisel, S. H. 2000. Choline: Needed for normal development of memory. *Journal of the American College of Nutrition* 19:528S–531S.

Sidebar: The Mental Merit of Mixed Meals

Christensen, L. et al. 1993. Effect of meal composition on mood. *Behavioral Neuroscience* 107:346–353.

Sizer, F., and E. Whitney. *Nutrition Concepts and Controversies*, 7th ed. Belmont, California: West/Wadsworth, 1997.

3 Healthy Fats That Power Your Brain

Dworkin, N. 1999. A reason to eat fat. *Psychology Today*, November. Online: www.findarticles.com.

Editor. 2000. DHA: The good-for-you fat. *Psychology Today*, March. Online: www.findarticles.com.

Editor. 1995. Mental vigor. *Prevention*, June, pp. 66–67.

2 Surprise Fluids for Peak Mental Fitness

Carper, J. 2000. A cool, juicy summer fruit juice packs a nutrition wallop. *USA Today Weekend*, July 23, p. 4.

Joshipura, K. J. et al. 1999. Fruit and vegetable intake in relation to risk of ischemic stroke. *Journal of the American Medical Association* 282:1233–1239.

4 Eating Plans to Sharpen Your Thinking

Blaun, R. 1996. How to eat smart. *Psychology Today*, May, pp. 34–44.

D'Amato, E. 1997. Food for what ails you. *Men's Health*, November, pp. 78–80.

Demontis, R. 2001. Mood food. *The Ottawa Sun*, April 22, p. S20.

Dye, L. et al. 2000. Macronutrients and mental performance. *Nutrition* 16:1021–1034.

Editor. 1998. Birth of a new "vitamin." *Prevention*, September, p. 53.

Lazor, D. 1994. Eat to win and be smarter, happier, sexier. *Cosmopolitan*, December, pp. 202–205.

Lloyd, H. M. 1994. Mood and cognitive performance effects of isocaloric lunches differing in fat and carbohydrate content. *Physiology and Behavior* 56:51–57.

McDonald, K. 2001. Food for thought. *Men's Health*, March, p. 78.

Pierre, C. 2001. The new science of eating to get smart. *Prevention*, July, pp. 122–129.

Sandmaier, M. 1996. Eat your way to a good mood: Can certain foods really make you feel better? *Good Housekeeping*, March, pp. 93–94.

A Berry for the Brain: The Amazing Fruit That Juices Up Your Mind

Editor. 1999. Health and research discoveries. *AARP Bulletin*, November. Online: www.elibrary.com.

McCord, H. 1999. Improve your memory with everyday food. *Prevention*, March, p. 50.

———.1999. The miracle berry. *Prevention*, June, pp. 122–127.

Iron and Boron: Brightest Mineral Superstars

Naghil, M. R. et al. 1996. The boron content of selected foods and the estimation of its daily intake among free-living subjects. *Journal of the American College of Nutrition* 15:614–619.

Nielson, F. H. 1988. Boron—An overlooked element of potential nutritional importance. *Nutrition Today*, January/February, pp. 4–7.

———.1998. The justification for providing dietary guidance for the nutritional intake of boron. *Biological Trace Element Research* 66:319–330.

Scrimshaw, N. S. 1991. Iron deficiency. *Scientific American*, October, p. 48.

Sizer, F., and E. Whitney. *Nutrition Concepts and Controversies*, 7th ed. Belmont, California: West/Wadsworth, 1997.

7 Brain-Protective Phytochemicals

Borek, C. 2001. Antioxidant effects of aged garlic extract. *Journal of Nutrition* 131:1010S–1015S.

Kim, H. et al. 2000. Attenuation of neurodegeneration-relevant modifications of brain proteins by dietary soy. *Biofactors* 12:243–250.

Lin, S. S. et al. 2000. Effects of ellagic acid by oral administration on N-acetylation and metabolism and 2-aminofluorene in rat brain tissues. *Neurochemical Research* 25:1503–1508.

Yan, J. J. et al. 2001. Protection against beta-amyloid peptide toxicity in vivo with long-term administration of ferulic acid. *British Journal of Pharmacology* 133:89–96.

Yoneda, T. et al. 1995. Antioxidant effects of "beta catechin." *Biochemistry and Molecular Biology International* 35:995–1008.

4 Easy Workouts to Pump Up Mental Fitness

Garcia, L. 2001. Fitness briefs. *Dallas Morning News*, June 15, p. 5C.

Perrig-Chiello, P. 1998. The effects of resistance training on well-being and memory in elderly volunteers. *Age and Aging* 27:469–475.

Smart Supplements: 10 Miracle Pills and Potions That Improve Mental Acuity

Barbagallo, S. G. 1994. Alpha-glycerophosphocholine in the mental recovery of cerebral ischemic attacks. An Italian multicenter clinical trial. *Annals of the New York Academy of Sciences* 717:253–269.

Blaun, R. 1996. How to eat smart. *Psychology Today*, May, pp. 34–44.

Curtis-Prior, P. et al. 1999. Therapeutic value of ginkgo biloba in reducing symptoms of mental decline. *The Journal of Pharmacy and Pharmacology* 51:535–541.

Editor. 2000. Can taking vitamins protect your brain? *Harvard Health Letter*, August. Online: www.findarticles.com.

Editor. 1998. Guide to the smart nutrients. *Natural Health*, March/April. Online: www.findarticles.com.

Editor. 2001. Herbal aid for exams. *The Mirror*, June 2, p. 14.

Gallia, K. 2001. Do you need a brain boost? *Natural Health*, March, p. 25.

Kanigel, R. 2000. Getting to the root of ginseng. *Health*, November/December, p. 75.

Lavalle, J. B. 2001. Discover alpha-GPC. *Let's Live*, June, pp. 66–68.

Sahelian, R. 1999. DMAE for brain health. *Better Nutrition*, April. Online: www.findarticles.com.

Tyler, V. 1998. Boost your brain and your libido. *Prevention*, June, pp. 91–93.

Train Your Brain and Sharpen Your Senses with These 16 Mental Exercises

Bowser, A. 1999. Cerebral fitness: How to get it, how to keep it. *Dermatology Times*, August, pp. 40–41.

Jaret, P. 1999. Brain boosters. Online: www.webmd.com.

Munson, M. et al. 1994. Brain boost. *Prevention*, August, pp. 28–29.

Zinczenko, D. 1994. Rocket science made easy. *Men's Health*, October, pp. 97–107.

Improve Your Performance with Mental Rehearsal

Altman, W. 1992. The mental edge. *U.S. News & World Report*, August 3, p. 50.

Hall, C. et al. 1995. Interference effects of mental imagery on a motor task. *British Journal of Psychology* 86:181–191.

Lynch, J. 1996. Mind over miles. *Runner's World*, May, pp. 88–92.

5 Ways to Make Smarter Decisions

Editor. 2001. How to develop your decision-making skills. Online: www. hooah4health.com.

Vaughn, L. 1985. How to make smarter decisions. *Prevention*, May, pp. 70–75.

Learn While You Sleep

Dunham, W. 2001. Study reveals how sleep helps brain development. Reuters News Service, April 26. Online: www.brain.com.

Neimark, J. 1995. It's magical. It's malleable. It's . . . memory. *Psychology Today*, January 11, pp. 44–51.

Segall, R. 2001. Sleep on it. *Psychology Today*, March, p. 18.

Sheff-Cahan, V. 1999. Snooze alarm sleep doc William Dement argues that too little shut-eye has become a national nightmare. *People*, October 4, p. 147.

Smith, S. 2001. Caught in a maze. *Psychology Today*, May, p. 20.

Wasowicz, L. 2001. Sleep is good for the brain. United Press International, April 26.

Sidebar: 9 Ways to Get Mentally Stimulating Sleep

Editor. 1993. Seven keys to the good life. *Tufts University Diet & Nutrition Letter*, August, p. 1.

LaForge, R. 1988. Helping the sandman. *Executive Health Report*, May, p. 8.

Ludington, A. 1996. Rest: How much is enough? *Vibrant Life*, March/April, pp. 4–6.

Nieman, D. C. 1995. Oh, for a good night's sleep. *Vibrant Life*, July/August, pp. 28–30.

Chapter 2: How to Manage Your Mood

Stock Your Pantry with These 13 Mood Foods

Barbor, C. 2001. Mood food. *Psychology Today*, January, p. 22.

Chatterjee, C. 1999. Depression: Fish food for your mood. *Psychology Today*, October, p. 22.

Holman, J. R. 1995. Foods that boost your moods. *Ladies Home Journal*, November, pp. 156–159.

Levine, H. 1998. Eat this! *Cosmopolitan*, February, pp. 240–243.

Lombard, C. B. 2000. What is the role of food in preventing depression? *The Medical Journal of Australia* 173:S104–S105.

McCord, H. 1998. Improve your mood with food. *Prevention*, August, p. 57.

Remerowski, G. 2001. Ah chocolate! Food of the gods. University Wire, February 6.

Sizer, F., and E. Whitney. *Nutrition Concepts and Controversies*, 7th ed. Belmont, California: West/Wadsworth, 1997.

Stuart, J. 2001. How to eat your way to happiness. *Independent*, June 7, p. 8.

Trankina, M. L. 1998. Choosing foods to modulate your moods. *The World & I*, March, p. 150.

The 6 Happy Hormones: Put Them to Work for You

Aeron Life Cycles. 2001. Progesterone cream list. Online: www.aeron.com.

Callahan, M. *DHEA: The Miracle Hormone*. New York: Penguin Books, 1997.

Editor. 1998. Depression in menopausal women could be testosterone deficiency, but no suitable testosterone products on market for women. *Medical Post*, June 16, p. 4.

Editor. 2001. Drug information. Online: www.pdr.net.

Editor. 1994. Natural progesterone. *Mid-Life Woman*, January, p. 7.

Editor. 1997. New antiaging hormone. *Flare*, September, pp. 90–95.

Editor. 2001. New products. Online: www.menopause-online.com.

Editor. 1996. Wild yam creams and natural progesterone. *Meno Times*, March, p. 16.

Gutfeld, G. 1994. Test-driving testosterone. *Men's Health*, November, pp. 50–51.

Munson, M. 1996. Can hormones make you happy? *Prevention*, March, pp. 90–97.

Schechter, D. 1999. Estrogen, progesterone, and mood. *Journal of Gender-Specific Medicine* 2:29–36.

Sheehy, G. 1997. DHEA: Does it hold the secret to youth? *The Natural Way*, January/February, pp. 38–42.

Smith, N. F. 1999. Do you need the menopause miracle? *Prevention*, January, pp. 116–121.

Get Healthy: Become an Optimist

Bruce, B. 1998. Is it time for an attitude adjustment? *USA Today Magazine*, September. Online: www.findarticles.com.

Eberlein, T. 1996. Think positive. *Good Housekeeping*, January, pp. 77–79.

Editor. 1999. Optimism may affect health as much as diet, exercise. *Patient-Focused Care and Satisfaction* 7:78–80.

Perlmutter, C. 1996. Think yourself healthy. *Prevention*, pp. 71–75, 146–149.

Chapter 3: Positive Psychology to Improve Your Frame of Mind

7 Ways to Catch Happiness

Easterbrook, G. 2001. Psychology discovers happiness. *The New Republic*, March, p. 5.

Epstein, R. 2001. Happiness reexamined. *Psychology Today*, January, p. 7.

Ferguson, S. 2001. Health: In search of joy. *Maclean's*, June 18, p. 36.

Morris, H. J. 2001. Happiness explained. *U.S. News & World Report*, September 3, p. 46.

Wellner, A. S. 2000. Happy days. *Psychology Today*, May. Online: www.findarticles.com.

Humor and Your Mental Health: 11 Ways to Laugh Away Your Problems

Dolan, M. B. 1994. Laughter: A daily trip to your internal pharmacy. *Caring* 13:38–40.

Du pré, A. 2001. Personal communication. August 8.

Leo, J. 1999. Chortle while you work. *U.S. News & World Report*, April 26, p. 19.

Seaward, B. L. 1992. Humor's healing potential. *Health Progress* 73:66–70.

Walsh, T. 2001. Funny heart protection. *Prevention*, April, p. 32.

Dream Up a Good Mood

Cartwright, R. et al. 1998. Role of REM sleep and dream affect in overnight mood regulation: A study of normal volunteers. *Psychiatry Research* 81:1–8.

Editor. 1999. Dreaming up a good mood. *Psychology Today*, September. Online: www.findarticles.com.

Editor. 1995. How to build a dream. *Psychology Today*, November, pp. 46–52.

Doom Your Gloom: 5 Supplemental Amino Acids to Lift Your Spirits

Balch, J. F., and P. A. Balch. *Prescription for Nutritional Healing*. New York: Avery Publishing Group, 1997.

Blomstrand, E. et al. 1991. Effect of branched-chain amino acid supplementation on mental performance. *Acta Physiologica Scandinavica* 143:225–226.

Editor. 2001. 5-HTP. *Natural Health*, July, p. 36.

2 Surprise Mood Boosters You've Never Heard About

Fugh-Berman, A. et al. 1999. Dietary supplements and natural products as psychotherapeutic agents. *Psychosomatic Medicine* 61:712–728.

Ohsugi, M. et al. 1999. Active-oxygen scavenging activity of traditional nourishing-tonic herbal medicines and active constituents of Rhodiola sacra. *Journal of Ethnopharmacology* 67:111–119.

Spasov, A. A. et al. 2000. A double-blind, placebo-controlled pilot study of the stimulating and adaptogenic effect of Rhodiola rosea SHR-5 extract on the fatigue of students caused by stress during an examination period with a repeated low-dose regimen. *Phytomedicine* 7:85–89.

———.The effect of the preparation rodakson on the psychophysiological and physical adaptation of students to an academic load. *Eksperimental'naia I Klinicheskaia Farmakologiia* 63:76–78.

Restore Your Mental Balance with 12 of the Most Promising Therapies

Castleman, M. 1997. Becoming unblued. *Mother Jones*, May 15, pp. 23–25.

Editor. 1994. High anxiety. *Chatelaine*, January, pp. 34–36.

Lang, S. 1994. Low-grade depression. *Good Housekeeping*, January, pp. 72–74.

Schrof, J. M. 1998. Married . . . with problems. *U.S. News & World Report*, January 19, p. 56.

Webster, D. 1995. Shrink to fit. *Men's Health*, April, pp. 76–78.

CHAPTER 4: HOW TO IMPROVE YOUR MEMORY

Snack Your Way to Better Recall: 5 Recipes That Enhance Memory

Gotthardt, M. 1999. Wake up with the shakes. *Men's Health*, May, pp. 108, 110.

Schwartz, J. 2001. Let food be your medicine. *Chatelaine*, April, pp. 74–80.

Wood, M. 2001. Folate and choline interplay investigated. *Agricultural Research*, March, p. 16.

Fight Forgetfulness: 8 Recommendations for Overcoming Mental Blips and Slips

Chillot, R. 1999. 25 tips to recharge your memory. *Prevention*, February, pp. 114–119.

Colino, S. 1994. 8 ways to sharpen your memory. *Redbook*, August, pp. 108–110.

Mitchell, E. 2000. The mind: Speak, memory as we age. *Time*, February 28, p. G1.

Ryan, M. 2001. How to keep your memory strong. *Parade*, June 24, pp. 12–14.

Tangley, L. 2000. Aging brains need fresh challenges to stay agile. *U.S. News & World Report*, June 5, p. 90.

Wray, H. 1999. Losing your mind? *U.S. News & World Report*, July 26, p. 44.

Zinczenko, D. 1994. Rocket science made easy. *Men's Health*, October, pp. 97–107.

Remember Names Like a Computer: 10 Proven Techniques

Gaut, D. R., and E. Perrigo. *Business and Professional Communication for the 21st Century.* Boston: Allyn and Bacon, 1998.

Golden, F. 2000. When to start fretting about forgetfulness. *Time*, June 12, p. 57.

Perrigo, Eileen. 2001. Personal communication, June 29.

Part 2: Quick and Easy Jump Starts

Chapter 5: Jump-Start Your Mental Powers

Sniff Your Way to Better Brainpower

Amodio, J. 1998. Mood makers. *Good Housekeeping*, November, pp. 53–54.

Eischen, N. 1998. Aromatherapy. *Countryside & Small Stock Journal*, July 17, p. 88.

Ilmberger, J. et al. 2001. The influence of essential oils on human attention. *Chemical Senses* 26:239–245.

Keville, K. 1996. Boost your brain power. *Vegetarian Times*, March. Online: www.findarticles.com.

Tobin, P. 1995. Aromatherapy and its application in the management of people with dementia. *The Lamp* 52:34.

Sit Up for Smarts

Editor. 1985. Boost your brainpower. *Prevention*, January, p. 137.

Get Smarter in 12 Minutes a Day

Johnson, K. A. 1995. What's IQ got to do with it? *Heart & Soul*, September 30. Online: www.ask.elibrary.com.

Padus, E. 1988. Brainpower. *Prevention*, July, pp. 107–108.

Wright, K. 1999. Why are you so smart? *Discover*, October. Online: www.find articles.com.

Zinczenko, D. 1994. Rocket science made easy. *Men's Health*, October, pp. 97–107.

Pass Exams with Flying Colors: 12 Foods to Avoid Before Taking a Test

Hamazaki, T. et al. 2000. Anti-stress effects of DHA. *Biofactors* 13:41–45.

————. 1996. The effect of docosahexaenoic acid on aggression in young adults. *Journal of Clinical Investigation* 97:1129–1134.

Lloyd, H. M. 1996. Acute effects on mood and cognitive performance of breakfasts differing in fat and carbohydrate content. *Appetite* 27:151–164.

Lloyd, H. M. et al. 1994. Mood and cognitive performance effects of isocaloric lunches differing in fat and carbohydrate content. *Physiology and Behavior* 56:51–57.

Ortega, R. M. et al. 1997. Dietary intake and cognitive function in a group of elderly people. *American Journal of Clinical Nutrition* 66:803–809.

Park, S. B. et al. 1994. Tryptophan depletion in normal volunteers produces selective impairments in learning and memory. *Neuropharmacology* 33:575–588.

Quick-Start Creativity: An Amazing Technique to Unleash Your Imagination

Persun, T. 2001. Personal communication. October 25.

The Cognition Enhancer You Can Drink Every Morning

Hogervorst, E. et al. 1999. Caffeine improves cognitive performance after strenuous physical exercise. *International Journal of Sports Medicine* 20:354–361.

Mitchell, P. J. et al. 1992. Effects of caffeine, time of day and user history on study-related performance. *Psychopharmacology* 109:121–126.

Rees, K. et al. 1999. The influences of age and caffeine on psychomotor and cognitive function. *Psychopharmacology* 145:181–188.

Smith, A. et al. 1994. Effects of breakfast and caffeine on cognitive performance, mood and cardiovascular functioning. *Appetite* 22:39–55.

————. 1994. Effects of evening meals and caffeine on cognitive performance, mood and cardiovascular conditioning. *Appetite* 22:57–65.

Get a Natural Brain Buzz: 2 Herbal Pep Pills to Stimulate Your Smarts

Espinola, E. B. et al. 1997. Pharmocological activity of guarana (Paullinia cupana Mart.) in laboratory animals. *Journal of Ethnopharmacology* 55:223–229.

Lieberman, H. R. 2001. The effects of ginseng, ephedrine, and caffeine on cognitive performance, mood, and energy. *Nutrition Reviews* 59:91–102.

Mayell, M. 1998. Healthy highs. *Natural Health*, July/August. Online: www.findarticles.com.

Zum Felde, A. 1998. Scientific support for the use of guarana. October 20. Online: www.symmetrix.ch.

Sidebar: *Ephedra: Too Dangerous to Recommend*
Ostgarden, J. 1995. Rocket fuel. *Bicycling*, July, pp. 92–93.

Turk, M. P. 1997. Ephedrine's deadly edge. *U.S. News & World Report*, July 7, p. 79.

The 2 Most Effective Alertness-Enhancing Drugs
DeNoon, D. 2001. Drug increases interest level in tasks, cuts back on brain "noise." WebMD Medical News, July 12. Online: www.webmd.com.

Editor. 1999. Draxis debuts Alertec for treatment of narcolepsy. *Worldwide Biotech*, July. Online: www.elibrary.com.

Editor. 2001. Drug information. Online: www.pdr.net.

Lang, S. 1998. Could you have attention deficit disorder? *Good Housekeeping*, August, pp. 153–154.

CHAPTER 6: JUMP-START YOUR MOOD

Acupuncture to Help Your Mood
Balch, J. F., and P. A. Balch. P. A. *Prescription for Nutritional Healing*. New York: Avery Publishing Group, 1997.

Editor. 1999. Pin down depression. *Psychology Today*, September. Online: www. findarticles.com.

12 Herbal Tranquilizers to Ease Your Mind
Bloomfield, H. H. *Healing Anxiety with Herbs*. New York: HarpersCollins Publishers, 1998.

Fugh-Berman, A. et al. 1999. Dietary supplements and natural products as psychotherapeutic agents. *Psychosomatic Medicine* 61:712–728.

Houck, C. 1998. Natural cures you can really trust. *Redbook*, May, pp. 106–109.

Mandile, M. N. 2001. Feel-good herbs. *Natural Health*, July, pp. 62–65, 102–104.

The 5 Newer and Least Risky Prescription Mood Drugs
Editor. 2001. Drug information. Online: www.pdr.net.

Instant Calm: Learn How in 30 Seconds

Balch, J. F., and P. A. Balch, *Prescription for Nutritional Healing*. New York: Avery Publishing Group, 1997.

Editor. 1993. Controlled breathing exercises. *National Women's Health Report*, May, p. 6.

CHAPTER 7: JUMP-START YOUR MEMORY

Oxygen and Your Brain: 4 Ways to Take a Breather and Enhance Your Memory

Goldstein, D. 1996. Oxygen bar. *Science World* 53:7.

Krop, H. D. et al. 1977. Neuropsychologic effects of continuous oxygen therapy. *Chest* 72:737–743.

Stephens, A. 2001. Grey matters. *The Mirror*, May 17, pp. 29–30.

Music: An Overlooked Way to Boost Your Recall Fast

Bender, M. 2001. Music that pumps up your brainpower. *Cosmopolitan*, April, p. 118.

Larkin, M. 2001. Music tunes up memory in dementia patients. *Lancet* 6: 47.

Memorization Made Easy: 6 Remarkable Mnemonic Techniques

Editor. 2001. Memory techniques and mnemonics. Online: www.mindtools.com.

Intelegen. 2000. Mnemonic techniques and specific memory tricks to improve memory, memorization. Online: www.brain.web-us.com.

Part 3: Preventing Problems

CHAPTER 8: STOP THE BRAIN DEPLETERS

Alcohol's Surprising Short-Term Effects on the Brain

Editor. 2000. This toast goes to your head. *Health*, November/December, p. 21.

Emsley, J. 1995. A dispassionate look at alcohol. *Consumers' Research Magazine*, July, pp. 19–24.

Oscar-Berman, M. et al. Impairments of the brain and behavior: The neurological effects of alcohol. *Alcohol Health & Research World*, January, pp. 65–75.

Schuckit, M. A. 1996. Alcohol, anxiety, and depressive disorders. *Alcohol Health & Research World*, March, pp. 81–85.

Danger Zone: These Nutritional Supplements Could Be Hazardous to Your Brain

Benzi, G. et al. 2001. Creatine as nutritional supplementation and medical product. *Journal of Sports Medicine and Physical Fitness* 41:1–10.

Editor. 2001. Mad cow disease and chondroitin sulfate. *Harvard Health Letter*, May, p. 3.

Editor. 2001. Staggering list of products made from cattle. Online: www.rense.com.

Wadman, M. 2001. New mad cow hideout: The medicine chest. *Fortune*, February 16. Online: www.fortune.com.

Why Some Weight-Loss Diets Make You Dumb

Brown, J. E. *The Science of Human Nutrition*. San Diego: Harcourt Brace Jovanovich, Publishers, 1990.

Green, M. W. et al. 1995. Impaired cognitive functioning during spontaneous dieting. *Psychological Medicine* 25:1003–1010.

Green, M. W. et al. 1998. Impairments in working memory associated with spontaneous dieting behavior. *Psychological Medicine* 28:1063–1070.

Polivy, J. 1996. Psychological consequences of dieting. *Journal of the American Dietetic Association* 96:589–592.

Sizer, F., and E. Whitney. *Nutrition Concepts and Controversies*, 7th ed. Belmont, California: West/Wadsworth, 1997.

Somer, E. 2001. Smart foods. WebMD Medical News. Online: www.webmd.com.

Pursue Lifelong Learning: 15 Actions to Keep Your Mind Smart and Supple

Miller, B. 1997. The quest for lifelong learning. *American Demographics*, March, pp. 20–21.

Rinegard, J. 2000. Enterprise careers: Distance learning sites. *InfoWorld*, March 10. Online: www.elibrary.com.

Slevin, C. 2000. Older students learn to keep brain active. *The Washington Times*, September 24, p. D2.

U.S. Department of Education. 1999. Participation in adult education in the United States: 1998–99. November. Washington, D.C.: Office of Educational Research and Improvement, U.S. Department of Education.

Chapter 9: Stop the Mood Depressors

The 5 Major Types of Depression: Know the Signs
16 Depression-Defeating Moves You Can Make Now

Gregory, D. 1996. Sex: Why you've gotta have it! *Heart & Soul*, March 31, 1996. Online: ask.elibrary.com.

Larson, D. E. (ed.) *Mayo Clinic Family Health Book*. New York: William Morrow and Company, Inc., 1990.

Maynard, R. 1997. An invisible killer. *Chatelaine*, March, p. 8.

Quattrocki, E. et al. 2000. Biological aspects of the link between smoking and depression. *Harvard Review of Psychiatry* 8:90–110.

Yapko, M. D. 1997. The art of avoiding depression. *Psychology Today*, May 15, pp. 37–38.

2 Blockbuster Antidepressants from Nature's Pharmacy

Colchamiro, R. 1998. Worting away depression. *American Druggist*, January, pp. 28–31.

Cowley, G. et al. The "sammy" solution. *Newsweek*, March, p. 65.

Editor. 1999. The happy pill. *Men's Health*, November, p. 48.

Sahelian, R. 1999. Brain boosters. *Let's Live*, August, pp. 40–43, 79.

Shearer, S. L., and G. K. Adams. 1993. Nonpharmacologic aids in the treatment of depression. *American Family Physician* 47:435–443.

Waltman, A. B. et al. 2000. Guide to natural health: Alternative medicine goes mainstream. *Psychology Today*, April, pp. 37–40, 42.

5 Ways to Chase Away Wintertime Blues

Attar-Levy, D. 1998. Seasonal depression. *Therapie* 53:489–498.

Brown, E. W. 1997. So sad to have SAD this winter. *Medical Update*, January 1, p. 4.

Editor. 1993. Women and depression: Seasonal affective disorder. *National Women's Health Report*, November 1, p. 4.

Lewy, A. J. 1998. Melatonin treatment of winter depression: A pilot study. *Psychiatry Research* 77:57–61.

Miller, A. L. 1998. St. John's wort (hypericum perforatum): Clinical effects on depression and other conditions. *Alternative Medicine Review* 3:18–26.

Sidebar: *From Here to Serenity: 29 Tips for Stress-Free Living*

Carpi, J. 1996. Stress . . . it's worse than you think. *Psychology Today*, January/February, pp. 34–37.

International Society of Sport Psychology Position Statement. 1992. Physical activity and psychological benefits. *The Physician and Sportsmedicine* 20:179–184.

Langer, S. 1995. Nutritionally coping with stress. *Better Nutrition*, July, pp. 42–44.

Lark, S. N. 1994. Strike back at high anxiety: Natural ways to stay calm in stressful times. *Vegetarian Times*, February, pp. 90–92.

Murray, F. 1992. The healthy approach to stress control. *Better Nutrition*, June, pp. 20–22.

Rapaport, W. S. 1993. He who laughs . . . lasts longer and lives better. *Diabetes in the News*, November/December, pp. 12–14.

CHAPTER 10: STOP THE MEMORY LOSERS

The 4 Main Dementias: What You Need to Know to Halt Memory Loss

Alzheimer's Society. 2001. Alzheimer's disease. Online: www.Alzheimer.ca.

Alzheimer's Society. 2001. Vascular dementia. Online: www.Alzheimer.ca.

Banazak, D. A. 1996. Difficult dementia: Six steps to control problem behaviors. *Geriatrics* 51:36–41.

Gross, J. S. 1997. Multi-infarct dementia: A common form of dementia associated with cerebrovascular disease. *Geriatrics* 52:95.

Hilton, C. 2000. Researchers monitoring AD risk in herpes patients. *Medical Post*, August 8. Online: www.elibrary.com.

Mylinski, N. P. 1997. New light on an old-age dementia. *The World & I*, November, p. 169.

Rosenfeld, I. 2001. Parkinson's sufferers—hang in there! *Parade*, August 12, pp. 12–13.

Top Defense Against Dementia: Avoid These 4 Memory-Damaging Toxins

Basky, G. 2001. MDs get mercury damage on film and find possible link to AD. *Medical Post*, May 1. Online: www.elibrary.com.

Editor. 2000. Lead exposure, laziness linked to Alzheimer's. Reuters News Service, May 3.

Editor. 1996. New Alzheimer's link. *Maclean's*, May 13, p. 31.

Editor. 2001. Prevention. Online: www.leadpoisoning-news.com.

Editor. 2001. Preventions. Online: www.herbaladvisor.com.

Environmental Protection Agency. 2001. Mercury poisoning. Online: www. epa.gov.

Graves, A. B. et al. 1990. The association between aluminum-containing products and Alzheimer's disease. *Journal of Clinical Epidemiology* 43:35–44.

Hatherill, J. R. 2000. Safer modes of pest control. *The World & I*, May, p. 164.

Helmuth, L. 2000. Pesticide causes Parkinson's in rats. *Science*, November 10. Online: www.elibrary.com.

Lamb, M. 2001. Chemical roulette. *Mother Earth News*, February, p. 66.

Miller, R. W. 1988. The metal in our mettle. *FDA Consumer*, December, pp. 24–27.

Nichols, M. 1995. Water worries: Studies suggest that aluminum may play a role in Alzheimer's. *Maclean's*, April 10, p. 45.

Saxe, S. R. et al. 1999. Alzheimer's disease, dental amalgram and mercury. *Journal of the American Dental Association* 130:191–199.

Soni, M. G. et al. 2001. Safety evaluation of dietary aluminum. *Regulatory Toxicology and Pharmacology* 33:66–79.

Wansbrough, G. 2000. Pesticides linked to Parkinson's disease: U.S. study. *Medical Post*, August 8. Online: www.elibrary.com.

Yokel, R. A. 2000. The toxicology of aluminum in the brain: A review. *Neurotoxicity* 21:813–828.

Caution: Do Too Much of This and Your Memory May Turn to Mush

Associated Press. 2001. Study: Hobbies can help slow Alzheimer's. August 13. Online: www.USAToday.com.

Foley, B. 2001. Too much television linked to dementia. March 7. Online: www. theage.com.

7 Memory Manglers and How to Outsmart Them

Bates, S. 1997. Getting to sleep away from home. *Nation's Business*, June, pp. 52–55.

Editor. 2001. Jet lag impairs memory, study says. *The Washington Times*, May 21, p. A8.

Lamb, M. 2001. Can emotions aid recall? *Psychology Today*, January. Online: www.findarticles.com.

McGeown, K. 2000. Pot may slow blood to brain, University of Iowa says. University Wire, March 30.

Morgan, P. (ed.). *The Female Body: An Owner's Manual.* Emmaus, Pennsylvania: Rodale Press, 1996.

Ricks, D. 2001. Bypass and brain deficit. *Newsday*, February 19, p. C3.

5 Types of Drugs That Can Destroy Your Memory

Editor. 2001. Drug information. Online: www.pdr.net.

Marshall, M. A. 2001. Danger in your medicine cabinet. *Cosmopolitan*, June, p. 158.

Be Kind to Your Mind: Stress and Memory

Berardelli, P. 1996. Chronic stress shrinks brains. *Insight on the News*, October 28, pp. 44–45.

Bremner, J. D. 1999. Does stress damage the brain? *Biological Psychiatry* 45:797–805.

4 Memory-Building Herbs You Can Grow in Your Own Garden

Perry, E. K. et al. 1999. Medicinal plants and Alzheimer's disease: From ethnobotany to phytotherapy. *Journal of Pharmacy and Pharmacology* 51:527–534.

Perry, S. 1997. Herbal teas. *Country Living*, September, pp. 78–80.

Rebhahn, P. 2001. Dangerous diet drinks. *Psychology Today*, March, p. 20.

Tyler, V. 2001. Herbal hope for Alzheimer's, cancer, and prostate disease. *Prevention*, March, p. 105.

Put Senility in Reverse with Phosphatidylserine (PS)

Editor. 1998. New formula offers help for ailing memories. *Worldwide Biotech*, February, p. 3.

Langer, S. 1998. Holding your remembers: Boosting memory with supplements. *Better Nutrition*, August. Online: www.findarticles.com.

Bring Back a Fading Memory with Memory-Boosting Zinc

Bhatnagar, S. et al. 2001. Zinc and cognitive development. *British Journal of Nutrition* 2:S139–S145.

Nakagawa, N. 1998. Studies on changes in trace elements of the brain related to aging. *The Hokkaido Journal of Medical Science* 73:181–199.

Part 4: Understanding Why

CHAPTER 11: THE MIND CONNECTIONS

Sidebar: *What's Your IQ?*

Editor. 2001. Intelligence tests. Online: www.brain.com.

Editor. 2001. IQ and intelligence. Online: www.brain.com.

Padus, E. 1988. Brainpower. *Prevention*, July, pp. 107–108.

Raise Smart Kids: 30 Recommendations

Aldridge, V. 2000. Brain storm. *The Dominion*, September 14, p. 9.

Begley, S. 2001. Are we getting smarter? *Newsweek*, April 23, p. 50.

Boodman, S. et al. 1995. What your baby really knows. *Redbook*, May, pp. 166–169.

Bower, B. 1999. Kids adopted late reap IQ increases. *Science News*, July 24. Online: www.findarticles.com.

Ceci, S. 2001. IQ intelligence: The surprising truth. *Psychology Today*, July, p. 46.

Cook, S. 1999. Report card on home schooling in U.S. *The Christian Science Monitor*, March 25, p. 3.

Editor. 1999. Music as brain builder. *Science*, March 26. Online: www.elibrary.com.

Editor. 1999. Your body: Thyroid alert. *Baby Talk*, December, p. 61.

Goff, K. G. 2000. Brainchild. *The Washington Times*, June 25, p. D1.

Green, F. E. 1999. Brain and learning research: Implications for meeting the needs of diverse learners. *Education*, July 15. Online: www.elibrary.com.

Hanser, S. B. et al. 1994. Effects of a music therapy strategy on depressed older adults. *Journal of Gerontology* 49:P265–P269.

Hertzog, B. 1995. Does exercise help make children smarter? *Sports Illustrated for Kids*, September, p. 10.

Kluger, J. et al. 2001. The quest for super kid geniuses are made, not born—or so parents are told. But can we really train baby brains, and should we try? *Time*, April 30, p. 50.

Kumar, A. M. et al. 1999. Music therapy increases serum melatonin levels in patients with Alzheimer's disease. *Alternative Therapies in Health and Medicine* 5:49–57.

Larkby, C. 1997. The effects of prenatal alcohol exposure. *Alcohol Health & Research World*, June 22, pp. 192–198.

Marcus, D. et al. 1999. How kids learn. *U.S. News & World Report*, September 13, p. 44.

McClelland, S. 2001. Life: Why dads matter: New studies show fathers' impact on child development. *Maclean's*, June 18, p. 34.

Neifert, M. 1999. Development: Raising a moral child's honesty, kindness, tolerance—who doesn't want to instill these qualities? *Parenting*, June, p. 90.

Polaneczky, R. 1996. How kids get smart: The surprising news. *Redbook*, March, pp. 102–107.

Rayl, A. J. S. 1995. Striking a neural chord: Musical links for scientists and mathematicians of tomorrow. *Omni,* December 22, p. 14.

Rusch, L. 1998. Ages & stages /3 to 5 years: Get moving, get smart. *Parenting*, August, p. 149.

Tsubata, K. 2001. 7 educational tips for the new year. *The Washington Times*, January 9, p. E5.

Wallis, C. 1998. How to make a better student: Their eight secrets of success. *Time*, October 19, p. 80.

Wickelgren, I. 1999. Nurture helps mold able minds. *Science*, March 19. Online: www.elibrary.com.

Williams, J. 2001. Analysis: Effects of day care on children. Talk of the Nation (NPR) transcript, April 24.

Zarrow, S. 1985. Bring out your child's talent. *Prevention*, June, pp. 52–57.

Your Brain on Music: 5 Reasons Why Your Mind Needs a Dose of Musical Medicine

Dess, N. K. 2000. Music on the mind. *Psychology Today*, September. Online: www.findarticles.com

Friedman, D. 1997. Drumming to the rhythms of life. *U.S. News & World Report*, June 9, p. 17.

Sari, H. 1999. Got pain? Got the blues? Try the music cure. *Prevention*, August, pp. 100–105.

Snyder, M. et al. 1999. Music therapy. *Annual Review of Nursing Research* 17:3–25.

Watkins, G. R. 1997. Music therapy: Proposed physiological mechanisms and clinical implications. *Clinical Nurse Specialist* 11:43–50.

White, J. M. 2001. Music as intervention: A notable way to improve patient outcomes. *Holistic Nursing Care* 36:83–92.

Winter, M. J. et al. 1994. Music reduces stress and anxiety of patients in the surgical holding area. *Journal of Post Anesthesia Nursing* 9:340–343.

Why You Should Master a Foreign Language

Blakesee, S. 1997. When an adult adds a language, it's one brain, two systems. *The New York Times*, July 15. Online: www.nytimes.com.

Colburn, D. 1997. Brain splits up language tasks by skills used, researchers report. *Minneapolis Star*, May 4, p. 3E.

Crispell, D. 1997. Speaking in other tongues. *American Demographics*, January, pp. 12–15.

Editor. 1998. Learning a language a great way to travel. *The Press*, January 19, p. 36.

Kim, K. H. S. et al. 1997. Distinct cortical areas associated with native and second languages. *Nature* 388:171–174.

Lane, E. 1998. The mother tongue. *Newsday*, August 8, p. C8.

Lundgren, C. 2000. Music helps BYU students learn foreign languages. University Wire, January 27.

Siegfried, T. 1997. Memory study has something familiar to say about language. *The Dallas Morning News*, March 31, p. 7D.

Sugeng, B. 1999. How one can become a good foreign-language learner. *Jakarta Post*, June 6. Online: www.elibrary.com.

Treays, R. *Understanding Your Brain*. Tulsa, Oklahoma: EDC Publishing, 1996.

His Brain/Her Brain: New Discoveries About How Men and Women Really Think

Allman, W. F. 1995. His brain, her brain. *U.S. News & World Report*, February 27, p. 15.

Editor. 1996. Grumpy old men. *Maclean's*, April 22, p. 31.

Howerter, M. E. 2001. Are men really brain damaged at birth? Online: www.brain.com.

Kleinwaks, R. et al. 1999. Your brain, explained. *Men's Health*, November, pp. 134–135.

Krueger, L. 1995. Brainstorm. *Chatelaine*, December, pp. 72–75.

Leo, J. 1995. Sex: It's all in your brain. *U.S. News & World Report*, February 27, p. 22.

Schrage, M. 1999. Why can't a woman be more like a man? It's all in your brain. *Fortune*, August 16, p. 184.

Society for Neuroscience. 1999. Gender and the brain. Online: www.brain.com.

Diagnosing Brain Disorders: 7 Tests Performed in Your Doctor's Office

American Academy of Neurology. 2001. Common neurological tests. Online: www.aan.com.

American Association of Neurological Surgeons. 2001. Glossary of Neurological Diagnostic Tests. Online: www.neurosurgery.org.

Brodin, M. B. *The Encyclopedia of Medical Tests*. New York: Pocket Books, 1997.

Editor. 2001. Cognitive tests. Online: www.webmd.com.

Larson, D. E. (ed.). *Mayo Clinic Family Health Book*. New York: William Morrow and Company, Inc., 1990.

CHAPTER 12: WHAT MAKES YOUR MOOD?

Sidebar: *7 Immune Boosters That May Protect Against Brain Bugs*

Chatterjee, C. 1999. Supplements: The illness fighter. *Psychology Today,* June, p. 26.

Editor. 1996. Depression at mid-life. *MidLife Woman*, January, pp. 1–4.

Editor. 2001. How serious is pneumonia? Online: www.webmd.com.

Izumoto, Y. et al. 1999. Schizophrenia and the influenza epidemics of 1957 in Japan. *Biological Psychiatry* 46:119–124.

Munk-Jorgensen, P. et al. 2001. Epidemiology in neurobiological research: Exemplified by the influenza-schizophrenia theory. *British Journal of Psychiatry Supplement* 40:S30–S32.

Pugliese, P. T. et al. 1998. Some biological actions of alkylglycerols from shark liver oil. *Journal of Alternative and Complementary Medicine* 4:87–99.

Ridley, T. 1999. Menopause and your mood. *Essence*, September, p. 56.

Romm, A. 2001. Do-it-yourself menopause remedies. *Prevention*, July, p. 139.

Rountree, R. 2000. Arming yourself to fight the flu. *Newsweek*, November 6, p. 88.

Shangold, M. 1990. Exercise in the menopausal woman. *Obstetrics and Gynecology* 75:53S–58S.

Slaven, L. et al. 1997. Mood and symptom reporting among middle-aged women: The relationship between menopausal status, hormone replacement therapy, and exercise participation. *Health Psychology* 16: 203–208.

Tyler, V. E. 1999. Five herbs that ease menopause. *Prevention,* March, pp. 94–97.

Washington, H. 1999. The infection connection. *Psychology Today*, August, pp. 43–44, 74.

Webb, D. 1999. Do you need a dose of "good" bacteria? *Prevention*, May, pp. 65–66.

Sidebar: *8 Ways to Cope with Toxic People*

McCafferty, M. F. 1998. You can dump toxic people from your life. *Cosmopolitan*, October, pp. 184–187.

Moore, M. 2000. Coping with toxic people. Online: www.life.ca/moore.

Get Religion: 5 Astounding Facts on Why the Faithful Are Less Depressed and More Fulfilled

Koenig, H. G. 1999. How does religious faith contribute to recovery from depression? *Harvard Mental Health Letter* 15:8.

Koenig, H. G. et al. 1992. Religious coping and depression among elderly, hospitalized medically ill men. *American Journal of Psychiatry* 149:1693–1700.

Matthews, D. A. et al. 1998. Religious commitment and health status. *Archives of Family Medicine* 7:118–124.

McCullough, M. E. et al. 1999. Religion and depression: A review of the literature. *Twin Research* 2:126–136.

CHAPTER 13: THE WORKINGS OF MEMORY

How Your Brain Records and Constructs Memories

Adderly, B. D. 1999. Mind body: Stay sharp! *Essence*, March, pp. 34, 37.

Begley, S. 2001. Memory's mind games. *Newsweek,* July 16, p. 52.

D'Esposito, M. 2000. Brain aging and memory. *Geriatrics,* June. Online: www.findarticles.com.

Farndon, J. *The Big Book of the Brain*. New York: Peter Bedrick Books, 2000.

Johnson, G. 2000. Memory/how it works. *Time*, June 12, p. 54.

Neimark, J. 1995. It's magical. It's malleable. It's . . . memory. *Psychology Today*, January 11, pp. 44–51.

Schacter, D. L. 2001. Why the brain forgets. *Natural Health*, October/November, pp. 67–71.

Sheppard, R. 2000. How we think. *Maclean's*, May, p. 42.

Treays, R. *Understanding Your Brain*. Tulsa, Oklahoma: EDC Publishing, 1996.

Yoffe, E. 1997. How quickly we forget. *U.S. News & World Report*, October 13, p. 52.

How Sharp Is Your Memory? Take This Quiz to Find Out

Alzheimer's Association. 2001. APOE gene testing. Online: www.alz.org.

Alzheimer's Association. 2001. Conducting an assessment. Online: www.alz.org.

Alzheimer's Association. 2001. The 7-minute screen. Online: www.alz.org.

Alzheimer's Society. 2001. The mini-mental state examination (MMSE)—a guide for people with dementia and their careers. March. Online: www.alzheimers. org.uk.

Chatterjee, C. 2001. The 15-minute diagnosis. *Psychology Today*, January, p. 26.

Editor. 2001. Memory quiz. (Memory assessment clinic of Bethesda, Maryland). Online: www.healthcentral.com.

Editor. 1998. New tests helpful in diagnosing Alzheimer's disease. *Geriatrics* 53:21–23.

Mendez, M. F. et al. 1992. Development of scoring criteria for the clock drawing task in Alzheimer's disease. *Journal of the American Geriatrics Society* 40:1095–1099.

Miller, S. 2000. You know something is wrong: Diagnosing Alzheimer's. July. Online: www.cbs.com.

Podolsky, D. 1993. The latest in testing—take out the high technology. *U.S. News & World Report*, November 22, p. 69.

Solomon, P. R. et al. 1998. Identification of the Alzheimer's disease patient in primary care practice: The 7-minute screen. Massachusetts Alzheimer's Disease Research Center, Eleventh Annual Scientific Poster Session, Boston, Massachusetts.

Is It Forgetfulness, or Is It Alzheimer's Disease? 10 Signs You Shouldn't Ignore

Alzheimer's Association. 2001. Symptoms. Online: www.alz.org.

Editor. 1997. Clinical practice guidelines: Early identification of Alzheimer's disease and related dementias. *Dermatology Nursing* 9:243–258.

5 Myths About the Aging Brain

Begley, S. 2001. The brain in winter. Online: www.msnbc.com.

Bowden, C. M. 1996. Aging brains are better. *Washington Informer*, January 17. Online: www.ask.elibrary.com.

Editor. 2001. Aging, memory, and the brain. *Harvard Health Letter*. Online: www.webpoint.com.

Editor. 2000. Science myths. *Discover*, February. Online: www.findarticles.com.

Hotz, R. L. 1999. A new wrinkle on our gray matter. *Los Angeles Times*, September 10. Online: www.brain.com.

Kluger, J. 2000. The battle to save your memory. *Time,* June 12. Online: www.time.com.

Part 5: Special Strategies to Help You Out

CHAPTER 14: DIFFERENT THERAPIES FOR SCARY CONDITIONS

Addiction: The Most Addictive Drugs and 5 Ways to Get Unhooked

American Cancer Society. 2001. Smoking statistics. Online: www.cancer.org.

Begley, S. 2001. How it all starts inside your brain. *Newsweek*, February 12, p. 40.

Myslinski, N. R. 1999. Addiction and the brain. *The World & I,* November, p. 162.

National Institute on Drug Abuse. 2001. Principles of drug addiction treatment. Online: www.nida.nih.gov.

Neimark, J. et al. 1994. Back from the drink. *Psychology Today*, September, pp. 46–53.

Rodgers, J. E. 1994. Addiction: A whole new view. *Psychology Today*, September, pp. 32–42.

Sherman, C. 1994. Kicking butts. *Psychology Today*, September, pp. 40–45.

6 Herbal Detoxifiers for Alcohol and Drug Addiction

Abrams, M. 1994. Herbal medicine. *Good Housekeeping,* March, pp. 111–112.

Apostolides, M. et al. 1996. How to quit the holistic way. *Psychology Today*, September, pp. 34–45.

Avants, S. K. et al. 2000. A randomized controlled trial of auricular acupuncture for cocaine dependence. *Archives of Internal Medicine* 160:2305–2312.

Carroll, K. M. et al. 1997. Nonpharmacologic approaches to substance abuse treatment. *The Medical Clinics of North America* 81:927–944.

Castleman, M. 1997. Liver let live: A natural remedy for liver disease has been ignored by mainstream medicine. *Mother Jones*, November 21, pp. 25–26.

Editor. 2001. Drug information. Online: www.pdr.net.

Fuller, J. A. 1982. Smoking withdrawal and acupuncture. *The Medical Journal of Australia* 1:28–29.

Geraci, R. 1999. Milk thistle. *Men's Health*, April, p. 46.

Keung, W. M. et al. 1998. Kudzu root: An ancient Chinese source of modern antidipsotropic agents. *Phytochemistry* 47:499–506.

Khatami, M. et al. 1982. Biofeedback treatment of narcotic addiction: A double-blind study. *Drug and Alcohol Dependence* 9:111–117.

Kurtzweil, P. 1996. Medications can aid recovery from alcoholism. *FDA Consumer*, May. Online: www.elibrary.com.

Lee, F. C. et al. 1987. Effects of Panax ginseng on blood alcohol clearance in man. *Clinical and Experimental Pharmacology and Physiology* 14:543–546.

Myrick, H. et al. 2001. New developments in the pharmacotherapy of alcohol. *American Journal on Addictions* 10:3–15.

Nestel, P. J. 1999. Isoflavones from red clover improve systemic arterial compliance but not plasma lipids in menopausal women. *Journal of Clinical Endocrinology & Metabolism* 84:895–898.

Sharma, K. et al. 1988. Rehabilitation of drug-addicted persons: The experience of the Nav-Chetna Drug De-addiction Center in India. *Bulletin of Narcotics* 40:43–49.

Southall, D. 1997. Complementary therapy to fight drug addiction. *Nursing Times* 93:48–49.

Tweed, V. 1999. Herbal remedy guide. *Saturday Evening Post*, March. Online: www.elibrary.com.

7 Top Lifestyle Strategies for Outwitting Alzheimer's Disease

Lemonick, M. D. et al. 2001. The nun study. *Time*, May 14, pp. 53–65.

Munson, M. et al. 1996. Clear thinking for life. *Prevention*, September, pp. 30–31.

2 Surprise OTC Medicines That Reduce Your Risk

Brody, J. E. 2001. New painkillers need closer look. *Minneapolis Star Tribune*, June 20, p. 6E.

Broe, G. A. et al. 2000. Anti-inflammatory drugs protect against Alzheimer disease at low doses. *Archives of Neurology* 57:1186–1591.

Editor. 1999. Alzheimer's disease: Seeking new ways to preserve brain function. *Geriatrics*, February. Online: www.elibrary.com.

Editor. 1998. Disposing of dementia. *The Economist*, October 24. Online: www.elibrary.com.

Editor. 2000. Ibuprofen reduces amyloid plaques. *Drug Discovery/Technology News*, August. Online: www.elibrary.com.

Evans, J. A. 1999. Pain pills that can save your life. *Prevention*, April, pp. 142–149.

Geier, T. 1996. Can aspirin help block Alzheimer's? *U.S. News & World Report*, September 16, p. 18.

Grieder, K. et al. 1996. Making our minds last a lifetime. *Psychology Today*, November 21, pp. 42–46.

Pennisi, E. 1998. Does aspirin ward off cancer and Alzheimer's? *Science*, May 22. Online: www.elibrary.com.

Smart Drugs

Editor. 1999. Alzheimer's disease: Seeking new ways to preserve brain function. *Geriatrics*, February. Online: www.elibrary.com.

Editor. 2001. Drug information. Online: www.pdr.net.

Life Extension Foundation. 2001. Age-associated mental impairment. Online: www.lef.org.

Future Alzheimer's Drugs You'll Be Hearing More About

Bachurin, S. et al. 2001. Antihistamine agent Dimebon as a novel neuroprotector and a cognition enhancer. *Annals of the New York Academy of Sciences* 939:425–435.

Freundlich, N. 2001. Arresting Alzheimer's. *Business Week*, June 11, p. 94.

Helmuth, L. 2000. An antibiotic to treat Alzheimer's? *Science*, September 17. Online: www.elibrary.com.

Hitt, E. 2001. Potential treatment for Alzheimer's identified. Reuters Health Information, September 17. Online: www.pdr.net.

Rubin, R. 2001. First study: Alzheimer's vaccine may be safe. Online: www.usatoday.com.

Travis, J. Possible Alzheimer's vaccine seems safe. *Science News*, July 15. Online: www.findarticles.com.

Huperzine A: The Miracle Memory Booster and Anti-Alzheimer's Agent

Bai, D. L. et al. 2000. Huperzine A, a potential therapeutic agent for treatment of Alzheimer's disease. *Current Medicinal Chemistry* 7:355–374.

Camps, R. et al. 2000. Huprine X is a novel high-affinity inhibitor of acetylcholinesterase that is of interest for the treatment of Alzheimer's disease. *Molecular Pharmacology* 57:409–417.

Dworkin, N. 1999. Restoring memory. *Psychology Today*, August, p. 28.

Editor. 1997. Hi-tech Pharmacal announces licensing of huperzine compound. *Worldwide Biotech*, August, p. 2.

O'Donnell, S. A. 1999. Ancient Chinese remedy: New hope for Alzheimer's. *Prevention*, June 6, p. 44.

Patocka, J. 1998. Huperzine A—an interesting anticholinesterase compound from the Chinese herbal medicine. *Acta Medica* 41:155–157.

Pilotaz, F. et al. 1999. Huperzine A: An acetylcholinesterase inhibitor with high pharmacological potential. *Annales Pharmaceutiques Francaises* 57:363–373.

Sun, Q. Q. 1999. Huperzine-A capsules enhance memory and learning performance in 34 pairs of matched adolescent students. *Zhongguo Yao Li Xue Bao* 20:601–603.

Zhang, R. W. et al. 1991. Drug evaluation of huperzine A in the treatment of senile memory disorders. *Zhongguo Yao Li Xue Bao* 12:250–252.

7 Other Amazing Anti-Alzheimer's Herbs

Kidd, P. M. 2000. A review of nutrients and botanicals in the integrative management of cognitive dysfunction. Online: www.thorne.com.

Ott, B. R. et al. 1998. Complementary and alternative medicines for Alzheimer's disease. *Journal of Geriatric Psychiatry and Neurology* 11:163–173.

Perry, E. K. 1999. Medicinal plants and Alzheimer's disease; from ethnobotany to phytotherapy. *Journal of Pharmacy and Pharmacology* 51:527–534.

Parkinson's Disease: The Best New Therapeutic Choices
Sidebar: Overlooked Nutrient for Parkinson's Disease

Brown, E. W. 1996. Pallidotomy: A surgical miracle for Parkinson's disease. *Medical Update*, September, pp. 2–3.

Editor. 2001. Basic information about Parkinson's disease. Online: www.apdapparkinson.com.

Editor. 2001. Drug information. Online: www.pdr.net.

Henkel, J. 1998. New treatments slow the onslaught of disease. *FDA Consumer*, July. Online: www.elibrary.com.

Holstein, W. J. 1999. Rewiring the brain. *U.S. News & World Report*, p. 52.

Rosenfeld, I. 2001. Parkinson's sufferers—hang in there! *Parade*, August 12, pp. 12–13.

Sweeney, P. J. 1995. Parkinson's disease: Managing symptoms and preserving function. *Geriatrics* 50:24–30.

Taggart, K. 2001. Deep brain stimulation aids Parkinson's patients for years. *Medical Post*, May 8. Online: www.elibrary.com.

CHAPTER 15: STROKE: IT DOESN'T HAVE TO HAPPEN

8 Recommendations to Prevent Strokes
5 Warning Signs of Stroke
Mini-Strokes: More Dangerous Than You Know

National Institute on Aging. 2001. Stroke: prevention and treatment. Online: www.nih.gov/nia.

National Stroke Association. 2001. What is a stroke/brain attack? Online: www.stroke.org.

Pechter, K. 1984. How to prevent a stroke. *Prevention*, May, pp. 57–62.

CHAPTER 16: THE MANY FACES OF ANXIETY

4 Anxiety Disorders

Broocks, A. et al. 1998. Comparison of aerobic exercise, clomipramine, and placebo in the treatment of panic disorder. *American Journal of Psychiatry* 155:603–609.

Dilsaver, S. C. 1989. Generalized anxiety disorder. *American Family Physician* 39:137–144.

Larson, D. E. (ed.). *Mayo Clinic Family Health Book*. New York: William Morrow and Company, Inc., 1990.

Life Extension Foundation. 2001. Disease therapies protocol. Online: www.lef.org.

Walley, E. J. et al. 1994. Management of common anxiety disorders. *American Family Physician* 50:1745–1755.

7 Natural Paths to Calm

Benjamin, J. et al. 1995. Double-blind, placebo-controlled, crossover trial of inositol treatment for panic disorder. *American Journal of Psychiatry* 152:1084–1086.

Benjamin, J.; G. Agam; J. Levine; Y. Bersudsky; et al. 1995. Inositol treatment in psychiatry. *Psychopharmocology Bulletin* 31:167–175.

Editor. 2001. A new natural relaxant. *Life Extension Magazine*, October. Online: www.lef.org.

Fux, M. et al. 1996. Inositol treatment of obsessive-compulsive disorder. *American Journal of Psychiatry* 153:1219–1221.

Gale Group. 2001. Sepia. *Gale encyclopedia of alternative medicine*. Online: www.findarticles.com.

Levine, J. 1997. Controlled trials of inositol in psychiatry. *European Neuropsychopharmacology* 7:147–155.

4 Nonaddictive Antianxiety Medications

Davidson, J. R. 2001. Pharmacotherapy of generalized anxiety disorder. *The Journal of Clinical Psychiatry* 62 (Supplement 11):46–50.

Editor. 2001. Drug information. Online: www.pdr.net.

The High Anxiety of Posttraumatic Stress Disorder: The Causes, The Cures

Anxiety Disorders Association of America. 2001. What is Post-Traumatic Stress Disorder? Online: www.adaa.org.

Cyr, M. et al. 2000. Treatment for post-traumatic stress disorder. *The Annals of Pharmacology* 34:366–376.

Flannery, R. B. 1999. Psychological trauma and post-traumatic stress disorder; a review. *International Journal of Emergency Mental Health* 1:135–140.

Foa, E. B. 2000. Psychosocial treatment of post-traumatic stress disorder. *The Journal of Clinical Psychiatry* 61:43–48.

Madison Institute of Medicine. 2001. What is PTSD? Online: www.ptsd.factsforhealth.org.

Morrison, J. *DSM-IV Made Easy: The Clinician's Guide to Diagnosis*. New York: The Guilford Press, 1995.

Pitts, C. D. 2001. Studies report paroxetine effective in treatment of PTSD. *American Family Physician*, June 15. Online: www.findarticles.com.

Platman, S. R. 1999. Psychopharmocology and post-traumatic stress disorder. *International Journal of Emergency Mental Health* 1:195–199.

Posttraumatic Stress Disorder Alliance. 2001. About PTSD. Online: www.ptsdalliance.com.

Sidebar: Novel Treatment for PTSD: Eye Movement Desensitization and Reprocessing (EMDR)

Chillot, R. 1994. Banish nightmarish memories with a wave of the hand. *Prevention*, December 1, p. 73–75.

Craig, J. 1996. Healing emotional trauma. *Chatelaine*, October 10, p. 190.

Editor. 2000. Overview and general description. Online: www.emdr.com.

Marano, H. E. 1994. Wave of the future. *Psychology Today*, July 1, pp. 22–25.

Chapter 17: Attention Deficit Hyperactivity Disorder (ADHD): Do You Have It?

Treatment Options

Barkley, R. A. 1999. Attention-deficit hyperactivity disorder. *Scientific American*, September. Online: www.sciam.com.

Challem, J. 2001. Technicolor health. Online: www.letsliveonline.com.

Craig, C. 1996. Clinical recognition and management of adult attention deficit hyperactivity disorder. *The Nurse Practitioner*, November, pp. 101–106.

Dykman, K. D. et al. 1998. Effect of nutritional supplements on attentional-deficit hyperactivity disorder. *Integrative Physiological and Behavioral Science* 33:49–60.

Editor. 2001. Attention deficit disorder. Online: www.tnp.com.

Editor. 2001. What causes ADD? Online: www.add.org.

Feingold Association. 2001. Some questions you may have. Online: www.feingold.org.

Haley, L. 2001. Double-blind study to test herbal therapy for ADD. *Medical Post*, March 13. Online: www.elibrary.com.

Hallowell, E. M. et al. 2001. The management of adult attention deficit disorder. Online: www.addult.org.

Hammer, C. 2001. What every beginner in ADD needs to know. Online: www.addult.org.

Hammer, C. 2001. The what, why, when, how and which of alternative treatments for ADD. Online: www.addult.org.

Heimann, S. W. 1999. Pycnogenol for ADHD? *Journal of the American Academy of Child and Adolescent Psychiatry* 38:357–358.

Kidd, P. M. 2000. Attention-deficit/hyperactivity disorder (ADHD) in children: Rationale for its integrative management. *Alternative Medicine Review* 5:402–428.

Lavalle, J. B. 1999. Diet and health among factors that shape treatment regimen. *Drug Store News*, January 11. Online: www.findarticles.com.

Life Extension Foundation. 2001. Attention deficit disorder. Online: www.lef.org.

Lyon, M. R. et al. 2001. Effect of the herbal extract combination Panax quinquefolium and ginkgo biloba on attention-deficit hyperactivity disorder: A pilot study. *Journal of Psychiatry and Neuroscience* 26:221–228.

Searight, H. R. 2000. Adult ADHD: Evaluation and treatment in family medicine. *American Family Physician*, November. Online: www.findarticles.com.

Shekim, W. O. et al. 1990. S-adenosyl-L-methionine (SAM) in adults with ADHD, RS: Preliminary results from an open trial. *Psychopharmacology Bulletin* 26:249–253.

CHAPTER 18: CREATVITY: A NEVER-ENDING GIFT

Creativity on the Job

Epstein, R. 1996. Capturing creativity. *Psychology Today*, July 17, pp. 41–46.

Gale Research. 1998. Creativity. *Gale Encyclopedia of Childhood & Adolescence*. Online: www.findarticles.com.

Gryskiewicz, S. S. 2000. Cashing in on creativity at work. *Psychology Today*, September. Online: www.findarticles.com.

Horne, J. A. 1988. Sleep loss and "divergent" thinking ability. *Sleep* 11:528–536.

Johnson, G. 1995. Many clues point to the nature of creativity, and it can be boosted. *Minneapolis Star Tribune*, September 13, p. 6E.

Levering, R. et al. *100 Best Companies to Work for in America*. New York: Penguin Books, 1994.

Perrine, S. 1994. The mind/body connection. *Men's Health*, September, pp. 62–69.

Schwambach, S. 2001. Personal communication.

Index

About the Author

Maggie Greenwood-Robinson, Ph.D., is one of the country's top health and medical authors. She has written numerous books on a wide range of topics, including nutrition, diet, weight loss, exercise, fitness motivation, osteoporosis, diabetes, skin care, women's hair loss, and herbs.

Her articles have appeared in *Let's Live, Physical Magazine, GreatLife, Shape Magazine, Christian Single Magazine, Women's Sports and Fitness, Working Woman, Muscle and Fitness, Female Bodybuilding and Fitness*, and many other publications. She is a member of the Advisory Board of *Physical Magazine* and has a doctorate in nutritional counseling.